VOCAL AGING

VOCAL AGING

Sue Ellen Linville, Ph.D.
Department of Speech Pathology and Audiology
Marquette University
Milwaukee, Wisconsin

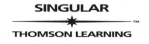

SINGULAR
THOMSON LEARNING

Australia • Canada • Mexico • Singapore • Spain • United Kingdom • United States

MW

SINGULAR

---✦--- ™

THOMSON LEARNING

Vocal Aging
by Sue Ellen Linville, Ph.D.

Business Unit Director:
William Brottmiller

Acquisitions Editor:
Marie Linvill

Editorial Assistant:
Kristin Banach

Executive Marketing Manager:
Dawn Gerrain

Channel Manager:
Tara Carter

Executive Production Manager:
Karen Leet

Production Editor:
Sandy Doyle

Library of Congress Cataloging-in-Publication Data
Linville, Sue Ellen.
Vocal aging / by Sue Ellen Linville.
p. ; cm.
Includes bibliographical references and index.
ISBN 1-56593-902-6 (soft cover : alk. paper)
1.Vocal cords—Aging.
2. Larynx—Aging. 3. Voice.
I. Title.
[DNLM: 1. Voice— physiology. 2. Aging— physiology. 3. Larynx— physiology. WV 501
QP306.L56 2000]
612.7'8—dc 21   00-034510

NOTICE TO THE READER

11/21/02

Contents

PREFACE

The topic of aging has been increasingly scrutinized in recent years. The baby boomers have moved into middle age and senior citizens are projected to make up an uncharacteristically large proportion of the population as the 21st century advances. This demographic shift has led to an explosion of new knowledge about aging reflected in conferences devoted exclusively to the topic and a plethora of new publications dealing with all aspects of normal and disordered aging.

The topic of aging also has captured the attention of researchers in the broad area of communication sciences and, more narrowly, in the specialization of normal voice production and voice disorders. This is evidenced by a substantial increase in the number of articles in scholarly journals devoted to issues related to the aging voice. Further, there have been a number of recent books dealing with comprehensive issues of communication problems in the elderly population, with chapters devoted specifically to vocal aging. However, as the knowledge base expands it becomes increasingly clear that an entire volume can be devoted exclusively to issues pertaining to the diagnosis and treatment of voice disorders in the elderly.

This book synthesizes existing knowledge on vocal aging. A problem inherent in an undertaking of this scope is determining the boundaries of the work. In this book I have limited discussion to current knowledge concerning processes directly and indirectly involved in aged voice both from a production and perception standpoint. I considered "normal" processes as well as clinical issues involved in diagnosis/treatment of vocal pathology in the elderly. These goals led to 17 chapters covering 5 broad topic areas (theoretical constructs, anatomic changes, physiologic alterations, acoustic/perceptual effects, and clinical issues).

Chapter 1 provides an introduction to the topic of aging in the broad sense. In this chapter general theories of aging are discussed. In addition, theories of vocal aging are presented. Writing this chapter was a humbling experience in that entire books have been written on aging theories in each of the individual disciplines covered (basic science, social science, behavioral science). To compensate for shortcomings inherent in representing a mountain of information in a single chapter, I refer the reader to numerous recent comprehensive volumes in which theories of aging are discussed at length. Discussing aging theories is advantageous, however, in that basic scientists and medical clinicians are exposed to social and behavioral perspectives that may be foreign to them (and vice versa). Such a discussion also provides a meaningful perspective from which the remaining chapters on the aging vocal mechanism might be viewed.

The 10 chapters that follow are devoted to changes in the speech production mechanism that occur normally during adulthood. Chapters 2 through 5 present age-related anatomic changes in the respiratory, laryngeal, supralaryngeal, and neuromuscular systems, respectively. Chapters 6 through 9 outline the impact of those anatomic changes on voice production in a relatively broad sense. Specifically, physiologic differences in speech breathing, vocal fold function, articulation, and speaking rate are considered. Chapters 10 and 11 focus on the impact of age-related anatomic and physiologic changes on the speech signal. That is, acoustic changes in the speech signal are described along with the significance of age-related acoustic changes to the listener.

Clinical issues are discussed in Chapters 12 through 17. An important factor in treating voice problems of the elderly involves distinguishing normal aging changes from disease processes. That distinction is frequently a difficult one and is discussed in Chapter 12. Much has been written of late on the unique aspects of professional voice use. Issues pertaining to the aging professional voice are considered in Chapter 13. Additional issues impacting on treatment decisions in older voice patients are prescription and nonprescription drug use and age-related endocrine changes. These topics are discussed in Chapters 14 and 15. The final two chapters of the book deal with strategies for treating voice disorders in the elderly. In Chapter 16, surgical treatments are considered. Chapter 17 focuses on special issues pertaining to voice therapy for elderly patients. To illustrate treatment strategies employed with elderly voice patients, case histories are included in Chapters 16 and 17.

I am indebted to the physicians and speech pathologists in the Department of Otolaryngology and Communication Sciences at the Medical College of Wisconsin for many of the case reports included in Chapters 16 and 17. In particular, I am indebted to Joan Kuhn, M.S., Director, Center for Communication and Swallowing Disorders, for compiling a list of potential cases and facilitating access to patient charts. I also am very appreciative of the contribution of Kerry Donovan, M.S. Without her diligent efforts sifting through patients' charts for countless hours and organizing the contents, presentation of many of these case studies would not have been possible.

I want to thank Dr. Tom Murry for his careful review of this manuscript. His thoughtful comments are most appreciated. I am indebted, as well, to Dr. Robert J. Toohill and Dr. Phillip K. Pellitteri for checking the accuracy of medical information in sections of the text. I am grateful, as well, to others who read various portions of the manuscript in preparation and offered valuable suggestions. I also want to thank the many colleagues and friends who offered support and encouragement along the way.

My husband Ron Ostrowski has been supportive and patient throughout the process. On more than one occasion he took up the slack in household tasks. He also served as computer consultant when interruptions in Internet access or software glitches threatened progress on the manuscript. I acknowledge his contributions with love and gratitude.

Theories of Aging

From early historical records, it is evident that people in all times have attempted to understand how people age. The present generation is merely the latest to look for explanations and undoubtedly future generations will do so as well. Most early models of aging reflected the broader views of the world held by that society. For example, according to ancient Hebrew scripture, the best predictor of longevity was obedience to God's commandments. Such obedience did not ensure long life, however, and variation was accepted as God's will. Throughout the early centuries, commentators repeatedly described the physical changes with aging (graying hair, stooped posture) and occasionally took note of increased wisdom and insight in the elderly. In virtually all early records, it is suggested that the indignities of old age relate to broader individual and relational purposes, although the specifics of such a relationship differs by time and culture. Although exceptions exist, these early explanations of aging tended to involve either moralistic prescriptions or individual reflection (Hendricks & Achenbaum, 1999).

Progressing beyond this early stage required refinement of statistical techniques and medical-technological development. Advances such as use of the microscope and X rays, as well as refinement of surgical, pharmaceutical, and psychiatric techniques allowed for differentiation of diseases/disabilities from normal changes over the life cycle. By the 1880s, technological advances had allowed biomedical researchers to begin to formulate descriptive compilations of the physical and pathological manifestations of growing older. By the beginning of the 20th century, a few scholars (Hall, 1922; Metchnikoff, 1903, 1907; Nascher, 1914) had ventured beyond descriptive compilations and begun to construct holistic theories of aging incorporating both biological and sociological perspectives (Hendricks & Achenbaum, 1999).

From the turn of the century up to World War II, holistic approaches to the study of aging prevailed in the United States. Nearly all fields of scholarly endeavor searched for a unifying theory in which knowledge from many disciplines could be subsumed into a single model. Many foundations and learned societies shared an interest in pooling resources to address issues of aging (Hendricks & Achenbaum, 1999). A significant achievement of this era was an edited volume (Cowdry, 1939) in which two differing views of aging were acknowledged that continue today; either aging is the result of degenerative processes or aging is a natural progression devoid of any particular pathology. Some view Cowdry's work as a benchmark for emphasizing the difficulty inherent in disentangling scientific data and social context (Hendricks & Achenbaum, 1999).

In postwar America, a combination of intellectual and institutional trends affected theory-building in gerontology. By that time, faculties at American universities had been organized into departments in which professional advancement required lengthy training beyond a bachelor's degree and publication of papers and books deemed acceptable by peers in that specific discipline. Institutions outside of academia (Veterans Administration, Rockefeller Foundation, National Science Foundation) reinforced the compartmentalization of information by choosing to invest more heavily in biomedical and natural science research than in research in the humanities or crossdisciplinary investigations. As a result, innovative theories usually evolved from work done within fields rather than from inquiries across disciplinary boundaries. Further, aging had not been identified as a major problem or issue in most disciplines at that time. Therefore, scientific interest in gerontology was sporadic and transitory, and scientists generally were more intent on pursuing other fields of inquiry (Hendricks & Achenbaum, 1999).

Modern interest in gerontology exploded in 1975 with the establishment of three agencies in the United States devoted to study in this area. Those agencies are the National Institute on Aging (National Institutes of Health); the Center on Aging (National Institute of Mental Health); and the Geriatric Research, Education and Clinical Centers Program (Veterans Administration). Research support from these agencies provided a major stimulus for research on aging in the United States and other nations as well (Birren, 1999; Brody, 1992). Undoubtedly, changes in the demographics of the world population led to establishment of these agencies. Currently, in most developed countries the proportion of the population aged 65 and over exceeds 10%. The relative size of the aging population in the United States is slightly lower than western European countries such as Sweden and Britain. This disparity is attributed to a more sustained postwar baby boom in the United States as well as a rejuvenating effect of immigration on population age structure (Grundy, 1992). Nonetheless, growth of the aged population in the United States in the 20th century has been dramatic. Although only 1 in 25 Americans exceeded 65 years of age in 1900, that proportion grew to 1 in 9 by 1984. The projected proportion of elderly Americans by 2050 is 1 in 5 (Cody, 1993).

Although interest in gerontology has exploded of late, there are those who feel that gerontological theory building still suffers from a lack of crossdisciplinary collaboration. Indeed, Hendricks and Achenbaum (1999) view recent major advancements in gerontology as limited to the area of measurement, as opposed to theory building. They point to a number of researchers at the National Institute on Aging who have devoted their careers to collecting "bits of data with precise calculations rather than pausing to theorize about the meanings of their findings" (p. 31). Hendricks and Achenbaum urge development of interdisciplinary models of aging that step beyond the medical model. Similarly, behavioral researchers have noted the lack of integrative theory on the psychology of aging despite a profusion of research findings pertaining to the psychological characteristics of aging (Birren & Birren, 1990; Birren & Schroots, 1996). Other writers, as well, point to the sheer diversity of explanations put forth to explain aging and conclude that aging is a very complex, dynamic process that can be understood in total only by considering many perspectives (Birren, 1999; Cavanaugh, 1999).

Despite differing opinions as to the best avenue to explore the phenomenon of aging, one fact is clear. With the explosion of the aging population, health care providers are increasingly called on to provide expert care to elderly patients. It has become more important than ever that clinicians understand normal physiological changes with aging to successfully recognize and treat disease processes affecting the elderly. It is important, as well, that health care providers consider psychological and cultural aspects of aging that influence general health in aged persons. In terms of voice disorders, awareness of the impact of aging on the human body as a whole gives clinicians a broader perspective into which voice production issues can be placed. In this chapter, the mystery of human aging is explored from various theoretical perspectives.

BIOLOGICAL THEORIES

Biological theories are among the oldest theories explaining the aging process. The theories are based on an immense amount of research on age-associated changes in organism function at both the molecular and systemic level. A thorough explanation of each of these theories is well beyond the scope of this chapter. For more comprehensive information on this topic, the reader is referred to several recent reviews (Cavanaugh, 1999; Clark, 1999; Davies, 1992b; Harmon, 1998). Biological theories fall into two general categories: those that explain aging on the basis of purposeful events and those that relate aging to the cumulative effect of a variety of random events on the organism. There are additional theories, as well, that incorporate various aspects of both of these classes.

Purposeful Event Theories

Purposeful event theories postulate that either genetic programming or hormonal changes direct the aging process. What these theories have in common is the premise that there is a "master plan" that governs the aging process (Cavanaugh, 1999).

Programmed Aging Theory

The theory of genetic control of aging is supported by the fact that there are characteristic species-specific life spans and that survival curves are relatively uniform within a species (Davies, 1992b). Further, there is evidence of species-specific patterns for causes of death. That is, the most common causes of death in elderly humans living in industrialized countries are vascular disease and malignancies (Smith, 1993). By comparison, causes of death in laboratory rodents are strain dependent and include kidney failure and malignancies not frequently associated with death in humans (Adams & Cory, 1991; Yu, Masoro, Murata, Bertrand, & Lynd, 1982). Additional support for genetic control of aging has been inferred from aging-like symptoms in a number of different genetic diseases in humans such as Werner syndrome, Hutchinson-Gilford syndrome, Cockayne syndrome, and Siep syndrome (Martin, 1978, 1982). Further, data extracted from the archives of life insurance companies indicate that the offspring of long-lived parents have a greater probability of living a long life span themselves (Davies, 1992b). However, evidence contrary to genetic programming is found in observations that individual members of a species die of various causes over a range of ages, that identical twins do not die at identical times, and that environmental factors can shorten life span (Cristofalo, Tresini, Francis, & Volker, 1999; Grundy, 1992). In addition, critics of genetic programming argue that such theories fail to account for evolution. That is, if genetically programmed cell death is to account for aging, then one must assume that aging was selected during the evolutionary process. However, older adults in the species failed to live long enough to allow for selection of aging by the process of evolution (Hayflick, 1994). An additional argument posed by critics of genetic programming concerns differences in life span recorded for different species with similar cellular and molecular constructs. The fact that these differences exist suggests that the critical variable in aging is not the genetic programming of the cells, themselves, but rather the manner in which the cells operate in different environmental niches (Davies, 1992a).

The Neuroendocrine Theory

The endocrine system has been considered by some to play a crucial role in why people age. Given the immense importance of the endocrine system to development and maturation in children, as well as metabolic regulation in adults, it makes sense that this system would be closely examined for potential contributions to aging. Further, recognition that the latter part of the life span is associated with a decline in homeostatic regulation in both humans and laboratory rodents has fueled study in this area (Finch & Seeman, 1999). Proponents of this theory argue that modifications of the internal environment in which cells live, regulated by the endocrine system, affect the rate of accumulation of DNA damage in cells with aging. Thus hormonal variables either hinder or facilitate repair of cellular damage and by so doing either promote or postpone aging (Davies, 1992a). Supporters of this theory also point out that in most species declining reproductive capacity, regulated by the endocrine system, predicts aging as strongly as does increased mortality rate (Cavanaugh, 1999). However, a problem with the endocrine theory is that hormonal changes with aging vary across gender within a species and those variations don't correspond to life expectancy. That is, women undergo more precipitous hormonal changes as they age but still live roughly 7 years longer than men. For this reason, some researchers have concluded that although hormonal changes correlate with aging processes, they probably are not responsible for those changes (Cavanaugh, 1999; Hayflick, 1994).

Random Event Theories

Random event theories postulate that aging is the end product of various forms of random damage over the life span. Specifics as to the nature of the random damage vary from theory to theory but include wear and tear, variations in energy expenditure, cross-linking of molecules that interferes with normal processes, oxidative stress effects to susceptible cells, imperfect repair of damaged cells, or immune system errors.

Wear and Tear Theory

According to the wear and tear theory of aging, death occurs because body systems and organs simply wear out (Whitbourne, 1996). In this view, human aging is seen as the cumulative effect of the abuse of everyday life. Critics see this theory as implausible as an explanation for the cause of aging, noting that although certain parts of the body (for instance joints) tend to wear out with aging, these observable changes more accurately describe aging outcomes. That is, wear and tear changes, such as arthritic joints, are an outcome of the aging process rather than an explanation for the process.

Rate of Living Theory

According to the rate of living theory, the total energy expenditure during a lifetime is genetically predetermined and, therefore, longevity depends on metabolic rate (Pearl, 1928). Thus, if the metabolic rate of an organism is reduced, that organism will have a lengthened life span and vice versa. Evidence for this theory derives from studies indicating that cold-blooded animals have reduced metabolisms and live longer at lower temperatures. Similarly, houseflies confined to containers that restrict movement to walking only (no flying) live 2½ times longer than controls, presumably because of the reductions in metabolic rate associated with elimination of flying (Balin & Allen, 1986). In addition, mammals that are induced to hibernate live longer than controls (Sacher, 1977). Although these observations support the hypothesis that metabolic rate, in some organisms, plays a role in aging, such observations do not identify the mechanism through which metabolism affects aging. Similarly, unidentified genetic factors may underlie the metabolic potential of a species (Cristofalo et al., 1999). In addition, it has been pointed out that many centenarian humans lead active lives, while many sedentary individuals die at a young age. Such an occurrence runs contrary to this theory (Cavanaugh, 1999).

Cross-Linking Theory

The cross-linking theory holds that changes at the cellular level are responsible for aging. Specifically, with aging, additional molecules called cross-links are added to cells that hold together parallel molecules composing the cell. The additional cross-links are thought to alter the characteristics of the cell. For instance, additional cross-links in collagen protein with aging increase rigidity and stiffness of skin cells. As a consequence, the skin of elderly adults is less soft and pliable than the skin of young adults. According to this theory, cross-links also occur in nucleic acids with aging. As nucleic acids are molecules that compose the genes, an increase in cross links theoretically would result in faulty genetic blueprints that are passed along as the cell divides. The shortcoming of this theory is that little is known currently about the mechanism of the cross-linking process and what causes cross-linking to occur. Also, it has yet to be demonstrated conclusively that cross-linking actually interferes with biological processes and causes faulty molecules to be produced (Cavanaugh, 1999).

Free Radical Theory

Proponents of the oxidative stress (free radical) theory contend that aging is the consequence of cumulative damage to cells by reactive oxygen (oxygen radicals) generated by mitochondria during cell metabolism as gaseous oxygen is converted to water. The specifics of the theory are explained by Clark (1999). Normally during cell metabolism, a small number of oxygen radicals escape from the reaction site and attack and seriously damage a wide range of cellular molecules. Indeed, the mitochondria, themselves, are frequently damaged resulting in decreased energy production within cells and compromised cell function. Furthermore, once mitochondria are damaged, leakage of oxygen radicals increases, compounding the damage to cells. Damage done by reactive oxygen to molecules necessary to operate cells can be enormous and involves protein molecules, lipid molecules, and DNA. It is damage to DNA that is of most concern in terms of aging. It has been estimated that the DNA in a single cell is "hit" by oxygen radicals tens of thousands of times per day. Interestingly, however, the DNA damage caused by oxygen radicals is not thought to produce cell mutations. Rather, mutations are thought to result most frequently from errors during the DNA repair process. With advancing age, the incidence of unrepaired oxidative injuries at the cellular level increases as the rate of production of oxygen radicals surpasses the effectiveness of prevention or repair of cellular damage, particularly to DNA. Proponents of the free-radical theory suggest that oxidative stress helps to explain differences in maximal life span across species, in that longer-lived species either generate less oxidative damage to begin with or have more effective prevention or repair mechanisms in place (Clark, 1999). However, perhaps the best evidence supporting the role of free-radicals in aging comes from studies suggesting that introduction of chemicals known to inhibit free-radicals (antioxidants) can prolong life by as much as 30% in non-human species. Further, there is some evidence that the administration of antioxidants delays the appearance of cancer, cardiovascular disease, immune system declines, and degenerative diseases of the central nervous system in humans (Hayflick, 1994).

Immune System Theory

The immune system has been studied extensively for possible relationships to aging because of its importance in protecting the body against foreign substances. The immune system theory is based on findings that the immune system of older adults is slower to build up defenses against specific diseases, even after vaccination (Lehtonen, Eskola, Vainio, & Lehtonen, 1990). This finding could explain why the elderly are more susceptible to certain infections (Abrams & Berkow, 1990). The immune theory also is supported by findings that aging reduces the body's ability to recognize organisms that are native to the individual, such as certain proteins. This decline in self-recognition ability can lead to autoimmune disorders such as rheumatoid arthritis (Weksler, 1990). A major unresolved issue with the immune system theory, however, is the extent to which some other process, such as age-related neuroendocrine system change, is actually responsible for immune system errors (Hayflick, 1994).

BEHAVIORAL THEORIES

The state of affairs in the behavioral sciences pertaining to theories of aging is generally more muddled than in biological science. This is due, in part, to greater diversity of research on aging in behavioral areas (Cavanaugh, 1999). In addition, much behavioral research has dealt with "aspects of aging" without examination of the significance of findings to the broader functioning and well-being of the aged person (Birren & Schroots, 1996).

Much early research into the psychology of aging dealt with differences in cognitive capacity with aging. These studies led to theories involving declines across a variety of cognitive processes, including attention, working memory, and processing speed (Cavanaugh, 1999). In some cases these theories provide powerful insight into the functional capacity of elderly persons. However, they do not address the more fundamental issues of why processing resources decline with aging. Further, they do not provide insight into the dynamics of age-related changes in these processes (Birren & Fisher, 1995; Birren & Schroots, 1996).

Psychological theories of aging also have addressed age-related changes in personality and identity. Much debate has centered on whether personality and identity remain stable across the life span or whether these constructs undergo systematic change (Cavanaugh, 1999). Some theorists have concluded that personality traits including neuroticism, extraversion, openness to experience, conscientiousness-undirectedness, and agreeableness-antagonism are stable across adulthood (McCrae & Costa, 1990). Others have proposed theories of dynamic, interactive growth of personality and identity during an individual's life span (Erikson, 1982; Kegan, 1982; Loevinger, 1976; Whitbourne, 1996) and stressed the utility of a life-course approach in developing public policy directed toward the elderly (Dobrof, 1990). It has been suggested, as well, that elderly individuals vary considerably both in the manner and the rate in which aging affects personality and identity (Birren & Schroots, 1996; Dobrof, 1990). Such an observation may explain much of the conflicting opinion about age-related changes in personality and identity. Certainly increased variability has been a very consistent finding across a wide range of physiologic, acoustic, and motor performance variables measured in elderly persons (Chapter 12).

Emerging theories concerning the psychology of aging focus on encouraging the replacement of chronological age as the sole criterion for assessing the significance of observed changes (Birren & Schroots, 1996). For example, according to the theory of gerodynamics, aging involves a series of transformations resulting from arrival at critical points in life. At these critical life points (bifurcation points), the individual undergoes change involving biological, behavioral, and social functioning. Thus, gerodynamics is the basis for the branching theory of aging in which aging results in patterns of stability and change across all levels of functioning analogous to a branching tree (Schroots, 1995a, 1995b). Interestingly, the recent trend in the field of psychology to get away from a view of aging based solely on chronological age parallels much current thinking about vocal aging (Chapter 12).

CULTURE AND AGING

Culture is a vital and pervasive force of humanity that molds a society's social and political institutions, ideals, and norms. It is generally defined in terms of shared basic value orientations and beliefs and by habits of living that are held in common (Luborsky & McMullen, 1999). Culture shapes the social settings, personal experiences, and living conditions of the elderly and contributes to many psychosocial and physical processes of aging. Culture also directs a society's attention to particular issues for study and instills particular notions of the correct way to conduct research on the topic of aging. That is, culture can foster a sort of intellectual blindfold by providing an underlying assumption about how things work that is taken for granted (Achenbaum 1978; Luborsky & McMullen, 1999; Luborsky & Sankar, 1993). For example, in the field of rehabilitation, long-held cultural assumptions supported the loss of physical function as a "normal" part of aging. This notion delayed recognition of the overall life-enhancing benefits of rehabilitation for the elderly (Becker & Kaufman, 1988).

The importance of societal influences on the process of aging has been well demonstrated through epidemiologic research. For instance, there is evidence of a link between mortality and social networks (Blazer, 1982; Seeman, Kaplan, Knudsen, Cohen, & Guralnik, 1987). There also is a suggestion that economic disadvantage exacerbates aging effects in certain segments of the population (Wilkins & Adams, 1983; Victor & Vetter, 1986). Even from a physiological perspective, societal adoption of cigarette smoking has been linked with earlier menopause in women (Willett et al., 1983). Clearly, considering a wide range of societal factors provides a broader perspective from which the complexities of the aging process might be better understood (Jeffreys, 1992).

Every culture includes unwritten expectations for proper behavior in individuals of a certain chronological age that have been referred to as sociocultural age. Sociocultural age involves a specific set of roles that are adopted by an individual in relation to other members of the culture to which they belong. Included in sociocultural age are behaviors and habits such as style of dress, customs, language, and interpersonal style. The extent to which a person demonstrates certain age-dependent behaviors expected by that culture forms the basis by which that individual is judged as socioculturally younger or older (Cavanaugh, 1999). From the perspective of voice production, apparent cultural stereotypes for "old voice" have been encountered in studies comparing speakers sounding young with those sounding old (Chapter 11). Also, the possibility has been raised that sociocultural factors influence speech rate in the elderly, although such a conclusion has yet to be substantiated empirically (Ramig, 1986). As pointed out by Hollien (1987), very little is currently known about the extent to which age-related voice changes contribute to stereotypic attitudes toward the elderly. Indeed, the entire realm of cultural influences on aged voice has yet to be investigated systematically and offers a fertile field for future research.

Culture has the potential to exert both positive and negative influences on individuals and communities. Culture can act positively by providing a sense of values and ideals. These values and ideals become particularly important when individuals face adversities, such as health problems, family problems, financial difficulties, and relationship conflicts. Under adverse conditions, culture can help to provide explanations for problems and offer guidelines for their resolution. However, culture also can be the source of considerable distress and hardship in times of adversity. It may set unrealistic goals and expectations for individuals or communities. Culture also devalues certain people or traits, provides negative stereotypes, and stigmatizes certain segments of the population (Luborsky & McMullen, 1999).

American culture places an extraordinarily high value on individualism, autonomy, and independence. In American society, full personhood (adulthood) is earned during the adult phase of life by being a responsible and productive worker, spouse, community member, and family member. To retain recognition as a self-determining, culturally competent, and complete person, an individual must retain competence in these areas. For individuals whose physical condition precludes their ability to meet social expectations (such as the frail elderly), there is a significant loss of esteem (Luborsky & McMullen, 1999). These cultural values produce a crisis of dependency in many American elders as they struggle to live independently (Albert & Cattell, 1994; Clark, 1972). A cultural value on independence also is linked to a reluctance of Americans to use adaptive devices to minimize the impact of physical impairments (Luborsky, 1994). In terms of communication competence, it is certainly possible that a cultural premium on autonomy and independence complicates acceptance of artificial larynges or augmentative communication devices by elderly patients whose lives stand to be improved by their use.

Looking inside American culture, it becomes important, as well, to consider the subculture of ethnicity and its impact on the aging process. The influence of ethnicity on aging is discussed at some length by Luborsky and McMullen (1999). Briefly, social gerontologists have become increasingly aware of the relationship of ethnic identity to aging. Questions scholars are addressing include: To what extent does ethnic group membership change the experience of old age? How is ethnic identity used by the elderly as a resource to cope with stresses encountered in later life? Do ethnic groups differ in the patterns of care they provide for older people? Questions such as these are difficult to answer, however, because ethnicity involves both conscious and unconscious beliefs and behaviors. In addition, ethnic identity is a "fluid" trait that people demonstrate to differing degrees and one that varies in individuals with variations in social, personal, cultural, and life span events. However, despite these conceptual difficulties, Luborsky and McMullen (1999) find little doubt that ethnic differences exist across a wide variety of life experiences, including reactions to illness (Suchman, 1964), responses to physical pain (Zborowski, 1969), variations in family configuration (Cohler & Grunebaum, 1981), patterns of alcohol consumption (Greeley, McCready,

& Theisen, 1980), beliefs about death (Kalish & Reynolds, 1976), patterns of institutionalization of the elderly (Markson, 1979), and interpretations of mental illness (Jenkins, Kleinman, & Good, 1991). Given the broad influence of ethnicity on many aspects of individual behavior, it is intriguing to consider the extent to which changes in voice with aging may be influenced by ethnic differences. The effect of ethnicity on voice changes with aging has yet to be investigated systematically. However, such differences may explain some of the variability researchers have encountered when measuring acoustic, physiologic, and perceptual voice parameters in elderly speakers (Chapter 12).

MODELS OF AGING VOICE

Relatively few scientists have attempted to propose models of aging voice, and any such models were presented as tentative. Hollien (1987) proposed the male–female coalescence model in which vocal changes with advanced age are viewed as a functional reversal of sex-oriented changes occurring at puberty. That is, whereas vocal changes occurring at puberty result in greater vocal dissimilarity in males and females, vocal changes following middle age result in greater similarity in male and female voices. This theory is intriguing, although Hollien (1987) applied it only to hormonally based changes in speaking fundamental frequency occurring at puberty and again at menopause (Chapter 10). Interestingly, the notion that the sexes become biologically more similar after middle age also fits data on age-related differences in glottal gap. Men develop glottal gaps for the first time relatively late in life, whereas women either maintain the same overall incidence of gap observed in young adulthood or demonstrate fewer gaps (Chapter 7). A question that remains, however, is the mechanism behind apparent coalescence of the sexes. Is this phenomenon strictly a response to hormonal differences or do broader genetic factors drive these differences?

Throughout this volume are indications that men show the effects of aging more dramatically in terms of voice (and speech) production than do women, although both demonstrate age-related changes. Evidence suggests that women show fewer aging effects in: onset/extent of laryngeal structure change (Chapter 3), fine motor control of laryngeal abductory/adductory movements (Chapter 8), tongue movements (Chapter 8), and speaking rate (Chapter 9). Speech breathing (Chapter 6) might be an exception to this pattern in that both sexes demonstrate significant age-related deterioration.

Many age-related voice changes might be explained by two physical factors: (1) loss of tissue elasticity and (2) muscle weakening. Increased stiffness of the thoracic cavity and loss of respiratory muscle strength impede the ability of the system to move air in and out during the breathing process, leading to reductions in vital capacity. Increased stiffness of laryngeal tissues accompanied by muscle weakening affect phonatory adjustments related to pitch level, pitch changing, vocal fold positioning, and intrinsic vocal fold vibratory characteristics. Articulatory changes attributed to these factors include slowed gestures, decreases in the extent of tongue and lip movement, and timing of supraglottic/glottic events in voiceless stop production. Further, it has been theorized that extrinsic laryngeal muscle weakening lowers laryngeal position and that weakened pharyngeal musculature shortens the duration of vocal fold vibration during the closure interval for voiced stop production in older speakers. A model of muscle weakening and tissue flaccidity also fits nicely with clinical observations that programs of general physical conditioning facilitate maintenance of vocal functioning into old age (Chapter 17). Such a model also explains some of the variability in age-related voice change (Chapter 12), if it is assumed that elderly individuals vary in the extent to which they engage in muscle conditioning activities.

A shortcoming of a "weakening and stiffening" theory is that it fails to account for gender differences in the process of vocal aging and, as noted previously, such differences can be significant. The mechanism(s) behind such gender differences still are unclear. In addition, this theory does not address the underlying cause of weakening and stiffening. Is a generalized loss of strength and elasticity in the speaking mechanism triggered by a disordered nerve supply or by changes in other bodily systems? A "weakening and stiffening" theory also fails to account for environmental factors such as medications, smoking, vocal use patterns, general health, and social/emotional variables that impact on voice. Further, potential cultural differences are not explained (Chapters 8, 11).

It is clear that a successful model of vocal aging must encompass biological, behavioral, and cultural elements. If the voice is the mirror of the soul, then, as such, aged voice reflects the psychological state of the speaker and the sociocultural environment in which an elderly individual functions. Remarkably little is known at present of the psychosocial/cultural aspects of voice production in the elderly. Of course, aged voice also derives from biological systems and is inextricably tied to any age-related changes in those systems. The challenge to future investigators is to ascertain the relative contributions of each of these elements to voice changes with aging and to be able to predict age-related voice change in an individual based on a set of characteristics unique to that person.

SUMMARY

This chapter presents varying views of the aging process from biological, psychological, and cultural perspectives. The biological sciences have uncovered a number of systems involved in the aging process. What remains in this field is to determine the relative contributions of a variety of biological mechanisms to the aging process. Biologists also must determine the nature of any interactions among systems that account for aging. In behavioral sciences, a similar deficiency is evident. Although age-related changes in basic cognitive processes have been identified, changes in information processing have yet to be linked with more holistic changes in thinking and identity that also have been uncovered. From a social science perspective, it is clear that aging cannot be understood without considering an individual's relationship with the larger culture. The fields of biology, psychology, and sociology all provide some insight into the mystery of aging. However, a complete explanation of aging awaits comprehensive crossdisciplinary efforts incorporating all aspects of the aging process.

How does vocal aging fit within the context of these larger issues? To what extent are anatomical and physiological changes within the larynx, respiratory system, and articulatory mechanism linked with biological mechanisms affecting other body systems? In what manner do behavioral changes alter aged voice production? How does the culture of aging in a given society affect voice production in elderly persons within that society? These are intriguing questions that have yet to be addressed. As the reader progresses through the chapters that follow it will be beneficial to consider these issues and reflect on the communication process as it fits within the larger realm of human aging.

REFERENCES

Abrams, W., & Berkow, R. (Eds.). (1990). *The Merck manual of geriatrics.* Rahwah, NJ: Merck Sharp & Dohme Research Laboratories.

Achenbaum, A. (1978). *Old age in the new land: The American experience since 1970.* Baltimore: Johns Hopkins Press.

Adams, J., & Cory, S. (1991). Transgenic models of tumor development. *Science, 254,* 1161–1167.

Albert, S., & Cattell, M. (1994). *Old age in global perspective: Cross-cultural and cross-national views.* New York: G. K. Hall.

Balin, A., & Allen, R. (1986). Mechanisms of biological aging. *Dermatological Clinics, 4,* 347–358.

Becker, G., & Kaufman, S. (1988). Old age, rehabilitation, and research: A review of the issues. *Gerontologist, 28,* 459–468.

Birren, J. (1999). Theories of aging: A personal perspective. In V. Bengtson & W. Schaie (Eds.), *Handbook of theories of aging* (pp. 459–471). New York: Springer Publishing Company.

Birren, J., & Birren, B. (1990). The concepts, models and history of the psychology of aging. In J. Birren & K. Schaie (Eds.), *Handbook of the psychology of aging (3rd ed.,* pp. 3–20). San Diego: Academic Press.

Birren, J., & Fisher, L. (1995). Aging and speed of behavior: Possible consequences for psychological functioning. *Annual Review of Psychology, 46,* 329–353.

Birren, J., & Schroots, J. (1996). History, concepts, and theory in the psychology of aging. In J. Birren & K. Schaie (Eds.), *Handbook of the psychology of aging (4th ed.,* pp. 3–23). San Diego: Academic Press.

Blazer, D. (1982). Social support and mortality in an elderly community population. *American Journal of Epidemiology, 115,* 684–694.

Brody, H. (1992). The aging brain. *Acta Neurologica Scandanavia* (Suppl.), *137,* 40–44.

Cavanaugh, J. (1999). Theories of aging in the biological, behavioral, and social sciences. In J. Cavanaugh & S. Whitbourne (Eds.), *Gerontology: An interdisciplinary perspective* (pp.1–32). New York: Oxford University Press.

Clark, M. (1972). An anthropological view of retirement. In F. Carp (Ed.), *Retirement* (pp. 117–156). New York: Human Sciences Press.

Clark, W. (1999). *A means to an end: The biological basis of aging and death.* New York: Oxford University Press.

Cody, R. (1993). Physiological changes due to age: Implications for drug therapy of congestive heart failure. *Drugs & Aging, 3,* 320–334.

Cohler, B., & Grunebaum, H. (1981). *Mothers, grandmothers and daughters: Personality and child care in three-generation families.* New York: Wiley.

Cowdry, E. V. (1939). *Problems of aging: Biological and medical aspects.* Baltimore: The Williams & Wilkins Company.

Cristofalo, V., Tresini, M., Francis, M., & Volker, C. (1999). Biological theories of senescence. In V. Bengtson & K. W. Schaie (Eds.), *Handbook of theories of aging* (pp. 98–112). New York: Springer Publishing Company.

Davies, I. (1992a). Aging and the endocrine system. In J. Brocklehurst, R. Tallis, & H. Fillit (Eds.), *Textbook of geriatric medicine and gerontology* (pp. 666–674). Edinburgh: Churchill Livingstone.

Davies, I. (1992b). Theories and general principles of aging. In J. Brocklehurst, R. Tallis, & H. Fillit (Eds.), *Textbook of geriatric medicine and gerontology* (pp. 26–60). Edinburgh: Churchill Livingstone.

Dobrof, R. (1990). Keynote address; A conceptual framework for research in aging: Revelations of the current decade. In E. Cherow (Ed.), *ASHA Reports No. 19. Proceedings of the Research Symposium on Communication Sciences and Disorders.* Rockville, MD: ASHA.

Erikson, E. (1982). *The life cycle completed: A review.* New York: Norton.

Finch, C., & Seeman, T. (1999). Stress theories of aging. In V. Bengtson & K. W. Schaie (Eds.), *Handbook of theories of aging* (pp. 81–97). New York: Springer Publishing Company.

Greeley, A., McCready, W., & Theisen, G. (1980). *Ethnic drinking subcultures.* New York: Praeger.

Grundy, E. (1992). The epidemiology of aging. In J. Brocklehurst, R. Tallis, & H. Fillit (Eds.), *Textbook of geriatric medicine & gerontology* (4th ed., pp. 3–20). Edinburgh: Churchill Livingstone.

Hall, G. S. (1922). *Senescence, the last half of life.* New York: D. Appleton & Company.

Harmon, D. (1998). Aging: Phenomena and theories. In D. Harmon, R. Holliday, & M. Meydani (Eds.), *Annals of the New York Academy of Sciences: Vol. 854. Towards prolongation of the healthy life span: Practical approaches to intervention* (pp. 1–7). New York: New York Academy of Sciences.

Hayflick, L. (1994). *How and why we age.* New York: Ballantine Books.

Hendricks, J., & Achenbaum, A. (1999). Historical development of theories of aging. In V. Berngtson & K. W. Schaie (Eds.), *Handbook of theories of aging* (pp. 21–39). New York: Springer Publishing Company.

Hollien, H. (1987). "Old voices": What do we really know about them? *Journal of Voice, 1,* 2–17.

Jeffreys, M. (1992). The elderly in society. In J. Brocklehurst, R. Tallis, & H. Fillit (Eds.), *Textbook of geriatric medicine and gerontology* (4th ed., pp. 971–979). Edinburgh: Churchill Livingstone.

Jenkins, J., Kleinman, A., & Good, B. (1991). Cross-cultural aspects of depression: Introduction. In J. Becker & A. Kleinman (Eds.), *Psychosocial aspects of depression* (pp. 67–97). Hillsdale, NJ: Lawrence Erlbaum.

Kalish, R., & Reynolds, M. (1976). *Death and ethnicity: A psychocultural study.* Los Angeles: Ethel Percy Andrus Gerontology Center, University of Southern California.

Kegan, R. (1982). *The evolving self.* Cambridge, MA: Harvard University Press.

Lehtonen, L., Eskola, J., Vainio, O., & Lehtonen, A. (1990). Changes in lymphocyte subsets and immune competence in very advanced age. *Journal of Gerontology: Medical Sciences, 45,* M108–M112.

Loevinger, J. (1976). *Ego development.* San Francisco: Jossey-Bass.

Luborsky, M. (1994). The cultural adversity of physical disability: Erosion of full adult personhood. *Journal of Aging Studies, 8,* 239–253.

Luborsky, M., & McMullen, C. (1999). Culture and aging. In J. Cavanaugh & S. Whitbourne (Eds.), *Gerontology. An interdisciplinary perspective* (pp. 65–90). New York: Oxford University Press.

Luborsky, M., & Sankar, A. (1993). Extending the critical gerontology perspective: Cultural dimensions. *The Gerontologist, 33,* 440–444.

Markson, E. (1979). Ethnicity as a factor in the institutionalization of the elderly. In D. Gelfand & A. Kutzik (Eds.), *Ethnicity and aging: Theory, research, and policy* (pp. 341–356). New York: Springer.

Martin, G. (1978). Genetic syndromes in man with potential relevance to the pathobiology of aging. *Birth Defects: Original Article Series, 14,* 5–39.

Martin, G. (1982). Syndromes of accelerated aging. *National Cancer Institute Monographs, 60,* 241–247.

McCrae, R., & Costa, P. (1990). *Personality in adulthood.* New York: Guilford.

Metchnikoff, E. (1903). *The nature of man: Studies in optimistic philosophy* (English translation edited by P. C. Mitchell). New York: G. P. Putnam's Sons.

Metchnikoff, E. (1907). *The prolongation of life: Optimistic studies.* New York: G. P. Putnam's Sons.

Nascher, I. (1914). *Geriatrics: The diseases of old age and their treatment including physiological old age, home and institutional care, and medico-legal relations.* Philadelphia: P. Blakiston's Son & Co.

Pearl, R. (1928). *The rate of living theory.* New York: A. A. Knopf.

Ramig, L. (1986). Aging speech: Physiological and sociological aspects. *Language and Communication, 6,* 25–34.

Sacher, G. (1977). Life table modification and life prolongation. In C. E. Finch & L. Hayflick (Eds.), *Handbook of the biology of aging* (pp. 582–638). New York: Van Nostrand Reinhold.

Schroots, J. (1995a). The fractal structure of lives: Continuity and discontinuity in autobiography. In J. Birren, G. Kenyon, J. Ruth, J. Schroots, & T. Svensson (Eds.), *Biography and aging: Explorations in adult development* (pp. 117–130). New York: Springer.

Schroots, J. (1995b). Gerodynamics: Toward a branching theory of aging. *Canadian Journal on Aging, 14,* 74–81.

Seeman, T., Kaplan, G., Knudsen, L., Cohen, R., & Guralnik, J. (1987). Social network ties and mortality among the elderly in the Alameda county study. *American Journal of Epidemiology, 126,* 714–723.

Smith, D. (1993). *Human longevity.* New York: Oxford University Press.

Suchman, E. (1964). Sociomedical variations among ethnic groups. *American Journal of Sociology, 70,* 328–329.

Victor, C., & Vetter, N. (1986). Poverty, disability and use of services in the elderly: Analyses of the 1980 General Household Survey. *Social Science & Medicine, 22,* 1087–1091.

Weksler, M. (1990). Protecting the aging immune system to prolong quality of life. *Geriatrics, 45,* 72–76.

Whitbourne, S. (1996). *The aging individual.* New York: Springer.

Wilkins, R., & Adams, O. (1983). Health expectancy in Canada, late 1970s: Demographic, regional and social dimensions. *American Journal of Public Health, 73,* 1073–1080.

Willett, W., Stampfer, M., Bain, C., Lipnick, R., Speizer, F., Rosner, B., Cramer, D., & Hennekens, C. (1983). Cigarette smoking, relative weight, and menopause. *American Journal of Epidemiology, 117,* 651–658.

Yu, B., Masoro, E., Murata, I., Bertrand, H., & Lynd, F. (1982). Life span study of SPF Fischer 344 male rats fed ad libitum or restricted diets: Longevity, growth, lean body mass, and disease. *Journal of Gerontology, 37,* 130–141.

Zborowski, M. (1969). *People in pain.* San Francisco: Jossey-Bass.

CHAPTER

2

Aging of the Respiratory System

As the power supply for voice, the respiratory system is central to the speech production process. Anatomic changes in the lungs, chest wall, and thoracic skeleton with aging lead to changes in the physiology of breathing. Age-related alterations in breathing physiology ultimately affect speech breathing (Chapter 6) and also impact the voice produced by elderly speakers.

In examining age-related changes in the respiratory system, it is important to distinguish changes that are a normal part of the aging process from changes that reflect the presence of disease. To fail to do so leads to mistreatment of otherwise healthy older individuals who might display normal age-related deterioration in lung function. In addition, it is important to separate changes strictly due to the passage of time from changes due to the effects of environmental factors, although such a distinction can be difficult to draw (Dhar, Shastri, & Lenora, 1976). For example, recent evidence suggests that one consequence of smoking is an enhancement of oxidative damage to lung tissue normally associated with aging. That is, elderly smokers experience the same oxidative damage observed in nonsmokers but to a greater extent (Lee et al., 1999).

After maturation, respiratory function declines progressively with increasing age in both men (age 25) and women (age 20). Although the mechanisms leading to diminished respiratory function are not completely understood, three factors stand out as important in the process: (1) decreased lung elasticity, (2) decreased strength of the respiratory muscles, and (3) increased stiffness of the thoracic cage (Mahler, 1983). In this chapter, structural changes in the respiratory system with aging are described and the impact of those changes on lung volumes and respiratory mechanics in elderly speakers is discussed. This information serves as an important foundation for understanding voice production in elderly speakers.

STRUCTURAL CHANGES

Lungs and Lower Airways

The lungs undergo marked anatomical changes as adulthood advances. The lungs of older persons at autopsy have been reported to be smaller, lighter in weight, and less elastic than those of younger adults (Richards, 1965; Rolleston, 1922). After ruling out airway obstruction, age-related dehydration has been mentioned as a causative factor in size reduction in the elderly (Macklin & Macklin, 1942).

Age changes also have been reported in the vascular tissue of the lungs. Blood vessel walls reportedly thicken with aging, although there is considerable variability among individuals in this regard (Richards, 1965). Several reports indicate that pulmonary venules and arterioles are less compliant in the elderly (Heath, 1964; Shephard, 1987) and capillary linings may become fibrotic due to collagen deposits or hyalinization (Lebowitz, 1988; Reddan, 1981; Shephard, 1987). It has been hypothesized that these changes result in increased resistance to diffusion of gas through the capillary walls because of increased vascular resistance (Robinson, 1964). Such an increase in resistance accounts for elevation of the alveolar-arterial oxygen (PO_2) gradient that has been observed with aging (Kenney, 1982; Lebowitz, 1988; Lynne-Davies, 1977; Pierce & Ebert, 1958).

Microscopic examination has revealed widening of the respiratory bronchioles and alveolar ducts as early as the third decade of life. Enlargement of these structures has been reported in almost all people, especially after age 40. This process has been labeled both "ductectasia" and "senile emphysema" (Brody & Thurlbeck, 1986; Thurlbeck, 1967, 1991). It is not certain whether enlargement of these terminal airways is due to aging alone or a combination of aging and environmental factors (Snider,

Kleinerman, Thurlbeck, & Bengali, 1985). Alveoli appear more flattened with age and have been reported to fuse as a consequence of disruption of adjacent walls and capillaries (Klocke, 1977; Pump, 1971; 1976; Thurlbeck, 1991). This results in fewer total alveoli and less total surface area for exchange of gases (Kahane, 1990). The decline in alveoli appears to be progressive from age 20 to age 80 (Thurlbeck, 1991) and results in declining available respiratory surface of the lung after age 20 at a rate of about 0.27 m²/yr (Klocke, 1977). Shephard (1987) projects that functional respiratory surface decreases from 75 m² in a young adult to 60 m² in a 70-year-old.

Changes in the bronchial tree with aging also have been reported. Gradual lowering of the bronchi and lungs within the thorax from young adulthood into old age has been observed (Merkel, 1902, cited in Macklin & Macklin, 1942). Lowering of respiratory structures has been attributed to weakened structural support, thinning of intervertebral discs, and reduced height of vertebral bodies (Kahane, 1981). The diameter of more distal bronchi decreases with aging, with the more proximal bronchi showing little age-related change other than cartilage calcification. Decreased diameter of distal bronchi, resulting in increased airway resistance, is believed to result from loss of elastic recoil of tissues (Gelb & Zamel, 1975; Kahane, 1990; Schmidt, Dickman, Gardner, & Brough, 1973).

Loss of elasticity of lung tissues is considered the most significant structural age-related change in the lungs (Mahler, 1983). Indeed, changes in elastic recoil characteristics in the fibrous connective tissues of the pulmonary system are the most intensely investigated aspect of lung morphology associated with aging (Rochet, 1991).

The elastic properties of the lung come from two separate components: tissue elasticity and surface forces. It has been estimated that surface forces account for 66%–75% of lung elasticity (Zemlin, 1988). Surface forces pertain to properties of the pulmonary alveolar epithelium that lines the alveoli. This fluid-coated lining creates a surface tension that causes the epithelium of the alveoli to behave like stretched elastic. That is, the pulmonary alveolar epithelium is constantly trying to shorten and resist further stretching. Although the reasons for loss of lung elasticity with aging are not fully understood and little information is available about the effect of aging on surface forces (Klocke, 1977), there is currently no convincing evidence that lung surface material is altered with age (Crapo, 1993; Lynne-Davies, 1977).

Tissue forces pertain to the highly elastic connective tissue (elastin and collagen) that forms a network throughout the lung and ensures that applied forces are distributed equally to all parts of the lung. Explanations for the decline in lung elasticity with age are usually attributed to changes in lung connective tissue (Crapo, 1993). Elastin and collagen fibers are arranged in a spiral fashion, resulting in an unfolding of this complex structure to accomplish inhalation (Pierce & Ebert, 1965). Early studies demonstrated that total lung elastin content increases with aging (Klocke, 1977). Subsequent studies specified that elastin content remains unchanged with advancing age in the cells composing the essential structure of the lungs (the parenchyma) while increasing in the pleura and septa and decreasing in the airway and blood vessels (Andreotti, Bussotti, Cammelli, Aiello, & Sampognaro, 1983; Brody & Thurlbeck, 1986; Campbell & Lefrak, 1984; Klocke, 1977; Pack & Millman, 1988; Pierce & Ebert, 1965; Thurlbeck, 1991). Parenchymal elastin in adults remains metabolically stable over the life span, with the number, length, and diameter of elastin fibers unchanged with age (Broody & Thurlbeck, 1986; Shapiro, Endicott, Province, Pierce, & Campbell, 1991; Thurlbeck, 1991). Changes in elastin with aging do not appear to explain the decrease in lung elasticity with age (Crapo, 1993).

Collagen may be more significant as a factor in lung elasticity than elastin (Crapo, 1993). Usually, collagen content of the lungs is reported to be constant with age when expressed per milligram of lung weight (Crapo, 1993), although changes have been reported when collagen solubility is considered (Brody & Thurlbeck, 1986). In the pleura, a decrease in the ratio of collagen to elastin from young adulthood to old age has been cited as an important factor, resulting in increased stiffness of the pleural membranes with aging (Pierce & Ebert, 1965). Increased stiffness of the pleural membranes makes it more difficult for the pleura to slide over each other, resulting in less efficient respiratory function (Comroe, 1965; Kahane, 1981).

Currently, there is no good explanation for age-related recoil property changes in collagen and elastic contents of the lungs. It is generally agreed that knowledge concerning age-related changes in connective tissue structure is incomplete and conflicting (Crapo, 1993; Murray, 1986; Pack & Millman, 1988).

Thorax

The thorax becomes increasingly rigid or stiff with aging, resulting in less movement in response to respiratory muscle forces. This increase in rigidity results from alterations in muscles of the chest wall, ribs, and costal joints (Kahane, 1981). The costal cartilages have been reported to undergo ossification and calcification with aging (Nascher, 1914; Norris & Landis, 1938). In fact, this process has been reported to begin as early as age 20 (Todd, 1942, cited by Kahane, 1981). Reportedly, the manubrium and body of the sternum fuse between age 30 and 80 in 10% of adults, resulting in immovable joints (Grant, 1972; Nascher, 1914).

The thorax also changes shape between young adulthood and old age (Macklin & Macklin, 1942). Around the age of 50 in females and a decade later in males, kyphosis of the thoracic spine begins, principally as a result of vertebral collapse due to osteoporosis (Fowler, 1985). Kyphosis also has been associated with alveolar emphysema (Macklin & Macklin, 1942). With senile kyphosis, the chest becomes concave, or "sunken in," as a result of compression of the vertebral bodies subsequent to thinning of the intervertebral disks (Kahane, 1981). Typically, the vertebral disk degeneration is greatest in the anterior aspect of the disk, causing the vertebral column to tip forward. The upper and middle thoracic regions of the vertebral column demonstrate pronounced curvature and the back becomes rounded, a state that is sometimes referred to as "dowager's hump" (Macklin & Macklin, 1942; Kahane, 1981, 1990). Compression of the vertebrae associated with senile kyphosis also has been reported to cause changes in the costovertebral joints, including flattening of the articular facets of the vertebrae (Nascher, 1914). This flattening alters the angle of inclination of the necks of the vertebrae and consequently restricts rib movement (Kahane, 1981). Senile kyphosis causes a narrowing of the anteroposterior dimension of the thorax and may affect the extent to which the lungs can be inflated during inhalation, although the direct effects of senile kyphosis on breathing are not completely known (Kahane, 1981, 1990).

The anteroposterior (A-P) diameter of the chest also has been reported to increase with aging (Brody & Thurlbeck, 1986; Edge, Millard, Reid, & Simon, 1964; Fowler, 1985; Macklin & Macklin, 1942; Rochet, 1991; Thurlbeck, 1967, 1991). In the extreme, this thoracic shape has been referred to as "barrel chest" (Macklin & Macklin, 1942). Although physicians may associate an increase in A-P diameter with the presence of emphysema, some increase in A-P diameter has been reported in elderly individuals having no sign of significant emphysema (Crapo, 1993). Macklin and Macklin (1942) hypothesized that barrel chest could be the result of age-related changes in the thoracic wall leading to inspiratory fixation or secondary to decreased lung elasticity with aging. These authors also note that barrel chests are not exclusively a province of the elderly, concluding that this condition may well be a pathological change rather than a normal aspect of aging.

Respiratory Muscles

Until recently, little data were available on age-related changes in respiratory muscles (Kahane, 1981, 1990). Early researchers reported weakening of respiratory muscles with advancing age beginning by age 30–40 (Dahr et al., 1976; McKeown, 1965). Similarly, Black and Hyatt (1969) asserted that both inspiratory and expiratory muscle forces lessened with aging. In contrast, Nascher (1914) suggested that muscle atrophy of significant degree occurs only with advanced age, although the precise age of such deterioration was not specified. More recently, Mizuno (1991) reported reductions with aging in the cross-sectional area of muscle fibers composing the internal intercostals. Similar muscle fiber reduction was also observed, although to a lesser degree, in the external intercostal muscle group.

Recently, investigators have begun to examine respiratory muscle strength in the elderly, employing a variety of static inspiratory and expiratory maneuvers that yield pressure measurements aimed at assessing overall respiratory muscle strength. Previously, such measures primarily had been used to quantify muscle weakness in patients with respiratory failure, malnutrition, or neuromuscular disease (Clausen, 1982). In a large scale study of 4,443 healthy (described as "ambulatory") volunteers ranging in age from 65 to 85, Enright and his associates found that measures of maximal respiratory pressure (MRP) decreased progressively after age 65, with larger age-related declines in men in comparison with women (Enright, Kronmal, Manolio, Schenker & Hyatt, 1994). However, because MRP measures provide information on the integrated functioning of groups of respiratory muscles rather than individual muscle function, additional studies were needed to shed light on age-related changes in specific muscles.

Tolep and his associates investigated possible age-related changes in the diaphragm by comparing maximum transdiaphragmatic pressure (Pdi_{max}) during maximal inspiratory efforts in 9 young and 10 elderly men. These investigators found that average Pdi_{max} values for the elderly group were 25% lower than those observed for young subjects (Tolep, Higgins, Muza, Criner, & Kelsen, 1995). The authors concluded that diaphragm strength is reduced in elderly individuals and suggested that elderly persons may be predisposed to diaphragm fatigue under conditions of increased ventilatory load. Using a somewhat different protocol, Polkey et al. (1997) also found lower Pdi_{max} values in 15 elderly subjects (10 male, 5 female), in comparison with 15 young subjects (10 male, 5 female). Although Polkey et al. (1997) concur that aging is associated with a reduction in diaphragm strength, they feel that the magnitude of that reduction is small.

FUNCTIONAL CHANGES

Life span changes in lung function have been categorized into four phases: (1) a growth period (up to age 11 or 12) during which lung function progressively increases, (2) a maturation period in adolescence when lung function accelerates disproportionately with growth, (3) a plateau period after maximal lung function is achieved beginning at approximately age 20 in women and 25 in men, and (4) a decline period (Mahler, Rosiello & Loke, 1986; Burrows, Cline, Knudson, Taussig, & Lebowitz, 1983). Changes in respiratory function during the decline period are not linear; the rate of decline is small in earlier years and accelerates with advancing age (Mahler, 1983).

As noted by Crapo (1993), changes in the functioning of the respiratory system with aging have been investigated employing two research design protocols: (1) cross-sectional studies in which groups of people of different ages are studied at one point in time and (2) longitudinal investigations in which the same group is studied over a long period of time. Both designs attempt to answer the question: When does declining respiratory function begin and what is the rate of decline? Cross-sectional studies predominate, probably because of difficulties inherent in following the same group of people for long periods of time. Cross-sectional studies are easier and less expensive to conduct than longitudinal studies and, with proper design, may yield data similar to longitudinal studies (Buist, 1982; Louis, Robins, Dockery, Spiro, & Ware, 1986). However, cross-sectional studies are prone to certain types of error. For instance, the height of a population may change over time, or individuals with better function may tend to live longer than their contemporaries, reducing apparent age-related effects. Although longitudinal studies avoid these pitfalls, they have problems of their own. For instance, individual subjects may learn to perform tests better or technician/instrument performance may change over time. While data on the effects of age on lung function vary considerably among individual studies, average cross-sectional and longitudinal results are generally quite similar (Crapo, 1993).

Lung Volumes

Vital capacity (VC) is the largest volume of air that can be expired from the lungs after maximum inspiration. It has been recognized for more than a century that VC decreases with age. The decline in VC has been reported as more rapid in men than women (Klocke, 1977; Knudson, 1991; Levitzky, 1984), although some studies have suggested that age declines in women may actually be more dramatic (Hoit & Hixon, 1987; Hoit, Hixon, Altman, & Morgan, 1989) if normalized values are utilized (VC/TLC; see Chapter 5). Average decreases in vital capacity on the order of approximately 26 mL/yr in men and 21 mL/yr in women have been reported (Klocke, 1977). Interestingly, in addition to the significance of VC to respiratory function, declining vital capacity with aging has been linked to general health. Specifically, an inverse relationship between vital capacity and probability of death within 10 years has been reported as well as a direct relationship between diminished vital capacity and likelihood of suffering a myocardial infarction (Dhar et al., 1976).

Total lung capacity (TLC) has been shown to decrease slightly over time when longitudinal data have been gathered (Crapo, 1993). However, TLC is highly correlated with height, and height also decreases in individuals with aging. When TLC has been examined in cross-sectional studies and normalized for height, both slight increases and decreases with aging have been reported, although most frequently no changes have been observed (Levitzky, 1984).

Residual volume (RV) is the amount of air left in the lungs after a maximum exhalation. Studies of age-related changes in RV and the RV/TLC ratio consistently have shown increases with age. Specifically, RV increases by a factor of about 40% between age 20 and age 70 (Lynne-Davies, 1977). In the young, RV is a static measure in which the outward recoil pressure of the respiratory system, mainly in the chest wall, is counterbalanced by the maximum pressure of expiratory muscles. That is, the limit of expiration in young individuals is established by a static balance of muscle and recoil forces. Most young subjects reach the limit quickly (2–4 sec) and no further volume change is apparent, even with continued effort. In the elderly, however, the limit of expiration is reached more slowly (10–15 sec), with decreasing flow tending to continue for as long as effort is continued (Leith & Mead, 1967). Increases in chest wall rigidity in the elderly produce a situation in which the expiratory muscles are not as effective in counterbalancing outward recoil pressures. RV in the elderly is no longer a static measure, as expiratory flow never falls to zero (Crapo, 1993). RV in the elderly must be determined in part by the length of time the subject can maintain an expiratory effort (Knudson, 1991).

Increases in RV with aging also are caused by changes in closing volume (CV). CV is the lung volume at which small airways start to close (Dhar et al., 1976). In the elderly, the small airways close during exhalation at higher lung volumes as a result of (1) loss of elastic recoil in the lungs, (2) a possible decrease in the recoil of the intrapulmonic airways, and (3) decreases in small airway diameter with age (Knudson, 1991; Mahler, 1983). Indeed, airway collapse has been reported to be the major factor limiting lung emptying in the elderly (Leith & Mead, 1967; Lynne-Davies, 1977).

Pulmonary Function Tests

The most commonly performed pulmonary function test is spirometry. Spirometry is performed during a forced VC maneuver and is displayed graphically as volume by time or flow by time (Crapo, 1993). With aging, maximum expiratory flow rates decrease, particularly at lower lung volumes, as illustrated in Figure 2–1 (Knudson, 1991; Knudson, Clark, Kennedy, & Knudson, 1977). At higher lung volumes, maximum flows decrease modestly with age. Age-related differences are most apparent at the end of the flow volume curve where progressively lower flows with aging are observed (Crapo, 1993; Knudson et al., 1977).

Currently, more information is available on age-related changes in VC and forced expiratory volume at 1 second (FEV_1) than other pulmonary function parameters (Crapo, 1993). It has been suggested that both VC and FEV_1 increase up to approximately age 20 in women and 25 in men (Burrows et al., 1983). After maturation, VC and FEV_1 change very little into the 30s, although interindividual variability is quite high (Crapo, 1993). It has been hypothesized that variability observed in cross-sectional studies on VC and FEV_1 during this plateau phase may represent subtle maturation-related increases in some people and subtle age-related declines in others (Knudson, 1991; Crapo, 1993). Following the plateau period, VC and FEV_1 begin to decline, with accelerated declines as age increases (Becklake & Permutt, 1979; Buist & Vollmer, 1988; Knudson, 1991; Schmidt et al., 1973). Ware et al. (1990) compared cross-sectional findings with longitudinal results and observed that although both methodologies showed accelerated decline with aging, the rate of loss accelerated more rapidly in the longitudinal model. Specifically, by age 75, the annual rate of loss of function in the longitudinal analysis was twice as great as the rate of loss observed in cross-sectional analysis. Interestingly, rates of decline have been observed to be greater in men than women, in tall people in comparison with short people, and in persons with larger baseline values (Crapo, 1993; Ware et al., 1990).

Control of Breathing

Respiratory control pertains to an individual's response to hypoxemia (lack of adequate oxygen in the blood) and hypercapnia (excessive carbon dioxide in the blood). Normal young adults respond to hypoxemia and hypercapnia with increases in respiratory rate, tidal volume, cardiac output, and blood pressure (Crapo, 1993). However, ventilatory and heart rate responses to hypoxemia and hypercapnia are diminished with aging (Kronenberg & Drage, 1973; Murray, 1986; Peterson, Pack, Silage, & Fishman, 1981). Specifically, the ventilatory response to hypercapnia in elderly men is reduced 40% in comparison with young men. Decreased responses to hypoxemia and hypercapnia have been attributed to decreased responses in tidal volume rather than to differences in responses of respiratory rate (Peterson et al., 1981). In addition, diminished heart rate responses to hypoxemia have been reported (Kronenberg

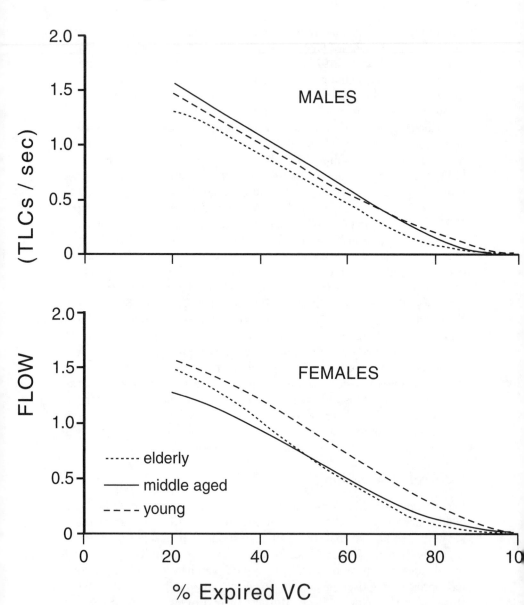

Figure 2–1. Maximum expiratory flow-volume curves for males and females as a function of chronological a group. Curves reflect only the effort-independent portions of performance. Flow is expressed as total lung capa ties per second and volume as percent of expired vital capacity to compensate for differences in physical size. *No* From "Effect of aging alone on mechanical properties of the normal adult human lung," by R. Knudson, D. Clark Kennedy, & D. Knudson, 1977, *Journal of Applied Physiology, 43,* p. 1058. Copyright 1977 by the American Physiologi Society. Reprinted by permission.

& Drage, 1973). Decreased response to hypoxemia and hypercapnia in the elderly cannot be explained by diminished muscle strength, differences in body size, or lung mechanics. It has been hypothesized that diminished respiratory drive in the elderly results from reductions in neuromuscular inspiratory output (Crapo, 1993; Mahler, 1983). Mahler (1983) suggests that the level of respiratory drive in elderly persons may prove inadequate to maintain adequate exchange of gases when an individual is stressed by either acute or chronic disease.

Aging and Exercise

Most people are aware of diminished physical fitness and performance as a result of aging. With exercise, requirements for oxygen are increased and decrement of function of the respiratory system may adversely affect or limit exercise capacity (Mahler, 1983). For example, it recently has been demonstrated that elderly men utilize greater diaphragmatic action along with more rapid, shallow breathing during exercise than do young men. It is hypothesized that this ventilatory pattern during exercise may be a consequence of thorax stiffening with advanced age (Teramoto, Fukuchi, Nagase, Matsuse, & Orimo, 1995). However, despite alterations in the ventilatory response to exercise in elderly persons relative to younger adults, ventilation during exercise in elderly persons is felt to be adequate for carbon dioxide elimination, even during maximal exercise (Grinton, 1994; Johnson, Badr, & Dempsey, 1994).

Exercise capacity (measured as maximum oxygen uptake) decreases with aging. Longitudinal studies generally show a slower rate of decline in oxygen uptake with age than do cross-sectional studies. Longitudinal studies also reveal that the decline in sedentary men occurs at twice the rate observed in physically active men (Crapo, 1993). Physical training may affect the rate of decline of exercise capacity, although no data are available on individuals with equivalent training levels, as older athletes tend to train with less intensity than do younger athletes (Makrides, Heigenhauser, & Jones, 1990).

Some investigators explain the decline in exercise capacity with aging as a consequence of alterations both in physiological function and physical activity (Rivera, Pels, Sady, Cullinane, & Thompson, 1989). Factors mentioned as possible contributors to the decline in exercise capacity include: (1) declining ability both to deliver and extract oxygen, (2) decreased maximum cardiac output, (3) decreased ventilation, (4) decreased muscle mass and strength, (5) reduced ability of the muscle to extract oxygen, (6) reduced ability to divert blood flow to the exercising muscle, and (7) diminished willingness to work to maximum levels.

SUMMARY

Respiratory function declines progressively with increasing age after maturation in both men and women. Although the mechanisms leading to diminished respiratory function are not understood completely, the factors of decreased lung elasticity, decreased respiratory muscle strength, and increased stiffness of the thorax appear to be important to the process.

The lungs in elderly persons are smaller, lighter, and less elastic than those of younger individuals. Microscopic examination has revealed widening of respiratory bronchioles and alveolar ducts, flattening/fusion of alveoli, and thickening of blood vessel walls. The lungs and bronchi lower within the thorax and the diameter of more distal bronchi decreases with aging.

Loss of elasticity of lung tissue is considered the most significant structural age-related change in the lungs. Although reasons for loss of lung elasticity with advancing age are not fully understood, there is little convincing evidence that lung surface material is altered with aging. Rather, declining lung elasticity is usually attributed to changes in lung connective tissue, although current knowledge concerning age-related changes in connective tissue is incomplete and conflicting.

The thorax becomes increasingly rigid or stiff with aging, resulting in less movement in response to respiratory muscle forces. The thorax also changes shape between young adulthood and old age. Changes such as kyphosis ("dowager's hump") and "barrel chest" have been reported.

Respiratory muscles have been reported to weaken with aging. Recently, measures of maximal respiratory pressure (MRP) have indicated that respiratory muscle strength decreases progressively after age 65, with larger age-related declines in men in comparison with women. In addition, investigations targeting diaphragm functioning using maximum transdiaphragmatic pressure measurements (Pdi_{max}) have revealed that diaphragm strength is reduced in elderly individuals.

Lung function also declines with aging in a nonlinear fashion. That is, the rate of decline is small in earlier years and accelerates with advancing age. Both cross-sectional and longitudinal designs have been used to investigate changes in lung functioning with aging and, although the effects of aging on lung function vary considerably among these studies, average cross-sectional and longitudinal results are generally quite similar.

Forced vital capacity (FVC) declines with age on the order of 26 mL/yr in men and 21 mL/yr in women. Declines in FVC are significant both for respiratory function as well as general health. In general, no changes in total lung capacity have been observed with aging. Residual volume (RV) increases by a factor of about 40% between age 20 and age 70. Declines in

RV with aging have been attributed both to increased in chest wall rigidity and to changes in closing volume of the lungs.

Pulmonary function tests have shown declines in maximum expiratory flow rate with aging, particularly at lower lung volumes. Both forced vital capacity (FVC) and forced expiratory volume at 1 second (FEV_1) decline with aging, with accelerated rates of decline as aging progresses. Longitudinal studies have shown twice as great a rate of decline in FVC and FEV_1 with aging than have cross-sectional studies. Rates of decline are greater in men than women, in tall people in comparison with short people, and in people with large baseline values.

Ventilatory responses to hypercapnia and hypoxemia are diminished with aging. It has been hypothesized that diminished respiratory drive in the elderly results from reductions in neuromuscular inspiratory output.

Exercise capacity decreases with aging, although ventilatory responses in elderly persons are felt to be adequate for carbon dioxide elimination, even during maximal exercise. Exercise capacity is tied to physical activity and may be improved with physical training, although data on physical training effects is incomplete at this time.

REFERENCES

Andreotti, L., Bussotti, A., Cammelli, D., Aiello, E., & Sampognaro, S. (1983). Connective tissue in aging lung. *Gerontology, 29,* 377–387.

Becklake, M., & Permutt, S. (1979). Evaluation of tests of lung function for "screening" for early detection of chronic obstructive lung disease. In P. T. Macklem & S. Permutt (Eds.), *The lung in transition between health and disease* (pp. 345–387). New York: Marcel Dekker.

Black, L., & Hyatt, R. (1969). Maximal respiratory pressures: Normal values and relationship to age and sex. *American Review of Respiratory Disease, 99,* 696–702.

Brody, J., & Thurlbeck, W. (1986). Development, growth and aging of the lung. In *Handbook of physiology* (Section 3) *The respiratory system:* Vol. 3. *Mechanics of breathing* (Part 1, pp. 355–386). Bethesda: American Physiological Society.

Buist, A. (1982). Evaluation of lung function: Concepts of normality. In D. H. Simmon (Ed.), *Current pulmonology* (Vol. 4, pp. 141–165). New York: John Wiley & Sons.

Buist, A., & Vollmer, W. (1988). The use of lung function tests in identifying factors that affect lung growth and aging. *Statistics and Medicine, 7,* 11–18.

Burrows, B., Cline, M., Knudson, R., Taussig, & Lebowitz, M. (1983). A descriptive analysis of the growth and decline of the FVC and FEV_1. *Chest, 83,* 717–724.

Campbell, E., & Lefrak, S. (1984). Physiologic processes of aging in the respiratory system. In S. W. Krechel (Ed.), *Anesthesia and the geriatric patient* (pp. 19–44). New York: Grune & Stratton.

Clausen, J. (1982). Maximal inspiratory and expiratory pressures. In J. Clausen (Ed.), *Pulmonary function testing guidelines and controversies* (pp. 187–191). Orlando: Grune & Stratton.

Comroe, J. (1965). Mechanical factors in breathing. In J. H. Comroe (Ed.), *Physiology of respiration.* Chicago: Year Book Medical Publishers.

Crapo, R. (1993). The aging lung. In D. A. Mahler (Ed.), *Pulmonary disease in the elderly patient: Vol. 63. Lung biology in health and disease* (pp. 1–25). New York: Marcel Dekker.

Dhar, S., Shastri, S., & Lenora, R. (1976). Aging and the respiratory system. *Symposium on Geriatric Medicine, Medical Clinics of North America, 60,* 1121–1139.

Edge, J., Millard, F., Reid, L., & Simon, G. (1964). The radiographic appearances of the chest in persons of advanced age. *British Journal of Radiology, 37,* 769–774.

Enright, P., Kronmal, R., Manolio, T., Schenker, M., & Hyatt, R. (1994). Respiratory muscle strength in the elderly: Correlates and reference values. *American Journal of Respiratory and Critical Care Medicine, 149,* 430–438.

Fowler, R. (1985). Ageing and lung function. *Age and Ageing, 14,* 209–215.

Gelb, A., & Zamel, N. (1975). Effect of aging on lung mechanics in healthy non-smokers. *Chest, 68,* 538–541.

Grant, J. (1972). *Grant's atlas of anatomy.* Baltimore: Williams & Wilkins.

Grinton, S. (1994). Respiratory limitations in the aging population. *Southern Medical Journal, 87,* S47–S49.

Heath, D. (1964). Structural changes in the pulmonary vasculature associated with aging. In L. Cander & J. H. Moyer (Eds.), *Aging of the lung* (pp. 70–76). New York: Grune & Stratton.

Hoit, J., & Hixon, T. (1987). Age and speech breathing. *Journal of Speech and Hearing Research, 30,* 351–366.

Hoit, J., Hixon, T., Altman, M., & Morgan, W. (1989). Speech breathing in women. *Journal of Speech and Hearing Research, 32,* 353–365.

Johnson, B., Badr, M., & Dempsey, J. (1994). Impact of the aging pulmonary system on the response to exercise. *Clinics in Chest Medicine, 15,* 229–246.

Kahane, J. (1981). Anatomic and physiologic changes in the aging peripheral speech mechanism. In D. S. Beasley & G. A. Davis (Eds.), *Aging communication processes and disorders* (pp. 21–45). New York: Grune & Stratton.

Kahane, J. (1990). Age-related changes in the peripheral speech mechanism: Structural and physiological changes. In E. Cherow (Ed.), *Proceedings of the research symposium on communication sciences and disorders and aging* (pp. 75–87). *ASHA Reports No. 19.* Rockville, MD: American Speech-Language-Hearing Association.

Kenney, R. (1982). *Physiology of aging: A synopsis.* Chicago: Year Book Medical Publishers.

Klocke, R. (1977). Influence of aging on the lung. In C. E. Finch & L. Hayflick (Eds.), *Handbook of the biology of aging* (pp. 432–444). New York: Van Nostrand Reinhold.

Knudson, R. (1991). Physiology of the aging lung. In R. G. Crystal & J. B. West (Eds.), *The lung* (pp. 1749–1759). New York: Raven Press.

Knudson, R., Clark, D., Kennedy, T., & Knudson, D. (1977). Effect of aging alone on mechanical properties of the normal adult human lung. *Journal of Applied Physiology: Respiratory, Environmental and Exercise Physiology, 43,* 1054–1062.

Kronenberg, R., & Drage, C. (1973). Attenuation of the ventilatory and heart rate responses to hypoxia and hypercapnia with aging in normal men. *Journal of Clinical Investigation, 52,* 1812–1819.

Lebowitz, M. (1988). Respiratory changes of aging. In B. Kent & R. N. Butler (Eds.), *Human aging research* (pp. 263–276). New York: Raven Press.

Lee, H., Lim, M., Lu, C., Liu, V., Fahn, H., Zhang, C., Nagley, P., & Wei, Y. (1999). Concurrent increase of oxidative DNA damage and lipid peroxidation together with mitochondrial DNA mutation in human lung tissues during aging—smoking enhances oxidative stress on the aged tissues. *Archives of Biochemistry & Biophysics, 362,* 309–316.

Leith, D., & Mead, J. (1967). Mechanisms determining residual volume of the lungs in normal subjects. *Journal of Applied Physiology, 23,* 221–227.

Levitzky, M. (1984). Effects of aging on the respiratory system. *Physiologist, 27,* 102–107.

Louis, T., Robins, J., Dockery, D., Spiro, A., & Ware, J. (1986). Explaining discrepancies between longitudinal and cross-sectional models. *Journal of Chronic Disease, 39,* 831–839.

Lynne-Davies, P. (1977). Influence of age on the respiratory system. *Geriatrics, 32,* 57–60.

Macklin, C., & Macklin, M. (1942). Respiratory system. In E. V. Cowdry (Ed.), *Problems of aging* (2nd ed., pp. 185–253). Baltimore: Williams and Wilkins.

Mahler, D. (1983). Pulmonary aspects of aging. In S. R. Gambert (Ed.). *Contemporary geriatric medicine* (Vol. 1). New York: Plenum Medical Books Corporation.

Mahler, D., Rosiello, R., & Loke, J. (1986). The aging lung. *Geriatric Clinics of North America, 2,* 215–225.

Makrides, L., Heigenhauser, G., & Jones, N. (1990). High intensity endurance training in 20- to 30- and 60- to 70-yr-old healthy men. *Journal of Applied Physiology, 69,* 1792–1798.

McKeown, F. (1965). *Pathology of the aged.* London: Butterworths.

Merkel, F. (1902). Atmungsorgane. In *Bardeleben's Handbuch der Anat. D. Menschen.* Jena: Fischer.

Mizuno, M. (1991). Human respiratory muscles: Fibre morphology and capillary supply. *European Respiration Journal, 4,* 587–601.

Murray, J. (1986). *Aging in the normal lung* (2nd ed.). Philadelphia: W. B. Saunders Co.

Nascher, I. L. (1914). *Geriatrics.* Philadelphia: Blakiston's Son and Co.

Norris, G., & Landis, H. (1938). *Diseases of the chest* (6th ed.). Philadelphia: W. B. Saunders Co.

Pack, A., & Millman, R. (1988). The lungs in later life. In A. P. Fishman (Ed.), *Pulmonary diseases and disorders* (pp. 79–90). New York: McGraw-Hill Book Company.

Peterson, D., Pack, A. Silage, D., & Fishman, A. (1981). Effects of aging on ventilatory and occlusion pressure responses to hypoxia and hypercapnia. *American Review of Respiratory Disease, 124,* 387–391.

Pierce, J., & Ebert, R. (1958). The elastic properties of the lungs in the aged. *Journal of Laboratory and Clinical Medicine, 51,* 63–71.

Pierce, J., & Ebert, R. (1965). Fibrous network of the lung and its change with age. *Thorax, 20,* 469–476.

Polkey, M., Harris, M. L., Hughes, P., Hamnegard, C., Lyons, D., Green, M., & Moxham, J. (1997). The contractile properties of the elderly human diaphragm. *American Journal of Respiratory and Critical Care Medicine, 155,* 1560–1564.

Pump, K. (1971). The aged lung. *Chest, 60,* 571–577.

Pump, K. (1976). Emphysema and its relationship to age. *American Review of Respiratory Diseases, 114,* 5–13.

Reddan, W. (1981). Respiratory system and aging. In E. L. Smith & R. C. Serfass (Eds.), *Exercise and aging: The scientific basis* (pp. 89–107). Hillside, NJ: Enslow.

Richards, D. (1965). Pulmonary changes due to aging. In R. Fenn & H. Rahn (Eds.), *Handbook of physiology* (pp. 1525–1529). Washington, DC: American Physiological Society.

Rivera, A., Pels, A., Sady, S., Cullinane, E., & Thompson, P. (1989). Physiological factors associated with the lower maximal oxygen consumption of master runners. *Journal of Applied Physiology, 66,* 949–954.

Robinson, S. (1964). Physical fitness in relation to age. In L. Cander & J. H. Moyer (Eds.), *Aging of the lung* (pp. 287–301). New York: Grune & Stratton.

Rochet, A. (1991). Aging and the respiratory system. In D. Ripich (Ed.), *Handbook of geriatric communication disorders* (pp. 145–163). Austin, TX: PRO-ED.

Rolleston, H. (1922). *Some medical aspects of old age.* London: MacMillan and Co., Ltd.

Schmidt, C., Dickman, M., Gardner, R., & Brough, F. (1973). Spirometric standards for healthy elderly men and women. 532 subjects ages 55 through 94 years. *American Review of Respiratory Diseases, 108,* 933–939.

Shapiro, S., Endicott, S., Province, M., Pierce, J., & Campbell, E. (1991). Marked longevity of human lung parenchymal elastic fibers deduced from prevalence of D-aspartate and nuclear weapons-related radiocarbon. *Journal of Clinical Investigation, 87,* 1828–1834.

Shephard, R. (1987). *Physical activity and aging* (2nd ed.). Rockville, MD: Aspen.

Snider, G., Kleinerman, J., Thurlbeck, W., & Bengali, Z. (1985). The definition of emphysema: Report of a National Heart, Lung, and Blood Institute, Division of Lung Diseases workshop. *American Review of Respiratory Diseases, 132,* 182–185.

Teramoto, S., Fukuchi, Y., Nagase, T., Matsuse, T., & Orimo, H. (1995). A comparison of ventilation components in young and elderly men during exercise. *Journals of Gerontology. Series A, Biological Sciences & Medical Sciences, 50A,* B34–B39.

Thurlbeck, W. (1967). The internal surface area of nonemphysematous lungs. *American Review of Respiratory Diseases, 95,* 765–773.

Thurlbeck, W. (1991). Morphology of the aging lung. In R. G. Crystal & J. B. West (Eds.), *The lung* (pp. 1743–1748). New York: Raven Press.

Todd, T. (1942). Skeleton, locomotor system and teeth. In E. V. Cowdry (Ed.), *Problems of ageing: Biological and medical aspects* (2nd ed.). Baltimore: Williams and Wilkins.

Tolep, K., Higgins, N., Muza, S., Criner, G., & Kelsen, S. (1995). Comparison of diaphragm strength between healthy adult elderly and young men. *American Journal of Respiratory and Critical Care Medicine, 152,* 677–682.

Ware, J., Dockery, D., Louis, T., Xu, X., Ferris, B., & Speizer, F. (1990). Longitudinal and cross-sectional estimates of pulmonary function decline in never-smoking adults. *American Journal of Epidemiology, 132,* 685–700.

Zemlin, W. (1988). *Speech and hearing science: Anatomy and physiology* (3rd ed.). Englewood Cliffs, NJ: Prentice-Hall.

CHAPTER

3

Aging of the Larynx

With aging, the larynx undergoes anatomical changes that impact on the voice produced by elderly speakers. Changes in the cartilages, muscles, connective tissues, glands, and vascular tissues within the larynx contribute to changes in the movement patterns of the vocal folds during voice production and alter the relationships among the varying forces impacting on a finely tuned sound generator.

As noted by Kahane (1987), several patterns are apparent in the research on aging of the larynx. First of all, substantial gender differences exist both in the onset and extent of age-related change in the laryngeal structures (Table 3-1). Changes begin at an earlier age in males and, in many cases, changes in the male larynx are more dramatic than those observed in the female larynx. In males, histologic changes in some tissues of the larynx begin by the third decade, with substantial evidence of such changes apparent by the fifth or sixth decades. In contrast, age-related changes begin in females after the fifth decade and those changes are less extensive than what occurs in males. Kahane (1987) also notes that tissues of the larynx age at varying rates and to varying extents. This results in an organ that can undergo substantial structural change before producing observable change in the voice. Differences in aging of the larynx as a function of race have not been examined specifically, although some similarity exists in data gathered on European and North American Anglos and Asians (Kahane, 1987).

Although much remains to be learned about the biology of the aging larynx, what has been learned to date offers insight into changes in voice that occur with aging. In this chapter age-related anatomical changes in the larynx are described.

LARYNGEAL CARTILAGES AND JOINTS

It has been documented that the structure of the laryngeal cartilages changes as an individual moves from young adulthood into old age. Both calcification and ossification have been reported in the hyaline cartilages of the larynx, including the cricoid and thyroid cartilages (Ardan, 1965; Chamberlain & Young, 1935; Hately, Evison, & Samuel, 1965; Kahane,

Table 3–1. Gender Differences in Aging of the Larynx

Laryngeal Structure	Nature of Aging Change	Gender Difference
Cartilages	Ossification/calcification	More extensive with earlier onset in males
Cricoarytenoid joint	General deterioration	More evident in males
Intrinsic muscles	Atrophy	Reported in males; limited data on females
Epithelium	Thickening	Progressive in males until 70; declines thereafter Progressive in females, particularly after age 70
Mucous glands	Degeneration	Reported in males; no data on females
Lamina propria	Degenerative changes Stiffer, more viscous tissue	Generally more extensive in males More evident in males
Macula flava	Degeneration of fibroblasts	No data on gender differences
Conus elasticus	Thinning of fibers; separation/ fragmentation of fiber bundles	Few changes observed in women
Thryoarytenoid muscle	Atrophy/degeneration	No data on gender differences
Innervation	Some evidence of disruption; Conflicting data reported	No data on gender differences
Vascular supply	Reduced blood vessel diameter Thickening of capillary walls	No data on gender differences

1981a; Keen & Wainwright, 1958; Roncallo, 1948). The arytenoid cartilages become partially ossified. That is, the apex and vocal processes
never ossify, whereas the body and muscular processes usually ossify
totally (Malinowski, 1967). The epiglottis, the only elastic cartilage in the
laryngeal framework, typically does not undergo ossification or calcification, although breakdown of elastic fibers in the epiglottis with aging has
been observed (Ferreri, 1959; Hommerich, 1972; Kahane, 1983b). On rare
occasions, however, a patient might be reported in whom partial transfor-
mation of the epiglottis had occurred (Ardran, 1965). Ossification has
been observed in both sexes, although it occurs earlier and is more extensive in males than in females. In males, laryngeal cartilage ossification
begins as early as the third decade of life, with changes in the thyroid and
cricoid cartilages beginning earlier than changes in the arytenoid cartilages. Typically, although no observable signs of ossification are present in
males at age 18, slight ossification is observable at age 27 and extensive
ossification is in evidence by age 81. In females, ossification begins to
appear in the fourth decade of life, with changes progressing at a slower
rate and to a lesser extent than changes observed in males (Kahane,
1981a, 1983a,1983b; Kahane & Beckford, 1991).

Each laryngeal cartilage displays its own pattern of ossification,
although it is rare for an entire cartilage to be transformed into bone
(Kahane, 1983a). Ossification in the thyroid cartilage begins in the inferior
cornu and spreads up the posterior lamina into the superior cornu.
Subsequently, ossification spreads anteriorly along the lamina of the thyroid cartilage. In the cricoid cartilage, the posterior lamina is the first to
show signs of ossification, with subsequent spread to adjacent areas. The
last area of the cricoid to ossify is the arch. In the arytenoid cartilages, the
central portion ossifies first and spreads peripherally, sparing the apex and
vocal process (Kahane, 1983b).

Kahane (1983b) indicates that it is possible to distinguish young
adults from elderly persons on the basis of extent of ossification, particularly in males. However, it is not possible to accurately estimate an individual's chronologic age from the extent of ossification once ossification is
well established. Nonetheless, the extent of ossification is felt to be a valuable marker of the biologic age of the larynx (Kahane, 1983b).
Interestingly, the degree of ossification of laryngeal cartilages also has
been associated with the presence of mineral deposits in the wall of the
aorta, suggesting that the extent of laryngeal cartilage ossification relates
to aging in other body systems (Noback, 1949).

Evidence of nonpathologic changes in laryngeal joints with aging has
been documented only fairly recently. To date, significant age-related
changes have been reported in the cricoarytenoid joint; the cricothyroid
joint has yet to be investigated. Interestingly, early writings suggested that

aging produced loosening of the cricoarytenoid joint with erosion of articular surfaces, although these reports were not supported by empirical evidence available at the time (Segre, 1971). Early light microscope investigations of the cricoarytenoid joint suggested that erosion with aging might
be fairly inconsequential (Kahane, 1983b). However, later investigations
on larger numbers of subjects revealed significant age-related changes in
the cricoarytenoid joint, particularly in males. Changes included thinning
of the articular surfaces, breakdown/disorganization of the collagen fibers
in the cartilage matrix, changes in the synovial membrane, and surface
irregularities (Kahane, 1990; Kahane & Hammons, 1987; Kahn & Kahane,
1986). Indeed, structural changes in the cricoarytenoid joint may lessen
the extent and approximation of the vocal folds as well as contribute to
loss of smoothness of vocal fold adjustments during phonation, increasing
the amount of breathiness or weakness in the voice, particularly in males
(Kahane, 1990).

A contrary view as to the significance of cricoarytenoid joint changes
with aging has been expressed by Casiano, Ruiz, and Goldstein (1994) following histopathologic laryngeal examinations. These authors concluded
that laryngeal changes other than those within the cricoarytenoid joint
may be more significant in determining voice quality in elderly speakers.
Disparity in the conclusions of Casiano et al. (1994) and Kahane (1988)
might be explained on the basis of differences in the size of the specimen
sample and the age range of the specimens examined. A relatively small
sample size (3 men and 4 women) coupled with a fairly restricted age
range of subjects (only 39 to 56 years for males) could have limited possible aging effects observed by Casiano and his associates (1994).

INTRINSIC LARYNGEAL MUSCLES

With the exception of the vocal folds, themselves, which are considered
later in this chapter, limited research has been conducted on age-related
changes in intrinsic laryngeal musculature. Among those researchers who
have examined intrinsic laryngeal muscle changes with aging, several have
stated that laryngeal muscles undergo regressive changes with increasing
age (Rodeno, Sanchez-Fernandez, & Rivera-Pomar, 1993). However, there
is no consensus as to the precise nature and extent of those changes. Some
researchers have indicated that all intrinsic muscles atrophy and that atrophy occurs equally in abductors and adductors (Carnevalle-Ricci, 1937,
reported by Kahane, 1990; Ferreri, 1959). Others have suggested that atrophy is greater in the abductor muscle than in adductor muscles (Bach,
Lederer, & Dinolt, 1941; Malmgren & Gacek, 1981). Specific atrophic

changes in muscles reported by Bach et al. (1941) included fatty infiltration, connective tissue interspersed between degenerating muscle fibers, unusual variation in cross-sectional area, loss of cross-striations, and an accumulation of debris in the cytoplasm. Interestingly, the cricothyroid has been reported to hypertrophy as it compensates for atrophy in other intrinsic muscles (Segre, 1971). Little information is available regarding gender differences in aging of intrinsic laryngeal muscles.

Atrophy of intrinsic laryngeal musculature has been attributed to disturbances in the vascular supply to the muscles. Specifically, reductions in blood supply resulting from narrowing of the arterial vessels have been implicated (Ferreri, 1959; Hommerich, 1972). A contrary view was expressed by Bach et al. (1941) who suggest that disturbances in the vasomotor fibers of sympathetic nerves supplying blood vessels result in undernourishment of laryngeal musculature and resultant atrophy.

VOCAL FOLDS

The vocal fold is a complex structure consisting of five distinct histologic layers (Hirano, 1974, 1981) including the epithelium, three subepithelial elastic and collagenous layers collectively called the lamina propria, and the thyroarytenoid muscle. The intermediate and deep layers of the lamina propria form the vocal ligament. Although knowledge of age-related changes in the vocal folds is incomplete, evidence indicates that a number of changes in these layers alter the biomechanical properties of the vocal folds. In addition, the length of the membranous vocal fold overall has been reported to shorten with aging in males, particularly after age 70 (Hirano, Kurita, & Sakaguchi, 1989). It is apparent, as well, that considerable variability exists in the rate and extent of age-related change in the vocal folds evidenced by occasional reports of minimal geriatric changes in vocal folds of females, even with very advanced chronological age (Hirano, Kurita, & Sakaguchi, 1988).

Epithelium and Mucous Glands

There is some disagreement in the literature regarding the age-related changes in the epithelium of the vocal folds (Kahane, 1981b; 1983a). Although several investigators have observed thickening of the laryngeal epithelium with aging (Eggston & Wolff, 1947; Hommerich, 1972), others have found no evidence of age-related changes (Hirano, Kurita, & Nakashima, 1983; Noell, 1962; Ryan, McDonald, & Devine, 1956). It has been suggested, as well, that mucosal thickness changes with aging may be gender-related. That is, in males, the thickness of the epithelium has been reported to increase until approximately age 70 and then decrease into advanced old age. In females, the epithelium has been reported to increase progressively with aging, particularly after the age of 70 (Hirano, Kurita, & Sakaguchi, 1989). Segre (1971) reported thinning and yellowing of the mucosa after middle age. In addition, Noell (1962) reported that with aging, the laryngeal epithelium attaches less firmly to the lamina propria underneath, a condition that could affect the structural support of the cover of the vocal fold and increase perturbation during phonation (Kahane, 1990).

Some of the age-related changes in the epithelium may be caused by atrophy of mucous glands in the laryngeal mucosa and the vestibular folds (Kahane, 1983a). Laryngeal glands, particularly those in the vestibular folds, play an important role in functioning of the vocal folds. Hydration of the vocal folds is recognized as important for the health of the epithelium, the structural integrity of the vocal fold cover, and the pliancy of the mucosal wave during phonation (Gracco & Kahane, 1989). It has been demonstrated that vocal fold vibration and voice quality can be adversely affected when laryngeal secretions are reduced. In addition, speakers report increased effort during phonation, vocal fatigue, and dryness of the vocal folds under such conditions (Bless & Shaikh, 1986; Finklehor, Titze, & Durham, 1988).

The number and density of subepithelial mucous glands appears to remain constant throughout life (Bak-Pedersen & Nielsen, 1986). However, age-related changes in composition of glands have been reported. In elderly men, Gracco and Kahane (1989) observed fatty infiltration of serous and mucous glands in the vestibular folds, accompanied by fibrotic changes in connective tissue and alterations in serous/mucous ratios. Atrophy of mucous acini (units of secretion) in the vestibular folds was reported to be a principal involuntional change that would result in decreased viscosity of laryngeal secretions and compromised protection/lubrication of the vocal folds. Similarly, Sato and Hirano (1998) concluded that age-related morphologic changes in laryngeal glands lessened lubrication of the vocal folds. Data are not available at present regarding gender differences in aging of mucous glands.

Age-related decline in vocal fold hydration has been implicated, to some extent, in voice changes observed in elderly speakers (Gracco and Kahane, 1989; Sato & Hirano, 1998). Gracco & Kahane (1989) concluded that drying of the epithelium of the vocal fold would increase the stiffness of the cover, possibly contributing to reported increases in fundamental frequency in elderly men. In addition, they noted that epithelial drying could increase instability of fundamental frequency, contributing to reported elevation of jitter levels (Chapter 10).

Lamina Propria

Three layers of connective tissue, referred to collectively as the lamina propria, lie under the epithelium of the vocal folds. Each layer has different mechanical properties. Together these layers have been shown to be essential to functioning of the vocal folds during voice production (Hirano, 1974). In addition to cellular structures (fibroblasts and macrophages), the lamina propria is composed of an extracellular matrix. The extracellular matrix consists of fibrous proteins (collagen and elastin) and interstitial proteins (proteoglycans and glycoproteins). The fibrous proteins provide the lamina propria with elasticity, whereas interstitial proteins are thought to affect viscosity, thickness of layers, fluid content, and density/size of collagen fibers (Gray, Titze, Chan, & Hammond, 1999; Pawlak, Hammond, Hammond, & Gray, 1996; Sato & Hirano, 1997). Proteoglycans (hyaluronic acid in particular) appear to play an important role in lamina propria biomechanics by affecting tissue viscosity; as the level of hyaluronic acid increases, tissue viscosity decreases. With decreased tissue viscosity, ease of phonation increases (Chan & Titze, 1999; Gray et al., 1999).

A variety of changes in the lamina propria with aging have been documented. When viewed through a scanning electron microscope, elastic fibers of the lamina propria in elderly individuals display irregular curvature accompanied by surface deposits resulting in a rough appearance (Ishii, Zhai, Akita, & Hirose, 1996). Atrophy of elastic fibers and mucosal thickening also have been reported (Hirano et al., 1989). In general, age-related changes in the lamina propria are more extensive in males than females (Kahane, 1990). Investigators also emphasize that histological changes in the lamina propria with aging vary considerably from individual to individual (Hirano et al., 1989).

Superficial Layer

In the superficial layer of the lamina propria, collagen fibers appear as small clusters and contribute to maintaining structural integrity within the layer (Ishii et al., 1996). Elastic fibers, composed of microfibrils and amorphous substances (elastin protein), give resilience and stiffness to the tissue. Changes in the superficial layer of the lamina propria with aging are among the most important in terms of resultant age-related voice changes (Sato & Hirano, 1997).

Early investigations revealed that the elastic tissues in the superficial layer thicken and become edematous with aging. Thickening is reported to increase progressively with aging in women, whereas in men thickness increases up to approximately age 70 and then begins to decrease in many cases. The extent to which edema is present with aging varies considerably among individuals (Hirano et al., 1983, 1989). Sato, Sakaguchi, Kurita, and Hirano (1992) noted degeneration, atrophy, and irregular fragmentation of elastic fibers in the superficial layer upon light microscope investigation. More recently, using a scanning electron microscope, Sato and Hirano (1997) observed disorganization, roughening of surfaces, and variations in size of elastic fibers in the superficial layer of the aged lamina propria. Further, transmission electron microscope examination revealed greater amounts of amorphous substance and fewer microfibrils in the superficial layer of aged vocal folds. Findings of fewer microfibrils indicate that the superficial layer of the lamina propria in elderly individuals ceases development and changes morphologically (Sato & Hirano, 1997). In addition, Sato and Hirano (1997) reported metabolic changes in aged elastic fibers, suggesting that replacement of elastic fibers in the superficial layer of the lamina propria occurs more slowly in elderly persons than in younger individuals.

The viscoelastic shear properties of the superficial layer of the lamina propria appear to increase with aging, particularly in males. That is, older men appear to have more elastic (stiffer) and more viscous vocal fold mucosa in comparison with younger men and women. An implication of this finding is that older men may need to expend more energy during phonation to compensate for a greater energy loss in their vocal fold tissues (Chan & Titze, 1999).

Intermediate Layer

In males, the intermediate layer of the lamina propria becomes thinner after age 40. In addition, the density of elastic fibers in this layer tends to decrease and show signs of atrophy, which alters the contour of the layer. After age 50, the elastic fibers frequently show fragmentation and breakdown, and the collagenous fibers tend to separate and become wavy. Bundles of elastic and collagenous fibers begin to lose the well-defined weave characteristic in younger men. In females, all of these changes are markedly less in evidence (Hirano et al., 1983, 1989; Kahane, 1983a, 1990; Kahane, Stadlan, & Bell, 1979).

Deep Layer

Changes in the deep layer of the lamina propria occur after the age of 50 in males. Around that time the layer begins to thicken. According to Hirano et al. (1989), that thickening is associated with an increase in the density of collagenous fibers in the deep layer. The increase in fiber density may be a result of fibers massing together or spreading apart in contrast to their usual tightly bound state (Kahane, 1990). Hirano et al. (1989) also describe the collagenous fibers in aged larynges as irregular in arrangement, running in a variety of directions. In contrast, collagenous fibers in young adults run roughly parallel to the edge of the vocal fold. As is the case with the intermediate layer, little change is observed in the deep layer of the lamina propria with aging in females (Hirano et al., 1983, 1989; Kahane, 1982, 1983a).

According to Kahane (1990), changes in the lamina propria with aging may contribute to bowing of the vocal folds and irregularities along the medial edge of the vocal fold in elderly individuals. A variety of acoustic changes in the voice could result from such structural changes, including aperiodicity in the signal and evidence of excessive air escape during phonation (Chapter 10).

Macula Flava

Maculae flavae are masses of dense elastic fibers located at the anterior and posterior ends of the vocal folds. These masses are a continuation of the intermediate layer of the lamina propria and appear to function as cushions, protecting the ends of the vocal fold from mechanical damage during vocal fold vibration (Hirano, 1981). The macula flava is important, as well, for the growth and development of the vocal ligament. In the adult, it controls the synthesis of fibrous components in the vocal ligament (Sato & Hirano, 1995).

To date, a limited number of studies have been reported in which age-related changes in the macula flava have been investigated. Sato and Hirano (1995) reported that the size of the macula flava does not change from young adulthood to old age. However, with aging, the number of fibroblasts in the macula flava declines, a process that appears to be a continuation of one begun after birth. That is, the number of fibroblasts declines progressively from birth to old age. These authors also found evidence that fibroblasts in aged macula flava have abnormal metabolism and undergo degeneration. With these age-related changes in the macula flava, a decrease in synthesis of fibrous components in the vocal fold mucosa would be expected and an increase in stiffness of the vocal fold would result. The changes in stiffness of the vocal fold resulting from age-related changes in macula flava are felt to be of sufficient magnitude to contribute to aging of the voice (Sato & Hirano, 1995). No mention is made of gender differences in the process of aging of the macula flava.

Conus Elasticus

Conus elasticus forms a support system of connective tissue for the vocal folds and the subglottal region. The structure consists of tightly packed collagenous and elastic fibers arranged in a linear pattern that extends from the superior border of the arch and lamina of the cricoid cartilage to the upper limits of the vocal fold. It has been suggested that conus elasticus helps to return the vocal folds to a state of equilibrium following displacement during vocalization (Kahane, 1983b).

Changes in conus elasticus with aging have been described in detail by Kahane (1983a, 1983b). In males, age-related changes begin after the age of 50 and become well-defined after the age of 60. Few age-related changes in the conus elasticus have been observed in women. In older males, the fibers of the conus elasticus are reported to be thinner than those observed in young males. In addition, the bundles of elastic and collagenous fibers in older males appear to be separated, fragmented, and to display a wavy pattern. Findings of separation and waviness suggest that the structural integrity of the fibers may have been compromised, much as what might occur if connections between fibers had broken down (Kahane, 1983b). Intramuscular septae also appeared to be fragmented in older males, with the number of fibroblasts among the connective tissue fibers reduced in comparison with younger males and females.

In females, the only age-related change in conus elasticus noted by Kahane (1983b) involves a reduction in the number of cells in collagenous fibers after the age of 50. Males demonstrate a similar reduction in cells, with the age-related reduction described as more striking.

Interestingly, Kahane (1983b) speculated that age-related changes in conus elasticus may be brought about by mechanisms similar to those that produce changes in the laryngeal cartilages. He noted that relative age-related changes in conus elasticus in both males and females tended to be proportional to the extent to which cartilages in the larynx had undergone ossification and calcification. That is, older larynges in which ossification and calcification had been more extensive tended also to exhibit greater morphologic change in conus elasticus.

According to Kahane (1983b), a consequence of age-related changes in conus elasticus may well be increased stiffness of the vibratory system, resulting in decreased sensitivity of the connective tissue wall to subglottal forces acting on the vocal folds. Increased stiffness would reduce the pliability of the vocal folds and contribute to increases in fundamental frequency observed in elderly men. In addition, breakdown of fibers of conus elasticus and the resulting loss of structural stability could explain irregularities in the vibratory pattern of the vocal folds in elderly speakers reflected in higher perturbation levels (Chapter 10).

Thyroarytenoid Muscle

The thyroarytenoid muscle (TA) undergoes significant changes with aging. These changes include atrophy, decrease in fiber diameter, and degeneration (Ferreri, 1959; Hommerich, 1972; Kersing, 1986; Sato & Tauchi, 1982). In addition, it has been reported that vocal fold musculature develops relatively late, but displays symptoms of aging at a fairly early age (Kersing, 1986). Histochemical studies of vocal fold muscle in elderly male speakers have shown that both Type 1 (slow twitch, high endurance) and Type 2 (fast twitch, low endurance) muscle fibers show age-related changes. The pattern of these changes is somewhat different for the two fiber types, however. Type 1 fibers show significant decreases in fiber number earlier in life (after age 60), whereas Type 2 fibers show significant declines only after age 70. Both fiber types show noticeably decreased numbers after age 80. No appreciable increases in fiber volume have been reported in Type 1 fibers with advanced aging. In Type 2 fibers, however, age-related declines in fiber number are accompanied by significant increases in fiber volume after age 70 (Sato & Tauchi, 1982).

Conflicting opinions have been expressed on the impact of age-related contractile changes in TA on aged voice. Research on age-related changes in the contractile properties of TA in baboons revealed only minor differences with aging. Specifically, TA muscles of older baboons contracted less rapidly and recovered from fatigue more slowly than did younger TA muscles. However, older muscles showed increased ability to develop maximum active tension in comparison with younger muscles. Dynamic stiffness and fatigue resistance were unaffected by aging (Mardini, McCarter, Neal, Wiederhold, & Compton, 1987). These findings led Mardini et al. (1987) to conclude that, in humans, changes in the morphology of the vocal folds or in laryngeal innervation, rather than age-related changes in the contractile properties of TA, may play a larger role in voice changes associated with aging. In contrast, Baker, Ramig, Luschei, and Smith (1998) concluded that reduced levels of TA muscle activity could contribute to hypophonia frequently observed in elderly speakers. This conclusion followed an EMG study of TA muscle activity in humans in which older speakers consistently demonstrated lower TA amplitudes than did young adult speakers.

INNERVATION AND VASCULAR SUPPLY

Only fairly recently has information begun to be gathered on age-related changes in innervation of the larynx. Malmgren and Ringwood (1988) found evidence of degeneration in the recurrent laryngeal nerve (RLN) of older rats, suggesting that mechanisms regulating nerve function may be disrupted with aging. In humans, the superior laryngeal nerve (SLN) exhibits declines in both the number and the diameter of axons in myelinated nerve fibers (Mortelliti, Malmgren, & Gacek, 1990). Similarly, the TA, posterior cricoarytenoid (PCA), interarytenoid (IA) and cricothyroid

(CT) muscles display distal axonal degeneration (Perie, St Guily, Callard, & Sebille, 1997). However, conflicting data regarding PCA innervation were reported by Gambino, Malmgren, & Gacek (1990). Those researchers observed no significant age-related changes in length of neuromuscular junctions or numbers of axonal terminal branches with aging in adults. Indeed, Gambino et al. (1990) concluded that neuromuscular junctions in the PCA are better preserved with aging than neuromuscular junctions in muscles in other parts of the body. They attributed the apparent youthfulness of the PCA to its relatively constant use throughout life in comparison with muscles with more variable activity, such as those in the limbs of the body. In summary, although some conflicting data has been reported, it appears that laryngeal nerve functioning may be disrupted with aging. Such changes would not be unexpected, given general patterns of nerve degeneration in elderly individuals (Weismer & Liss, 1991).

As noted by Kahane (1990), changes in the blood supply to the laryngeal nerves have been reported as early as the fifth decade. Age-related changes include reductions in blood vessel diameter and thickening of walls of capillaries (Ferreri, 1959; Hommerich, 1972).

SUMMARY

The larynx undergoes anatomical changes with aging that affect the voice produced by elderly speakers. Both calcification and ossification have been reported in the hyaline cartilages of the larynx, a process that occurs earlier and to a greater extent in males than females. Similarly, the cricoarytenoid joint, particularly in elderly males, shows evidence of thinning of articular surfaces, breakdown/disorganization of collagen fibers in the cartilage matrix, changes in the synovial membrane, and surface irregularities.

Limited research on intrinsic laryngeal musculature other than the vocal folds, themselves, suggests that laryngeal muscles undergo regressive changes with increasing age. Changes include fatty infiltration, connective tissue interspersed between degenerating muscle fibers, unusual variation in cross-sectional area, loss of cross-striations, and an accumulation of debris in the cytoplasm. The cricothyroid has been reported to hypertrophy as it compensates for atrophy in other intrinsic muscles.

There is some disagreement in the literature regarding age-related changes in the epithelium of the vocal folds. Although several investigators observed thickening of the laryngeal epithelium, others found no evidence of age-related changes. There also is some suggestion that the epithelium may increase in thickness in males up to age 70 and then decrease with more advanced old age. In females, the epithelium may increase progressively with aging, particularly after age 70. The epithelium also may attach less firmly to the lamina propria underneath, affecting the structural support of the cover of the vocal fold. Atrophy of mucous glands in the laryngeal mucosa could contribute to age-related changes in the epithelium by reducing secretions that keep the vocal folds hydrated, at least in males. Data is not available currently regarding age-related changes in mucous glands in females.

A variety of changes in the lamina propria with aging have been documented. Age-related changes in the lamina propria are more extensive in males than in females. In the superficial layer, elastic tissues thicken and become edematous. In females, thickening increases progressively with aging, whereas in males thickness increases up to approximately age 70 and then begins to decrease. Edema in the superficial layer is variable among individuals. Elastic fibers degenerate, atrophy, and show evidence of irregular fragmentation. In addition, microfibrils decrease in number, with amorphous substance increasing. In elderly men, the mucosa stiffens and becomes more viscous in comparison with younger men and women.

The intermediate layer of the lamina propria becomes thinner after age 40 in males. The density of elastic fibers also decreases in this layer. In addition, elastic fibers show evidence of atrophy, fragmentation, and breakdown, as collagenous fibers separate and become wavy. Finally, elastic and collagenous fibers become unwoven.

Changes in the deep layer of the lamina propria occur after age 50 in males. Changes include thickening associated with increasing density of collagenous fibers. Collagenous fibers also become irregular in their arrangement. As is the case with the intermediate layer, little change has been observed in the deep layer with aging in females.

The size of the macula flava does not change with aging, although the number of fibroblasts in the macula flava does decline progressively from birth to old age. There also is evidence that fibroblasts in aged macula flava have abnormal metabolism and undergo degeneration. Such changes decrease synthesis of fibrous components in the vocal fold mucosa, increasing the stiffness of the vocal fold.

Changes in conus elasticus begin after the age of 50 in males and become well-defined after age 60. Few age-related changes in conus elasticus have been observed in women. In older males, fibers of conus elasticus become thin and bundles of elastic/collagenous fibers separate and become wavy, suggesting that the structural integrity of the fibers has been compromised. It has been speculated that age-related changes in conus elasticus are brought about by mechanisms similar to those producing changes in laryngeal cartilages. Age-related changes in conus elasticus might be expected to increase the stiffness of the vibratory system, making the connective tissue wall less sensitive to subglottal forces impacting the vocal folds.

Age-related changes in the thyroarytenoid muscle include atrophy, decrease in fiber diameter, and degeneration. Opinions are divided as to the significance of changes in thyroarytenoid contractile properties on voice changes associated with aging in humans.

Although some conflicting data has been reported, it also appears that laryngeal nerve functioning may be disrupted with aging. Such a conclusion stems from evidence of recurrent laryngeal nerve degeneration (in rats) as well as declines in both the number and diameter of axons in the superior laryngeal nerve (in humans). Similarly, several intrinsic laryngeal muscles have been reported to display distal axonal degeneration. Changes in the blood supply to laryngeal nerves also have been reported to occur as early as the fifth decade.

REFERENCES

Ardran, G. (1965). Calcification of the epiglottis. *British Journal of Radiology, 38,* 592–595.

Bach, A., Lederer, F., & Dinolt, R. (1941). Senile changes in the laryngeal musculature. *Archives of Otolaryngology, 34,* 47–56.

Bak-Pedersen, K., & Nielsen, K. (1986). Subepithelial mucous glands in the adult human larynx. *Acta Otolaryngologica (Stockholm), 102,* 341–352.

Baker, K., Ramig, L., Luschei, E., & Smith, M. (1998). Thyroarytenoid muscle activity associated with hypophonia in Parkinson disease and aging. *Neurology, 51,* 1592–1598.

Bless, D., & Shaikh, A. (1986). *The effects of atropine on voice production.* Presented at the Meeting of Wisconsin Medical Society of Otolaryngology, Milwaukee, WI.

Carnevalle-Ricci, R. (1937). Osservazioni isopatologiche sulla laringe nella senescenza. *Archivo Italiano di Otologia, Rhinologia e Laringologia, 49,* 1.

Casiano, R., Ruiz, P., & Goldstein, W. (1994). Histopathologic changes in the aging human cricoarytenoid joint. *Laryngoscope, 104,* 533–538.

Chamberlain, W., & Young, B. (1935). Ossification (so-called "calcification") of normal laryngeal cartilages mistaken for foreign bodies. *American Journal of Roentgenology, 33,* 441–450.

Chan, R., & Titze, I. (1999). Viscoelastic shear properties of human vocal fold mucosa: Measurement methodology and empirical results. *Journal of the Acoustical Society of America, 106,* 2008–2021.

Eggston, A., & Wolff, D. (1947). *Histopathology of the ear, nose, and throat.* Baltimore: Williams & Wilkins.

Ferreri, G. (1959). Senescence of the larynx. *Italian General Review of Oto-Rhino-Laryngology, 1,* 640–709.

Finklehor, B., Titze, I., & Durham, P. (1988). The effect of viscosity changes in the vocal folds on the range of oscillation. *Journal of Voice, 1,* 320–325.

Gambino, D., Malmgren, L., & Gacek, R. (1990). Age-related changes in the neuromuscular junctions in the human posterior cricoarytenoid muscles: A quantitative study. *Laryngoscope, 100,* 262–268.

Gracco, C., & Kahane, J. (1989). Age-related changes in the vestibular folds of the human larynx: A histomotphometric study. *Journal of Voice, 3,* 204–212.

Gray, S., Titze, I., Chan, R., & Hammond, T. (1999). Vocal fold proteoglycans and their influence on biomechanics. *Laryngoscope, 109,* 845–854.

Hately, B., Evison, G., & Samuel, E. (1965). The pattern of ossification in the laryngeal cartilages: A radiological study. *British Journal of Radiology, 38,* 585–591.

Hirano, M. (1974). Morphological structure of the vocal cord as a vibrator and its variations. *Folia Phoniatrica, 26,* 89–94.

Hirano, M. (1981). *Clinical examination of voice.* New York: Springer-Verlag.

Hirano, M., Kurita, S., & Nakashima, T. (1983). Growth, development and aging of human vocal fold. In D. Bless & J. Abbs (Eds.), *Vocal fold physiology: Contemporary research and clinical issues.* San Diego: College-Hill Press.

Hirano, M., Kurita, S., & Sakaguchi, S. (1988). Vocal fold tissue of a 104-year-old lady. *Annual Bulletin RILP, 22,* 1–5.

Hirano, M., Kurita, S., & Sakaguchi, S. (1989). Ageing of the vibratory tissue of human vocal folds. *Acta Otolaryngologica (Stockholm), 107,* 428–433.

Hommerich, K. (1972). Der alternde Larynx: Morphologische Aspekte. *Hals Nasen Ohrenaerzte, 20,* 115–120.

Ishii, K., Zhai, W., Akita, M., & Hirose, H. (1996). Ultrastructure of the lamina propria of the human vocal fold. *Acta Otolaryngologica (Stockholm), 116,* 778–782.

Kahane, J. (1981a). Age-related histological changes in the human male and female laryngeal cartilages: Biological and functional implications. In V. Lawrence (Ed.), *Transcripts of the ninth symposium: Care of the professional voice* (pp. 11–20). New York: The Voice Foundation.

Kahane, J. (1981b). Anatomic and physiologic changes in the aging peripheral speech mechanism. In D. Beasley & G. A. Davis (Eds.), *Aging, communication processes and disorders* (pp. 21–45). New York: Grune & Stratton.

Kahane, J. (1982). Age-related changes in the elastic fibers of the adult male vocal ligament. In V. Lawrence (Ed.), *Transcripts of the eleventh symposium: Care of the professional voice* (pp. 116–122). New York: Voice Foundation.

Kahane, J. (1983a). Postnatal development and aging of the human larynx. *Seminars in Speech and Language, 4,* 189–203.

Kahane, J. (1983b). A Survey of age related changes in the connective tissues of the adult human larynx. In D. Bless & J. Abbs (Eds.), *Vocal fold physiology: Contemporary research and clinical issues* (pp. 44–49). San Diego: College-Hill Press.

Kahane, J. (1987). Connective tissue changes in the larynx and their effects on voice. *Journal of Voice, 1,* 27–30.

Kahane, J. (1988). Age related changes in the human cricoarytenoid joint. In O. Fujimura (Ed.), *Vocal physiology: Voice production, mechanisms, and functions* (pp. 145–157). New York: Raven Press.

Kahane, J. (1990). Age-related changes in the peripheral speech mechanism: Structural and physiological changes. *Proceedings of the research symposium on communicative sciences and disorders and aging. ASHA Reports, No. 19* (pp. 75–87). Rockville, MD: American Speech-Language-Hearing Association.

Kahane, J., & Beckford, N. (1991). The aging larynx and voice. In D. Ripich (Ed.), *Handbook of geriatric communication disorders* (pp. 165–186). Austin, TX: PRO-ED.

Kahane, J., & Hammons, J. (1987). Developmental changes in the articular cartridge of the human circoarytenoid joint. In T. Baer, C. Sasaki, & K. Harris (Eds.), *Laryngeal function in phonation and respiration* (pp. 14–28). San Diego: College-Hill Press.

Kahane, J., Stadlan, E., & Bell, J. (1979, November). *A histological study of the aging human larynx.* Scientific exhibit, Annual meeting of the American Speech-Language-Hearing Association, Atlanta, GA.

Kahn, A., & Kahane, J. (1986). India ink pinprick assessment of age-related changes in the cricoarytenoid joint (CAJ) articular surfaces. *Journal of Speech and Hearing Research, 29,* 536–543.

Keen, J., & Wainwright, L. (1958). Ossification of the thyroid, cricoid and arytenoid cartilages. *South African Journal of Laboratory and Clinical Medicine, 4,* 83–108.

Kersing, W. (1986). Vocal musculature, aging and developmental aspects. In J. Kirchner (Ed.), *Vocal fold histopathology* (pp. 11–16). San Diego: College-Hill Press.

Malinowski, A. (1967). The shape, dimensions and process of calcification of the cartilaginous framework of the larynx in relation to age and sex in the Polish population. *Folia Morphologica (Warsaw), 26,* 118–128.

Malmgren, L., & Gacek, R. (1981). Histochemical characteristics of muscle fiber types in the posterior cricoarytenoid muscle. *Annals of Otology, Rhinology, and Laryngology, 90,* 423–429.

Malmgren, L., & Ringwood, M. (1988). Aging of the recurrent laryngeal nerve: an ultrastructural morphometric study. In O. Fujimura (Ed.), *Vocal physiology: Voice production, mechanisms and function* (pp. 159–180) New York: Raven Press.

Mardini, I., McCarter, R., Neal, G. D., Wiederhold, M., & Compton, C. (1987). Contractile properties of laryngeal muscles in young and old baboons. *American Journal of Otolaryngology, 8,* 85–90.

Mortelliti, A., Malmgren, L., & Gacek, R. (1990). Ultrastructural changes with age in the human superior laryngeal nerve. *Archives of Otolaryngology Head and Neck Surgery, 116,* 1062–1069.

Noback, G. (1949). Correlation of stages of ossification of the laryngeal cartilages and morphologic age changes in other tissues and organs. *Journal of Gerontology, 4,* 329.

Noell, G. (1962). On the problem of age related changes of the laryngeal mucosa. *Archiv fuer klinische und experimentelle Ohren-Nasen-und Kehlkopfheilkunde, 179,* 361–365.

Pawlak, A., Hammond, T., Hammond, E., & Gray, S. (1996). Immunocytochemical study of proteoglycans in vocal folds. *Annals of Otology, Rhinology, & Laryngology, 105,* 6–11.

Perie, S., St Guily, J., Callard, P., & Sebille, A. (1997). Innervation of adult human laryngeal muscle fibers. *Journal of Neurological Sciences, 149,* 81–86.

Rodeno, M., Sanchez-Fernandez, J., & Rivera-Pomar, J. (1993). Histochemical and morphometrical ageing changes in human vocal cord muscles. *Acta Otolaryngologica (Stockholm), 113,* 445–449.

Roncallo, P. (1948). Researches about ossification and conformation of the thyroid cartilage in men. *Acta Otolaryngologica, 36,* 110–134.

Ryan, R., McDonald, J., & Devine, K. (1956). Changes in laryngeal epithelium: Relation to age, sex and certain other factors. *Mayo Clinic Proceedings, 31,* 47–52.

Sato, K., & Hirano, M. (1995). Age-related changes of the macula flava of the human vocal fold. *Annals of Otology, Rhinology and Laryngology, 104,* 839–844.

Sato, K., & Hirano, M. (1997). Age-related changes of elastic fibers in the superficial layer of the lamina propria of vocal folds. *Annals of Otology, Rhinology and Laryngology, 106,* 44–48.

Sato, K., & Hirano, M. (1998). Age-related changes in the human laryngeal glands. *Annals of Otology, Rhinology & Laryngology, 107,* 525–529.

Sato, K., Sakaguchi, S., Kurita, S., & Hirano, M. (1992). A morphological study of aged larynges. *Larynx Japan, 4,* 84–94.

Sato, T., & Tauchi, H. (1982). Age changes in human vocal muscle. *Mechanisms of Ageing and Development, 18,* 67–74.

Segre, R. (1971). Senescence of the voice. *Eye, Ear, Nose & Throat Monthly, 50,* 62–68.

Weismer, G. & Liss, J. (1991). Speech motor control and aging. In D. Ripich (Ed.), *Handbook of geriatric communication disorders* (pp. 205–225). Austin, TX: PRO-ED.

4

Aging of the Supralaryngeal System

The supralaryngeal system consists of the entire vocal tract above the level of the larynx, including the articulators used in speech production. Anatomic and physiologic changes in these structures with aging could produce measurable changes in speech as well as biologic functions served by the mechanism. In this chapter, anatomic changes that occur with aging in the facial skeleton, mastication/facial muscles, temporomandibular joint, oral cavity, tongue, pharynx, and soft palate are described. In addition, alterations in biologic functions served by these supralaryngeal structures, as currently understood, are reviewed. In terms of speech production, current knowledge as to measurable changes in articulation and speech intelligibility with aging are presented in Chapter 8. Changes in resonance with aging are discussed in Chapter 10.

CRANIOFACIAL SKELETON AND MUSCULAR SYSTEM

Structural Changes

Facial Bones

It has been recognized for some time that the adult craniofacial skeleton continues to grow throughout adulthood, although the pattern of growth and the consistency of findings of growth is open to some question (Kahane, 1981). Some investigators have reported increasing dimensions up to age 60, followed by declining dimensions (Goldstein, 1936; Hellman, 1927). Others have reported increasing dimensions throughout adulthood (Hooton & Dupertuis, 1951; Lasker, 1953). In one investigation no age-related pattern of growth in the adult craniofacial skeleton could be identified (Moore, 1955). Interestingly, a recent investigation limited to anthropometric measurement of interpupillary distance indicates that females, in particular, show an increase in this facial parameter during adulthood. However, it is unclear whether such an increase is related to growth of the craniofacial skeleton or changes in the soft tissues of the orbital region (Pointer, 1999).

Perhaps the most impressive evidence for continuing growth of the craniofacial skeleton in adulthood comes from Israel (1973). This investigator studied 36 men and 26 women longitudinally for periods of 13 to 28 years (mean = 19.48 years). He completed a series of measurements of skeletal structures from two cephalograms per subject taken at young adult and older adult age levels. From these measurements, Israel determined that the cranial and facial skeletons continue to grow throughout adulthood. Indeed, growth was noted even into old age. This growth pattern was described by Israel as a pattern of "symmetrical enlargement," which tended to be uniform across all areas. Thus, the proportionate relationship among component parts of the craniofacial skeleton was maintained during the growth process. The absolute magnitude of the growth that was documented was small: on the order of 3%–5% in the facial region during the 20-year interval from the middle third to the sixth decade of life. Although Israel's data suggest that craniofacial enlargement typifies the aging process, Kahane (1981) noted that additional data are needed from the sixth to ninth decades, in particular, to confirm that an enlargement trend continues into the oldest age ranges.

In addition to the issue of growth of the craniofacial skeleton, attention also has been paid to the question of resorption of both the upper and lower alveolar ridges with aging. Although loss of alveolar bone secondary to loss of dentition has been characterized as a "well-known" phenomenon, the rate at which resorption occurs varies considerably among individuals and all the factors relating to such loss have yet to be identified (Adams, 1991). Friedman and Costantino (1990) characterize the extent of alveolar resorption following loss of dentition as down to or below the level where the root tips of the teeth had been located, or a loss of over 50% of the total mandibular height. Although the wearing of dentures is generally believed to delay resorption, evidence in this regard is conflicting. Reportedly, poorly fitted dentures actually might accelerate resorption (Zarb & MacKay, 1988). Interestingly, periodontal resorption in elderly individuals also has been reported when all teeth remain (Friedman & Costantino, 1990).

Loss of dentition also has been linked with the size of the mandibular jaw angle (gonial angle). Ohm and Silness (1999) report that the gonial angle in edentulous patients is larger, on average, than in patients with no tooth loss. Partially dentate patients have jaw angle sizes between those of the other two groups.

Facial Muscles

Muscles of the facial region, particularly those in the circumoral region, are important for swallowing as well as for speech production. During swallowing, muscles in this area provide for an adequate lip seal as well as preparation of the bolus. These muscles also assist in the articulation of consonants and vowels. Other muscles in the facial region are important for facial expression, a visual parameter that contributes to nonverbal conveyance of message meaning during the communication process. Excellent reviews of early literature on age-related changes in facial musculature are provided by Kahane (1981, 1990).

Human perioral muscles (orbicularis oris, levator labii, zygomaticus) normally include both Type I (slow twitch) and Type II (fast twitch) muscle fibers, with Type II accounting for at least 50% of the fibers (Schwarting, Schroder, Stennert, & Goebel, 1982). Although there is no direct evidence that this balance changes with aging in perioral muscles, there are reports of a disproportionate decline in Type II fibers in limb and abdominal muscles (Doherty, Vandervoot, & Brown, 1993; Tomonaga, 1977). If similar declines occur in oral musculature, then speed of response in these muscles could decline with aging, in comparison with sustained contraction ability (Wohlert & Smith, 1998).

Reported changes in the facial muscles with aging include loss of tone, muscle atrophy, decreased elasticity, decreased blood supply, and breakdown of collagenous fibers. In addition, facial expressions in elderly individuals are reportedly less pronounced than those observed in younger adults as a result of smoothing of natural folds of the face. Smoothing of facial folds occurs as a consequence of shrinkage of connective tissues attaching muscle fibers to skin in the facial area, in conjunction with reductions in muscle tone in facial muscles themselves (Leveque, Corcuff, de Rigal, & Agache, 1984; Pitanguy, 1978).

In addition to changes in the musculature and connective tissues in the facial area, the skin of the face loses elasticity with aging and the subcutaneous layer of fat under the skin of the face is depleted. Also, the collagenous fibers in the dermis of the skin break down, resulting in wrinkles and skin redundancy over the facial skeleton (Brown, 1951; Gordon, 1978).

Functional Changes

Clearly, changes in the muscles, connective tissues, and epithelium in the facial region with aging have a dramatic impact on facial appearance. The considerable interest in rejuvenation of the older face through plastic surgery is testament to such aging effects. Indeed, the extent to which aging of facial structures affects functioning of facial muscles is likely to be less significant than cosmetic concerns (Kahane, 1981, 1990).

Although age-related changes in facial muscles might primarily result in cosmetic alterations, changes in lip posture and tone with aging have been mentioned as possible factors contributing to observations of labial spill of saliva in elderly individuals (Baum & Bodner, 1983). Evidence regarding age-related changes in lip muscle function is conflicting, however. Wohlert (1996a) examined correlations of electromyographic (EMG) activity among paired sites surrounding the lips (upper lip, lower lip, right side, left side, diagonal pairs) as a measure of muscle coupling during oral movements. Regardless of age, women showed the same pattern of uniformly high correlations among all EMG sites, indicating functional coupling of all lip areas during these nonspeech tasks. Wohlert (1996a) concluded that muscular functioning of the lips in women during a variety of nonspeech oral tasks including lip protrusion and chewing are relatively unaffected by the aging process. These findings are in agreement with earlier studies showing generally synergistic co-contraction in oral musculature in normal, nongeriatric subjects (Folkins, Linville, Garrett, & Brown, 1988; Moore, 1993; Smith, 1989; Wohlert & Goffman, 1994). In addition, these findings suggest that aging does not affect the motor control strategy employed by women in performing chewing and protrusion tasks, activities that utilize a relatively restricted range of lip configurations.

In contrast, reflex responses in the perioral system have been reported to decrease in old age, at least in women. Specifically, lower lip sites of women 67–85 years of age demonstrate fewer reflex responses, decreased amplitude of such responses, and longer latency from stimulation to onset of response in comparison with young women. In addition, older women display much higher average EMG values during protrusion and chewing than do young women. Speculated causes for higher average EMG values in elderly women include: (1) resistance of oral musculature to age-related degeneration observed in other muscle systems in the body, (2) age-related reinnervation of oral musculature following loss of motor neurons with aging so that the remaining motor units are fewer in number but produce greater firing amplitudes, (3) a greater number of active motor units in older women to compensate for less effective contraction of muscle fibers, (4) loss of skin elasticity requiring muscles to work harder, (5) loss of insulating fat in skin tissue making signals appear larger, or (6) more pronounced protrusion gestures and tighter lip seals during chewing in older women (Wohlert, 1996a, 1996b).

Aging also appears to affect perioral strength. When asked to press their lips together with maximum effort, 10 elderly adults (collapsed across gender) produced significantly lower levels of pressure than did young adults. However, perioral endurance, measured as the length of time an individual maintains 50% of their own maximum bilabial compression pressure, did not differ significantly in young and elderly persons (Wohlert & Smith, 1998). The observed disparity between muscle strength and endurance in elderly persons provides support for the hypothesis mentioned previously that Type I muscle fibers, which are involved in sustained muscle contraction, are differentially retained with aging in lip musculature.

Significant declines in both upper and lower lip spatial acuity also have been reported with aging in both men and women. Interestingly, lip tactile acuity threshold values for young women are significantly lower (greater acuity) than those for young men, although that gender difference disappears in elderly persons. When elderly groups were subdivided in young-elderly (66–75 years) and older-elderly (76–85 years) it was apparent that declines in lip spatial acuity begin early in old age; young elderly subjects did not differ significantly from older elderly subjects, although the older group did show some tendency for further deterioration. Observed age-related declines in spatial acuity at the lips have been attributed to peripheral declines in receptor density and/or age-related changes in lip tissue composition (Wohlert, 1996c; Wohlert & Smith, 1998).

Lip function during swallowing in elderly patients has not been investigated directly. However, there is evidence that peak suction pressure, which is likely to reflect, in part, the strength of the lip seal, is the same during a single swallow event in young and elderly individuals. However, during forced repetitive swallow, peak suction pressure does not tend to increase as much in elderly as in young individuals. This finding is felt to reflect a decline in reserve capacity with aging. That is, elderly persons are performing at or near their maximum capacity during normal conditions and have less reserve strength to call on during swallowing activities that require more strenuous or repetitive muscle activity (Nilsson, Ekberg, Olsson, & Hindfelt, 1996).

TEMPOROMANDIBULAR JOINT

The temporomandibular joint (TMJ) primarily functions to chew and grind food during mastication. During speech production, the TMJ alters jaw position and, therefore, affects oral resonance. In addition, the TMJ, through mandibular movement, affects the articulatory characteristics of certain phonemes and participates in coarticulatory patterns during speech production.

Structural Changes

Temporomandibular Joint

The TMJ undergoes extensive changes with aging, including alterations in the mandibular condyle and the glenoid fossa. Interestingly, women have been reported to display changes in the TMJ with aging more frequently than do men (Oberg, Carlsson, & Fajers, 1971; Weisengreen, 1975). Age-related changes in the mandibular condyle are described at some length by Kahane (1981). The major change in the mandibular condyle and glenoid fossa is referred to as regressive remodeling. This process, associated with loss of dentition and changes in supporting structures for the teeth with aging, consists of removal of bone from the condyle, which reduces its height and resets the articulating surface at a lower level. Additional changes in these structures include gradual reduction in the size of the mandibular condyle, thinning of the glenoid fossae, and flattening of the articular surfaces of the joint (Vaughn, 1943).

Recent investigations involving large numbers of autopsy specimens have indicated that changes in the TMJ involving the articular disc, the articular capsule, and posterior disc attachment also are part of the normal aging process (Akerman, Rohlin, & Kopp, 1984; Nannmark, Sennerby, &

Haraldson, 1990; Pereira Junior, Lundh, & Westesson, 1996; Stratmann, Schaarschmidt, & Santamaria, 1996). Significant changes in the articular capsule and posterior disc attachments with aging include: (1) a decrease in the number of fibroblasts in the lateral capsule and posterior disc attachment, (2) an increase in dense connective tissue (fibrosis) in the posterior disc attachment, and (3) diminished blood supply in the central posterior disc attachment. In addition, articular disc thinning with subsequent bone exposure as well as disc perforation have been reported as a consequence of physiological wear and tear during the normal aging process (Stratmann et al., 1996). Previously, disc thinning and perforation were believed to occur most frequently in association with degenerative and/or inflammatory disease (Blackwood, 1969).

Many investigators have commented on the difficulty in distinguishing histologically between a joint that can be regarded as aged and one that has become pathologically involved (de Bont, Boering, Liem, Eulderink, & Westesson, 1986; Pereira et al., 1996; Scapino, 1983). Several histological changes believed to be age-related also are considered a pathologic sign associated with abnormal disc position, findings that point out the difficulty in separating pathology from age-related physiologic processes. However, although degenerative changes in TMJ are highly correlated with disc displacement, such changes do not always occur with disc displacement. Further, degenerative changes also occur in cases without disc displacement. So, despite the difficulty of such distinctions, some investigators appear to be broadening the definition of normal aging with regard to the TMJ to include degenerative changes previously classified only as pathological (Pereira Junior et al., 1996).

Mastication Muscles

Changes in mastication muscles with aging have not received a great deal of research attention (Kahane, 1990; McComas, 1998). Early investigators reported that mastication muscles lose strength in elderly individuals as a result of atrophy (Greenfield, Shy, Alvord, & Berg, 1957; MacMillan, 1936). Also, with changes in the location of muscle attachments as a result of resorption/remodeling of bone, muscles such as the masseter and temporalis are less efficient in raising the mandible with advanced age (Baum & Bodner, 1983). More recently, age-related changes in the masseter and medial pterygoid muscles have been studied using computed tomography (Newton, Abel, Robertson, & Yemm, 1987). Findings confirm that cross-sectional area and density of both muscles declines significantly with advancing age, with the changes occurring equally in both men and women.

Functional Changes

With loss of muscle strength in mastication muscles with aging, a reduction in masticatory force and skill with aging might be expected (Newton et al., 1987). Indeed, Kaplan (1971) reported that biting force declines from 300 lb/sq inch in young adults to 50 lb/sq inch in the elderly. Although biting force and chewing efficiency may decline with aging, maximal bite force varies considerably among the elderly as a function of dentition status (Tsuga, Carlsson, Osterberg, & Karlsson, 1998). Chewing efficiency also declines with aging, although the extent to which this decline is directly the result of TMJ and masticatory muscle changes is unclear, as chewing efficiency also is linked to the status of dentition (Adams, 1991; Carlsson, 1984; Feldman, Kapur, Alman, & Chauncey, 1980). In contrast, maximum velocity of jaw movement does not appear to decline between young adulthood and the mid-60s (Nagasawa, Yuasa, Tamura, & Tsuru, 1991).

Elderly persons also report symptoms of dysfunction of the mastication system. In a sample of 194 70-year-old patients in Sweden, 74% reported symptoms including tenderness to palpation, deviations of the mandible, and TMJ sounds. In addition, 7% reported functional pain (Agerberg & Osterberg, 1974). Such findings may not seem surprising given the plethora of histological changes in TMJ with aging that have been identified, many of which have been described as "severe" (Nannmark et al., 1990). Interestingly, however, patient awareness of symptoms of TMJ dysfunction actually decreases from age 70 to 85, especially in men (Osterberg, Carlsson, Wedel, & Johansson, 1992). That is, cross-sectional and longitudinal research on large numbers of patients has indicated that reports of TMJ dysfunction (impaired mobility, muscle pain, movement pain, impaired function) decline after age 70. This finding is felt to reflect acceptance by older subjects of gradual impairment of bodily functions, with functioning of the masticatory system included.

ORAL CAVITY

The oral cavity consists of the region delimited laterally and anteriorly by the alveolar processes and teeth, posteriorly by the palatoglossal arch, superiorly by the hard and soft palates, and inferiorly by the tongue. Changes in this region with aging are numerous and primarily involve the epithelia, mucous membranes, salivary glands, and dentition. Changes in sensory functions also have been reported.

Structural Changes

Mucous Membrane

The oral mucosa has been reported to undergo changes with aging, with such changes most apparent after age 70 (Kahane, 1990). Changes include loss of elasticity, thinning, and deterioration of attachments of epithelium to connective tissue and bone. In addition, the surface of the mucosa has been reported to develop roughened areas thought to be associated with age-related changes in chewing patterns and bolus manipulation during swallowing (Klingsberg & Butcher, 1960; Squire, Johnson, & Hoops, 1976).

There is some difference of opinion as to whether observed changes in the oral mucosa in elderly individuals can be considered solely a part of the normal aging process. Several writers note that environmental factors have been observed to produce changes in the oral mucosa similar to those reported to be age-related. Such environmental factors include prolonged periods of smoking, mastication, poorly fitting or inadequately maintained prostheses, and ingestion of a variety of medications (Baum, 1984a, 1984b; Breustedt, 1983; Ofstehage & Magilvy, 1986). Sonies (1991) concluded that if major changes occur in the oral mucosa of elderly individuals, such changes are the result of drugs, disease, or pathological conditions instead of the aging process. As support for this position, she cites observations of healthy, nonsmoking elderly persons with excellent oral hygiene in whom few changes in the oral mucosa have been found. Similarly, Cruchley et al. (1994) concluded that oral mucosal density changes are not associated with aging per se, but are associated with smoking history.

Salivary Glands

The three major pairs of salivary glands are the parotid, submandibular, and sublingual. Minor salivary glands include the labial, palatal, and buccal. Histological changes in both the parotid and submandibular salivary glands have been reported with aging. These changes include increases in the proportion of fat and fibrovascular tissue as well as reductions in the volume of acini (Scott, 1977a, 1977b, 1977c, 1979, 1987; Scott, Flower, & Burns, 1987). No change in the number of ducts has been reported. These changes mean that increasing age results in progressive replacement of parenchyma with connective tissue and fat. Similar loss of parenchyma has been reported with aging in the minor saliva glands, although loss of acini in those glands was accompanied by increased fibrovascular tissue as opposed to fatty degeneration (Drummond & Chisholm, 1984; Scott, 1980, 1987; Syrjanen, 1984).

In addition to loss of functional parenchyma, it also appears that the salivary glands show an age-related drop in the synthesis of proteins. The rate of protein synthesis in the parotid acinar cells declined by 60% with advanced age in rats (Kim, 1987). Although it is yet unproven that such decreases also occur in humans, an age-related decrease in the concentration of some organic components in saliva provides indirect evidence that humans experience a similar phenomenon (Vissink, Spijkervet, & Van Nieuw Amerongen, 1996).

The composition of saliva is subject to age-related changes, although those changes appear to be limited to organic components. That is, inorganic components of saliva such as sodium, potassium, chloride, phosphate, and calcium appear to be relatively stable across age levels. Organic components of saliva include amylase, total protein, sIgA, and acidic proline-rich proteins. Although these organic proteins appear to remain stable across age levels in parotid gland saliva, sIgA secretions in mucous labial saliva appear to be reduced by two-thirds with aging. Reductions in sIgA secretions have implications for immune system functioning in the aged. In addition, secretion of mucins from mucous glands also is reduced with age. Declining mucous secretions may have clinical implications for elimination of microorganisms from the oral cavity. Reductions in these defense systems in the elderly can make the oral soft tissues more susceptible to environmental factors, resulting in mucosal inflammation (Vissink et al., 1996).

Dentition

An excellent review of changes in dentition with aging is provided by Adams (1991). As noted by Adams, although tooth loss has been frequently mentioned as a characteristic sign of oral cavity aging, there is no biological reason why a person's teeth shouldn't last a lifetime. The teeth do undergo change with aging, however. The enamel becomes harder and less porous as a result of fluoride accumulation. Also, the enamel becomes darker in older teeth as organic material from saliva is absorbed or as the enamel becomes more translucent, allowing the yellow color of dentine to become more visible. With aging, enamel also is lost to erosion or abrasion, although the extent to which this occurs varies depending on factors such as diet, habits of occlusion, and disease processes. Interestingly, dentine hypersensitivity, which typically might be experienced between the ages of 35 to 50 years, declines as a symptom after middle age because of secondary dentine formation. Cracking of the enamel, particularly in the crowns of the incisors, also is frequently observed in the elderly. However, such cracks may not be a phenomenon of aging but may simply be more visible in the older population because of staining.

The major change to dentine with aging involves mineral deposits within the dentinal tubules in a regular pattern from the apex of the tooth crownward. In fact, this change occurs in such a predictable pattern that it can be used in forensic work to estimate an individual's age. The additional mineral deposits make the dentine very brittle, posing a hazard for the retention of teeth into old age.

The risk of caries in the elderly appears to be somewhat of a mixed bag (Powell, 1998). On one hand, the incidence of root caries is reported to be higher in the elderly in comparison with younger persons because of gingival recession, poor oral hygiene, and a generally softer diet. On the other hand, continual deposits of dentine on the periphery of the pulp with aging afford better protection of the pulp. Interestingly, although tooth loss in the elderly tends to be linked more with periodontal disease than caries, evidence for this conclusion is not entirely clear-cut. For instance, it has been noted that the lower anterior teeth tend to remain remarkably resistant to loosening, even after posterior teeth have been lost. In fact, anterior teeth may wear away to a substantial degree as a result of their firm support (Adams, 1991).

Sensory Innervation

Information on changes in oral cavity sensation with advancing age is limited. It has been reported that sensory innervation to the oral cavity is reduced with aging (Truex, 1940). In addition, oral form, pressure, and touch discrimination, as well as the ability to sense vibration, have been reported to decline (Calhoun, Gibson, Hartley, Minton, & Hokanson, 1992; Canetta, 1977), although oral form discrimination losses may be shape-specific (Calhoun et al., 1992). Touch discrimination losses in the oral region appear to be relatively minimal (Stevens & Choo, 1996). Temperature sensing ability, perception of food viscosity, and sharp versus soft discrimination do not appear to be affected significantly by aging (Calhoun et al., 1992; Weiffenbach, Tylenda, & Baum, 1990).

There appears to be a high degree of individual variability in oral cavity sensitivity decline, with some people of very advanced age (80 and above) maintaining responses identical to young adults (Calhoun et al., 1992). Findings of increased variability of performance in elderly individuals certainly are not unique to the realm of oral sensation (Chapter 12).

In summary, researchers recognize that considerably more study of oral sensory function with aging is necessary. It has been suggested that the effect of age on oral sensitivity may be more complex than a simple dulling of sensation with advanced age (Baum, Caruso, Ship, & Wolff, 1991).

Functional Changes

Salivation

Saliva serves a number of purposes in addition to maintaining moisture in the oral cavity. Saliva helps to soften food, assist in bolus formation, prevent mechanical damage from dentures, cleanse the oral tissues, and remineralize teeth. In addition, saliva acts as a solvent and may play a role in taste perception. Dysfunction of salivary glands results in numerous problems, including oral dryness, dysphagia, oral discomfort, and increased susceptibility for dental caries and oral infections (Vissink et al., 1996).

An extensive review of the literature on age-related changes in salivary secretion is provided by Vissink et al. (1996). According to these reviewers, approximately 25% of elderly persons experience oral dryness (xerostomia) and related complaints. Interestingly, saliva flow rate has been shown to be lower in women than men across age levels. Conflicting findings have been reported on age-related changes in saliva flow within the same gender. Several studies have found no relationship between saliva flow rate and age. This is true both for stimulated and unstimulated flow rates (Ben-Aryeh, Miron, Szargel, & Gutman, 1984; Ben-Aryeh et al., 1986; Heintze, Birkhed, & Bjorn, 1983; Parvinen & Larmas, 1982; Shern, Fox, & Li, 1993). A smaller number of researchers report reduced salivary flow rate with aging (Navazesh, Mulligan, Kipnis, Denny, & Denny, 1992; Percival, Challacombe, & Marsh, 1994). Methodological variations among these studies may contribute to contradictory findings and make interpretation of findings difficult. It appears, however, that healthy elderly persons have sufficient salivary capacity to keep the oral tissues moist, although they may require additional stimulation to do so. Vissink et al. (1996) conclude that the frequently mentioned subjective complaint of oral dryness in elderly persons is often related to a disease process rather than the normal aging process. According to these authors, the major cause of oral dryness in the elderly is the use of drugs such as antiarrhythmics, diuretics, antihypertensives, and antidepressants, all of which can substantially reduce unstimulated salivary flow rates (Chapter 14). Oral dryness also can be experienced as a negative side effect of radiotherapy of the head or neck area or as a symptom of systemic disease such as Sjogren syndrome (Vissink, Panders, Gravenmade, & Vermey, 1988).

Dentition

It would be expected that tooth loss in elderly persons compromises masticatory performance, particularly in individuals for whom acceptable artificial dentition is not in place. However, masticatory performance (reduction of food per fixed number of strokes) has been shown to remain constant between the ages of 25 and 75 years for persons with complete or only partially compromised natural dentition. In contrast, individuals with "compromised" dentition show declines in masticatory performance regardless of age and also demonstrate a willingness to accept a larger particle size for swallowing than do persons with uncompromised dentition (Feldman et al., 1980; Sonies, 1991).

Oral Sensation and Swallow Function

The fact that temperature detection ability appears to remain stable with aging suggests that an elderly person is no more likely than a young person to mistakenly ingest food that is at an inappropriate temperature. Although acknowledging that temperature detection is not altered with aging, Calhoun et al. (1992) concluded that age-related changes in oral sensation still could have implications for swallow function in elderly individuals. They cite declines in touch sensitivity and oral form discrimination as evidence that elderly persons are disadvantaged in appreciation of the size and shape of ingested material and therefore could be less competent than younger persons in bolus formation. However, early direct investigation of age-related changes in the oral phase of swallow revealed no changes, even in advanced old age (Blonsky, Logemann, Boshes, & Fisher, 1975). It appears that additional research is needed to determine conclusively the extent to which observed declines in oral sensation with aging translate into meaningful changes in swallow function.

TONGUE

The tongue is an important organ for swallow function and taste. Significant changes in these biological functions with aging have been reported.

Structural Changes

Epithelium

Reportedly, aging results in thinning of the epithelium of the tongue, particularly in the central portion (Kahane, 1990; Sasaki, 1994). In addition, fissuring of the tongue surface has been reported in more than 50% of persons over the age of 65, with veins on the undersurface of the tongue becoming more prominent (Klein, 1980).

Taste buds are found within the epithelial lining of the tongue, most commonly on the tongue tip and dorsum and relatively rarely in the mid-portion of the tongue (Williams, Warwick, Dyson, & Bannister, 1989). Studies in which morphological changes in taste buds with aging have been investigated have resulted in conflicting findings (Sonies, 1991). Some investigators have reported age-related changes in taste buds found primarily near the anterior portion of the tongue, called fungiform papillae (Kaplan, 1971; Satoh & Seluk, 1988). Also, changes have been reported in taste buds located at the tongue tip and on the dorsum of the tongue, called filiform papillae (Kaplan, 1971). Reportedly, these papillae decrease both in number and size with the process beginning earlier in females (40–45 years) than in males (50–60 years). Other investigators, however, have found no anatomical changes in papillae that are correlated with aging alone (Azzali, Gennari, Maffei, & Ferri, 1996; Kullaa-Mikkonen, Koponen, & Seilonen, 1987; Mavi & Ceyhan, 1999; Miller, 1988; Mistretta, 1989).

Muscles

Limited information is available on age-related changes in tongue musculature. According to Kahane (1990), investigators reported atrophy of tongue muscles with increasing age as early as 1934. In addition, deposits of starchlike proteins (amyloids) in the aged tongue have been reported (Yamaguchi, Nasu, Esaki, Shimada, & Yoshiki, 1982). Recent investigation has confirmed age-related atrophy in tongue musculature, along with progressive fatty infiltration (lipomatosis) beginning in the second and third decade of life. Reportedly, fatty infiltration begins in the body, root, and tip of the tongue (Bassler, 1987). In addition, lipid pigment (lipofuscin) granules have been found in tongue muscles in increasing quantities with advancing age in both males and females (Dayan, Abrahami, Buchner, Gorsky, & Chimovitz, 1988).

Nerve Supply

No direct experimental investigations of sensory or motor innervation of the tongue have been conducted, although functional losses in tongue movement and sensation have been documented. Such losses are described in the next section.

Functional Changes

Tongue Movement

Significant changes in motor function have been reported in the tongue with aging. Recent ultrasound observation of tongue movements during mastication led investigators to the conclusion that tongue motor skills in the elderly decline in comparison with young adult persons (Koshino, Hirai, Ishijima, & Ikeda, 1997). Similarly, when strength and endurance of the tongue were measured using a pressure transducer, tongue strength was observed to decline after age 79. Tongue endurance did not change appreciably with aging (Crow & Ship, 1996). Also, investigation of maximum lingual isometric and swallowing pressures at three lingual sites (tip, blade, and dorsum) revealed that although swallowing pressures remain similar across the life span, overall pressure reserve declines with age. Thus, elderly persons may work harder to produce adequate swallowing pressures and may be at higher risk for swallowing problems if stressed by illness (Robbins, Levine, Wood, Roecker, & Luschei, 1995). It has been reported, as well, that as many as 63% of elderly persons with no symptoms of dysphagia display difficulties in the oral phase of swallowing (ingesting, controlling, and delivering the bolus) relative to young persons (Ekberg & Feinberg, 1991).

Taste

Changes in taste with aging have been investigated quite extensively. Although many investigators have reported that elderly persons are poorer at taste perception than are younger persons (Bischmann & Witte, 1996; Cowart, Yokomukai, & Beauchamp, 1994; Matsuda & Doty, 1995; Schiffman, Gatlin, Frey, et al., 1994; Schiffman, Gatlin, Sattley-Miller, et al., 1994; Stevens, Cruz, Hoffman, & Patterson, 1995), other research has failed to find significant age-related changes in taste perception (Drewnowski, Henderson, Driscoll, & Rolls, 1996; Walter & Soliah, 1995; Weiffenbach et al., 1990). When specific taste sensations have been examined as a function of age, contradictory findings have been reported for age-related changes in sweet and salt perceptions (Drewnowski et al., 1996; Matsuda & Doty, 1995; Stevens et al., 1995; Walter & Soliah, 1995). In contrast, studies examining perception of bitterness yield consistent findings of age-related declines in sensitivity (Cowart et al., 1994; Schiffman, Gatlin, Frey, et al., 1994). It may be that these contradictory findings are related to reports of considerable variability in taste sensitivity among elderly individuals (Stevens et al., 1995). Also, it has been suggested that age-related alterations in taste perception are much less dramatic than the loss of acuity that occurs with senses such as vision and hearing (Easterby-Smith, Besford, & Heath, 1994). Interestingly, older persons appear to be less sensitive to taste stimuli in food, as opposed to dissolved in water, because of the masking effects of multiple tastes in food (Stevens, 1996). It has been reported, as well, that dietary supplements, such as zinc, improve taste acuity in the elderly (Prasad et al., 1993).

Tongue Sensation

Changes in sensitivity of the tongue with aging to sensations unrelated to taste also have been reported, although such changes appear to be limited. That is, elderly persons have shown declines in localized pressure sensitivity on the dorsum of the tongue in comparison with young adults (Weiffenbach et al., 1990). However, elderly individuals performed no differently from young adults when asked to indicate when two separate calipers were detected (two-point discrimination) on the mucosa of the midline anterior tongue. Similarly, no age-related changes were observed in the ability to distinguish sharp from soft sensations, the direction of passive tongue movements, and thermal sensations (Calhoun et al., 1992).

PHARYNX AND SOFT PALATE

Structural Changes

Epithelium

Aging effects on the epithelium of the pharynx and soft palate have not been investigated extensively. Although the pharyngeal epithelium has been reported to thin with increasing age (Ferreri, 1959), age-related changes in the epithelium are not believed to be extensive (Kahane, 1990). Sensation in the pharyngeal region is reported to diminish progressively with advancing age, however, which may contribute to the development of dysphagia and aspiration in the elderly (Aviv et al., 1994; Caruso & Max, 1997). The only study relating to epithelial changes in the soft palate with aging involved thermal sensitivity testing at the juncture of the hard and soft palate. No aging effects were observed (Calhoun et al., 1992).

Muscles

Conflicting evidence exists concerning muscular changes in the pharynx with aging, at least with respect to alterations in pharyngeal cross-sectional area. Early research suggested that pharyngeal musculature weakens with aging resulting in dilation of the pharynx (Kiuchi, Sasaki, Arai, & Suzuki, 1969; Zaino & Benventano, 1977). Similarly, investigators reported loss of tone in elderly pharyngeal musculature followed by atrophy (Sheth & Diner, 1988). An additional investigation led to the conclusion that the mean percentage of different types of muscle fibers in the pharyngeal constrictor muscles and the mean diameter of the muscle fibers does not change significantly with aging, although aging leads to increased variability in fiber diameters. The increased variability is thought to be a consequence of age-related atrophy and compensatory hypertrophy (Leese & Hopwood, 1986). More recently, investigators found no correlation between pharyngeal cross-sectional area and age in 181 adults ranging in age from 21 to 69 years, although pharyngeal compliance (collapsibility) increased with aging in males, suggesting loss of muscle tone (Huang et al., 1998).

Interestingly, the number of neurons present in the myenteric plexus at the junction of the pharynx with the esophagus has been reported to decline significantly after age 70, accompanied by an increase in the size of remaining neurons (Meciano Filho, Carvalho, & deSouza, 1995). Although such nerve cell declines relate directly only to esophageal disorders in the elderly (Filho et al., 1995), similar declines in neuronal density in the pharyngeal musculature, if present, could explain reports of loss of pharyngeal motor function in elderly persons.

Little empirical data are available on aging of the soft palate musculature (Kahane, 1990). Atrophy of the tensor and levator palatini as well as the uvula have been reported, although it has been suggested that the greatest age-related change occurs in the tensor palatini (Tomoda, Morii, Yamashita, & Kumazawa, 1984). Such an age-related change would have limited significance for speech production, although it could affect eustachian tube function in the elderly (Kahane, 1990).

Functional Changes

Swallowing abnormalities have been observed more commonly in elderly persons than young persons. Such abnormalities may involve pharyngeal functioning and reportedly include such parameters as pharyngeal peristalsis, temporal aspects of oropharyngeal swallow, and pharyngoesophageal segment abnormalities (Ekberg & Feinberg, 1991; Frederick, Ott, Grishaw, Gelfand, & Chen, 1996; Robbins, Hamilton, Lof, & Kempster, 1992; Tracy et al., 1989). Interestingly, however, functional pharyngeal abnormalities observed in elderly persons do not correlate well with presenting symptoms. That is, pharyngeal abnormalities may be present in elderly individuals, yet not explain the swallowing problems of the patient. Conversely, elderly persons without symptoms of swallowing problems may have pharyngeal function abnormalities during swallowing (Frederick et al., 1996). Perhaps this lack of correspondence can be explained by the fact that normal age-related changes in pharyngeal functioning are relatively minor and therefore not likely to correspond with significant swallowing difficulties. Indeed, it has been suggested that major changes in swallowing duration in elderly individuals indicate underlying disease rather than normal aging (Sonies, Parent, Morrish, & Baum, 1988). Similarly, Frederick et al. (1996) concluded that age-related changes in pharyngeal functioning, in the absence of disease, are minor.

Little information is available on functional changes in the soft palate with aging. Jones (1994) commented that the soft palate may not make contact with the posterior pharyngeal wall in elderly individuals because of atrophy of muscle tissue. However, there appears to be little evidence to support claims of significant functional loss of soft palate elevation associated with normal aging (Hoit, Watson, Hixon, McMahon, & Johnson, 1994).

SUMMARY

Structural changes with aging have been reported both in the facial bones and the facial muscles. Facial bones have been reported to continue to grow into old age, although the magnitude of that growth is fairly modest. Resorption of bone in both the upper and lower alveolar ridges also has been documented. Age-related changes in facial muscles include loss of tone, atrophy, loss of elasticity, decreased blood supply, and breakdown of collagen fibers.

Loss of function associated with facial muscle changes with aging has been limited. Although cosmetic changes in elderly persons are a principal effect, elevated average EMG values during nonspeech lip movements have been documented in elderly women. In addition, there is evidence that peak suction pressures during forced repetitive swallowing do not increase as much in elderly as in young individuals.

Reportedly, the TMJ undergoes extensive changes with aging, including regressive remodeling of the mandibular condyle and glenoid fossa, fibrosis/blood supply reductions in disc attachments, articular disc thinning, and disc perforation. However, many investigators have commented on the difficulty in distinguishing histologically between a TMJ that is aged and one that has become pathologically involved. Mastication muscles undergo atrophy with aging and also lose efficiency as a result of changes in the location of muscle attachments.

Biting force and chewing efficiency appear to decline in the elderly. However, maximum velocity of jaw movement does not appear to be affected by aging, at least into the mid 60s. Although elderly persons report symptoms of dysfunction in the mastication system, patient awareness of such symptoms actually decreases from age 70 to the mid 80s, especially in men. This finding is believed to reflect acceptance of older subjects of gradual impairment of bodily functions.

The oral mucosa reportedly undergoes changes with aging including: (1) loss of elasticity, (2) thinning, (3) deterioration of attachments of epithelium/connective tissue to bone, and (4) roughening of the mucosal surface. Writers differ in their view as to whether these observed changes reflect normal aging or are a consequence of drugs, disease, or pathological conditions. Histological changes with aging also have been reported in the salivary glands. These changes include loss of parenchyma, decline in protein synthesis, and alterations in saliva composition. Dental structures also undergo changes with aging, although tooth loss per se is not an inevitable consequence of aging. Dental changes that are linked with aging include hardening, loss of porosity, erosion, and cracking of enamel. The major change in dentine involves mineral deposits within the dentinal tubules, which results in increased brittleness. The incidence of root caries is reportedly higher in the elderly, with continual deposits of dentine on the periphery of the pulp with aging decreasing the risk of caries there. Limited information is available on loss of oral sensation with aging. Although there may be limited loss of oral form discrimination as well as pressure and touch discrimination, such changes appear to be minimal and considerable variability in performance in elderly persons has been observed.

Loss of salivary function with aging has been reported to result in symptoms including oral dryness, dysphagia, oral discomfort, and increased susceptibility for dental caries and oral infection. Masticatory performance in elderly individuals is reported to remain unaffected by aging as long as dentition remains complete or only partially compromised. Some investigators have concluded that loss of oral sensation with aging may impact on swallow function in elderly individuals. However, early direct investigation of the oral phase of swallow in elderly individuals would suggest that any changes in oral sensation with aging do not significantly alter swallow function.

Changes in the epithelium of the tongue with aging include thinning and fissuring of the tongue surface. Findings with regard to age-related changes in taste buds are conflicting. Some investigators report decreases in the number and size of taste buds, whereas others find no anatomical changes in taste buds associated with aging. Atrophy and fatty infiltration of tongue muscles and deposits of amyloids in the aged tongue have been reported. In addition, an increased quantity of lipid pigment granules also has been found in elderly tongue muscles.

Significant declines in tongue strength have been reported in the elderly, although tongue endurance does not change appreciably with aging. Also, lingual pressure reserves during swallowing decline with aging, although maximum tongue pressures during swallow events remain stable over the life span. Although several investigators report that elderly persons are poorer at taste perception than are younger persons, other research has failed to find significant age-related changes in taste perception. Contradictory findings have been reported for age-related changes in sweet and salt perception while bitterness perception appears to show consistent declines in sensitivity with aging. Age-related changes in sensitivity of the tongue to pressure sensations also have been reported.

The epithelium of the pharynx and soft palate has been reported to thin with aging, although not extensively. In addition, pharyngeal sensation is reported to diminish progressively with advancing age. Pharyngeal musculature has been reported to weaken and lose tone with aging. Although the mean percentage of different types of muscle fibers within the pharyngeal constrictor muscles and the diameter of fibers present remains unchanged in the elderly, the elderly display increased variability in fiber diameters in comparison with young adults. Little information is available on aging of soft palate musculature, although atrophy of the tensor and levator palatini muscles as well as the uvula have been reported.

Swallowing abnormalities in elderly persons linked to changes in pharyngeal peristalsis, temporal aspects of oropharyngeal swallow, and pharyngoesophageal segment abnormalities have been reported. Interestingly, however, pharyngeal abnormalities observed in elderly persons do not correlate well with symptoms the elderly person experiences.

REFERENCES

Adams, D. (1991). Age changes in oral structures. *Dental Update, 18,* 14–17.

Agerberg, G., & Osterberg, T. (1974). Maximal mandibular movements and symptoms of mandibular dysfunction in 70-year old men and women. *Swedish Dental Journal, 67,* 147–163.

Akerman, S., Rohlin, M., & Kopp, S. (1984). Bilateral degenerative changes and deviation in form of temporomandibular joints: An autopsy study of elderly individuals. *Acta Odontologica Scandinavica, 42,* 205–214.

Aviv, J., Martin, J., Jones, M., Wee, T., Diamond, B., Keen, M., & Blitzer, A. (1994). Age-related changes in pharyngeal and supraglottic sensation. *Annals of Otology, Rhinology and Laryngology, 103,* 749–752.

Azzali, G., Gennari, P., Maffei, G., & Ferri, T. (1996). Vallate, foliate and fungiform human papillae gustatory cells. An immunocytochemical and ultrastructural study. *Minerva Stomatologica, 45,* 363–379.

Bassler, R. (1987). Histopathology of different types of atrophy of the human tongue. *Pathology, Research and Practice, 182,* 87–97.

Baum, B. (1984a). Normal and abnormal oral status in aging. *Annual Review of Gerontology and Geriatrics, 4,* 87–105.

Baum, B. (1984b). The dentistry-gerontology connection. *Journal of the American Dental Association, 109*, 899–900.

Baum, B., & Bodner, L. (1983). Aging and oral motor function: Evidence for altered performance among older persons. *Journal of Dental Research, 62*, 2–6.

Baum, B., Caruso, A., Ship, J., & Wolff, A. (1991). Oral physiology. In A. Papas, L. Niessen, & H. Chauncey (Eds.), *Geriatric dentistry: Aging and oral health* (pp. 71–82). St. Louis: Mosby.

Ben-Aryeh, H., Miron, D., Szargel, R., & Gutman, D. (1984). Whole saliva secretion rates in old and young healthy subjects. *Journal of Dental Research, 63*, 1147–1148.

Ben-Aryeh, H., Shalev, A., Szargel, R., Loar, A., Laufer, D., & Gutman, D. (1986). The salivary flow rate and composition of whole and parotid resting and stimulated saliva in young and old healthy subjects. *Biochemical Medicine and Metabolic Biology, 36*, 260–265.

Bischmann, D., & Witte, K. (1996). Food identification, taste complaints, and depression in younger and older adults. *Experimental Aging Research, 22*, 23–32.

Blackwood, H. (1969). Pathology of the temporomandibular joint. *Journal of the American Dental Association, 79*, 118–124.

Blonsky, E., Logemann, J., Boshes, B., & Fisher, H. (1975). Comparison of speech and swallowing function in patients with tremor disorders and in normal geriatric patients: A cinefluorographic study. *Journal of Gerontology, 30*, 299–303.

Breustedt, A. (1983). Age-induced changes in the oral mucosa and their therapeutic consequences. *International Dental Journal, 33*, 272–280.

Brown, A. (1951). Surgical restorative art for the aging face: Note on artistic anatomy. *Journal of Gerontology, 8*, 173–190.

Calhoun, K., Gibson, B., Hartley, L., Minton, J., & Hokanson, J. (1992). Age-related changes in oral sensation. *Laryngoscope, 102*, 109–116.

Canetta, R. (1977). Decline in oral perception from 20 to 70 years. *Perceptual Motor Skills, 45*, 1028–1030.

Carlsson, G. (1984). Masticatory efficiency: The effect of age, the loss of teeth, and prosthetic rehabilitation. *International Dental Journal, 34*, 93–97.

Caruso, A., & Max, L. (1997). Effects of aging on neuromotor processes of swallowing. *Seminars in Speech & Language, 18*, 181–192.

Cowart, B., Yokomukai, Y., & Beauchamp, G. (1994). Bitter taste in aging: Compound-specific decline in sensitivity. *Physiology and Behavior, 56*, 1237–1241.

Crow, H. & Ship, J. (1996). Tongue strength and endurance in different aged individuals. *Journals of Gerontology. Series A. Biological Sciences & Medical Sciences, 51*, M247–M250.

Cruchley, A., Williams, D., Farthing, P., Speight, P., Lesch, C., & Squier, C. (1994). Langerhans cell density in normal human oral mucosa and skin: Relationship to age, smoking and alcohol consumption. *Journal of Oral Pathology & Medicine, 23*, 55–59.

Dayan, D., Abrahami, I., Buchner, A., Gorsky, M., & Chimovitz, N. (1988). Lipid pigment (lipofuscin) in human perioral muscles with aging. *Experimental Gerontology, 23,* 97–102.

de Bont, L., Boering, G., Liem, R., Eulderink, F., & Westesson, P. (1986). Osteoarthritis and internal derangement of the temporomandibular joint: A light microscopic study. *Journal of Oral Maxillofacial Surgery, 44,* 634–643.

Doherty, T. Vandervoot, A., & Brown, W. (1993). Effects of ageing on the motor unit: A brief review. *Canadian Journal of Applied Physiology, 18,* 331–358.

Drewnowski, A., Henderson, S., Driscoll, A., & Rolls, B. (1996). Salt taste perceptions and preferences are unrelated to sodium consumption in healthy older adults. *Journal of the American Dietetic Association, 96,* 471–474.

Drummond, J., & Chisholm, D. (1984). A qualitative and quantitative study of the ageing human labial salivary glands. *Archives of Oral Biology, 29,* 151–155.

Easterby-Smith, V., Besford, J., & Heath, M. (1994). The effect of age on the recognition thresholds of three sweeteners: Sucrose, saccharin and aspartame. *Gerodontology, 11,* 39–45.

Ekberg, O., & Feinberg, M. (1991). Altered swallowing function in elderly patients without dysphagia: Radiologic findings in 56 cases. *American Journal of Roentgenology, 156,* 1181–1184.

Feldman, R., Kapur, K., Alman, J., & Chauncey, H. (1980). Aging and mastication: Changes in performance and in the swallowing threshold with natural dentition. *Journal of the American Geriatrics Society, 28,* 97–103.

Ferreri, G. (1959). Senescence of the larynx. *Italian General Review of Oto-Rhino-Laryngology, 1,* 640–709.

Folkins, J., Linville, R., Garrett, J., & Brown, C. (1988). Interactions in the labial musculature during speech. *Journal of Speech and Hearing Research, 31,* 253–264.

Frederick, M., Ott, D., Grishaw, E., Gelfand, D., & Chen, M. (1996). Functional abnormalities of the pharynx: A prospective analysis of radiographic abnormalities relative to age and symptoms. *American Journal of Radiology, 166,* 353–357.

Friedman, C., & Costantino, P. (1990). Facial fractures and bone healing in the geriatric patient. *Head and Neck Diseases in the Elderly. Otolaryngologic Clinics of North America, 23,* 1109–1119.

Goldstein, M. (1936). Changes in dimensions and form of the face and head with age. *American Journal of Physical Anthropology, 22,* 37–89.

Gordon, H. (1978). Rhytidectomy. *Clinics in Plastic Surgery, 5,* 97–107.

Greenfield, J., Shy, G., Alvord, E., & Berg, L. (1957). *Atlas of muscle pathology in neuromuscular diseases.* Edinburgh: Livingstone.

Heintze, U., Birkhed, D., & Bjorn, H. (1983). Secretion rate and buffer effect of resting and stimulated whole saliva as a function of age and sex. *Swedish Dental Journal, 7,* 227–238.

Hellman, M. (1927). Changes in the human face brought about by development. *International Journal of Orthodontics, 13,* 475–516.

Hoit, J., Watson, P., Hixon, K., McMahon, P., & Johnson, C. (1994). Age and velopharyngeal function during speech production. *Journal of Speech and Hearing Research, 37,* 295–302.

Hooton, E., & Dupertuis, C. (1951). Age changes and selective survival in Irish males. In *American Association of Physical Anthropology: Studies in physical anthropology, no. 2.* New York: Wenner-Gren Foundation.

Huang, J., Shen, H., Takahashi, M., Fukunaga, T., Toga, H., Takahashi, K., & Ohya, N. (1998). Pharyngeal cross-sectional area and pharyngeal compliance in normal males and females. *Respiration, 65,* 458–468.

Israel, H. (1973). Age factor and the pattern of change in craniofacial structures. *American Journal of Physical Anthropology, 39,* 111–128.

Jones, B. (1994). The pharynx. Disorders of function. *Radiologic Clinics of North America, 32,* 1103–1115.

Kahane, J. (1981). Anatomic and physiologic changes in the aging peripheral speech mechanism. In D. Beasley & G. A. Davis (Eds.). *Aging: communication processes and disorders* (pp. 21–45). New York: Grune & Stratton.

Kahane, J. (1990). Age-related changes in the peripheral speech mechanism: Structural and physiological changes. *Proceedings of the Research Symposium on Communication Sciences and Disorders and Aging, ASHA Reports no. 19* (pp. 75–87), Rockville, MD: American Speech-Language-Hearing Association.

Kaplan, H. (1971). The oral cavity in geriatrics. *Geriatrics, 26,* 96–102.

Kim, S. (1987). Protein synthesis in salivary glands as related to aging. In D. Ferguson (Ed.), *The aging mouth* (pp. 96–110). Basel: Karger.

Kiuchi, S., Sasaki, J. Arai, T., & Suzuki, T. (1969). Functional disorders of the pharynx and esophagus. *Acta Oto-laryngologica Suppl (Stockholm), 256,* 1–30.

Klein, D. (1980). Oral soft tissue changes in geriatric patients. *Bulletin of the New York Academy of Medicine, 56,* 721–727.

Klingsberg, J., & Butcher, E. (1960). Comparative histology of age changes in oral tissues of rat, hamster and monkey. *Journal of Dental Research, 39,* 158–169.

Koshino, H., Hirai, T., Ishijima, T., & Ikeda, Y. (1997). Tongue motor skills and masticatory performance in adult dentates, elderly dentates, and complete denture wearers. *Journal of Prosthetic Dentistry, 77,* 147–152.

Kullaa-Mikkonen, A., Koponen, A., & Seilonen, A. (1987). Quantitative study of human fungiform papillae and taste buds: Variation with aging and in different morphological forms of the tongue. *Gerodontics, 3,* 131–135.

Lasker, F. (1953). The age factor in bodily measurements of adult male and female Mexicans. *Human Biology, 25,* 50–63.

Leese, G., & Hopwood, D. (1986). Muscle fibre typing in the human pharyngeal constrictors and oesophagus: The effect of ageing. *Acta Anatomica (Basel), 127,* 77–80.

Leveque, J., Corcuff, P., de Rigal, J., & Agache, P. (1984). In vivo studies of the evaluation of physical properties of the human skin and aging. *International Journal of Dermatology, 23,* 322–329.

MacMillan, H. (1936). Anatomy of the throat, mylohyoid region and mandible in relation to retention of mandibular artificial dentures. *Journal of the American Dental Association, 23,* 1435–1442.

Matsuda, T., & Doty, R. (1995). Regional taste sensitivity to NaCl: Relationship to subject age, tongue locus and area of stimulation. *Chemical Senses, 20,* 283–290.

Mavi, A., & Ceyhan, O. (1999). Bitter taste threshold and its relation to number of circumvallate papillae in the elderly. *Aging* (Milano), *11*, 61–63.

McComas, A. (1998). Oro-facial muscles: Internal structure, function and ageing. *Gerodontology*, 15, 3–14.

Meciano Filho, J., Carvalho, V., & deSouza, R. (1995). Nerve cell loss in the myenteric plexus of the human esophagus in relation to age: A preliminary investigation. *Gerontology, 41,* 18–21.

Miller, J. (1988). Human taste bud density across adult age groups. *Journal of Gerontology: Biological Sciences, 43,* B26–B30.

Mistretta, C. (1989). Anatomy and neurophysiology of the taste system in aged animals. In C. Murphy, W. Cain, & D. Hegsted (Eds.), *Nutrition and the chemical senses in aging: Recent advances and current research needs* (pp. 277–290). New York: New York Academy of Sciences.

Moore, C. (1993). Symmetry of mandibular muscle activity as an index of coordinative strategy. *Journal of Speech and Hearing Research, 36,* 1145–1157.

Moore, S. (1955). *Hyperostosis Cranii.* Springfield, IL: Charles C. Thomas.

Nagasawa, T., Yuasa, Y., Tamura, H., & Tsuru, H. (1991). Mandibular reaction time to auditory and visual signals in young and elderly subjects. *Journal of Oral Rehabilitation, 18,* 69–74.

Nannmark, U., Sennerby, L., & Haraldson, T. (1990). Macroscopic, microscopic and radiologic assessment of the condylar part of the TMJ in elderly subjects: An autopsy study. *Swedish Dental Journal, 14,* 163–169.

Navazesh, M., Mulligan, R., Kipnis, V., Denny, P. A., & Denny, P. C. (1992). Comparison of whole saliva flow rates and mucin concentrations in healthy Caucasian young and aged adults. *Journal of Dental Research, 71,* 1275–1278.

Newton, J., Abel, E. W., Robertson, E., & Yemm, R. (1987). Changes in human masseter and medial pterygoid muscles with age: A study by computed tomography. *Gerodontics, 3,* 151–154.

Nilsson, H., Ekberg, O., Olsson, R., & Hindfelt, B. (1996). Quantitative aspects of swallowing in an elderly nondysphagic population. *Dysphagia, 11,* 180–184.

Oberg, T., Carlsson, G., & Fajers, C. (1971). The temporomandibular joint: A morphological study on human autopsy material. *Acta Odontologica Scandinavica, 29,* 349–384.

Ofstehage, J., & Magilvy, K. (1986). Oral health and aging. *Geriatric Nursing, 7,* 238–241.

Ohm, E., & Silness, J. (1999). Size of the mandibular jaw angle related to age, tooth retention and gender. *Journal of Oral Rehabilitation, 26,* 883–891.

Osterberg, T., Carlsson, G., Wedel, A., & Johansson, U. (1992). A cross-sectional and longitudinal study of craniomandibular dysfunction in an elderly population. *Journal of Craniomandibular Disorders, 6,* 237–245.

Parvinen, T., & Larmas, M. (1982). Age dependency of stimulated salivary flow rate, pH, and lactobacillus and yeast concentrations. *Journal of Dental Research, 61,* 1052–1055.

Percival, R., Challacombe, S., & Marsh, P. (1994). Flow rates of resting whole and stimulated parotid saliva in relation to age and gender. *Journal of Dental Research, 73,* 1416–1420.

Pereira Junior, F., Lundh, H., & Westesson, P. (1996). Age-related changes of the retrodiscal tissues in the temporomandibular joint. *Journal of Oral Maxillofacial Surgery, 54*, 55–61.

Pitanguy, I. (1978). Ancillary procedures in face lifting. *Clinics in Plastic Surgery, 5*, 51–69.

Pointer, J. (1999). The far interpupillary distance. A gender-specific variation with advancing age. *Ophthalmic & Physiological Optics, 19*, 317–326.

Powell, L. (1998). Caries prediction: A review of the literature. *Community Dentistry & Oral Epidemiology, 26*, 361–371.

Prasad, A., Fitzgerald, J., Hess, J., Kaplan, J., Pelen, F., & Dardenne, M. (1993). Zinc deficiency in elderly patients. *Nutrition, 9*, 218–224.

Robbins, J., Hamilton, J., Lof, G., & Kempster, G. (1992). Oropharyngeal swallowing in normal adults of different ages. *Gastroenterology, 103*, 823–829.

Robbins, J., Levine, R., Wood, J., Roecker, E., & Luschei, E. (1995). Age effects on lingual pressure generation as a risk factor for dysphagia. *Journals of Gerontology. Series A. Biological Sciences & Medical Sciences, 50*, M257–M262.

Sasaki, M. (1994). Histomorphometric analysis of age-related changes in epithelial thickness and Langerhans cell density of the human tongue. *Tohoku Journal of Experimental Medicine, 173*, 321–336.

Satoh, Y., & Seluk, W. (1988). Taste threshold, anatomical form of fungiform papillae and aging in humans. *Journal of Nihon University School of Dentistry, 30*, 22–29.

Scapino, R. (1983). Histopathology associated with malposition of the human temporomandibular joint disc. *Oral Surgery, Oral Medicine, Oral Pathology, 55*, 382–397.

Schiffman, S., Gatlin, L., Frey, A., Heiman, S. Stagner, W., Cooper, D., & Erickson, R. (1994). Taste perception of bitter compounds in young and elderly persons: Relation to lipophilicity of bitter compounds. *Neurobiology of Aging, 15*, 743–750.

Schiffman, S., Gatlin, L., Sattely-Miller, E., Graham, B., Heiman, S., & Stagner, W. (1994). The effect of sweeteners on bitter taste in young and elderly subjects. *Brain Research Bulletin, 35*, 189–204.

Schwarting, S., Schroder, M., Stennert, E., & Goebel, H. (1982). Enzyme histochemical and histographic data on normal human facial muscles. *Journal of Oto-Rhino-Laryngology and Its Related Specialities, 44*, 51–59.

Scott, J. (1977a). Degenerative changes in the histology of the human submandibular salivary gland occurring with age. *Journal de Biologie Buccale, 5*, 311–319.

Scott, J. (1977b). A morphometric study of age changes in the histology of the ducts of human submandibular salivary glands. *Archives of Oral Biology, 22*, 243–249.

Scott, J. (1977c). Quantitative age changes in the histological structure of human submandibular salivary glands. *Archives of Oral Biology, 22*, 221–227.

Scott, J. (1979). The proportional volume of mucous acinar cells in normal human submandibular salivary glands. *Archives of Oral Biology, 24*, 479–481.

Scott, J. (1980). Qualitative and quantitative observations on the histology of human labial salivary glands obtained post mortem. *Journal de Biologie Buccale, 8*, 187–200.

Scott, J. (1987). Structural changes in salivary glands. *Frontiers in Oral Physiology, 6,* 40–62.

Scott, J., Flower, E., & Burns, J. (1987). A quantitative study of histological changes in the human parotid gland occurring with adult age. *Journal of Oral Pathology, 16,* 505–510.

Shern, R., Fox, P., & Li, S. (1993). Influence of age on the secretory rates of the human minor salivary glands and whole saliva. *Archives of Oral Biology, 38,* 755–761.

Sheth, N., & Diner, W. (1988). Swallowing problems in the elderly. *Dysphagia, 2,* 209–215.

Smith, A. (1989). Neural drive to muscles in stuttering. *Journal of Speech and Hearing Research, 32,* 252–264.

Sonies, B. (1991). The aging oropharyngeal system. In D. Ripich (Ed.), *Handbook of geriatric communication disorders* (pp. 187–203). Austin, TX: PRO-ED.

Sonies, B., Parent, L., Morrish, K., & Baum, B. (1988). Durational aspects of the oral-pharyngeal phase of swallow in normal adults. *Dysphagia, 3,* 1–10.

Squire, C. Johnson, N., & Hoops, R. (1976). *Human oral mucosa.* London: Blackwell Scientific Publications.

Stevens, J. (1996). Detection of tastes in mixture with other tastes: Issues of masking and aging. *Chemical Senses, 21,* 211–221.

Stevens, J., & Choo, K. (1996). Spatial acuity of the body surface over the life span. *Somatosensory & Motor Research, 13,* 153–166.

Stevens, J., Cruz, L., Hoffman, J., & Patterson, M. (1995). Taste sensitivity and aging: High incidence of decline revealed by repeated threshold measures. *Chemical Senses, 20,* 451–459.

Stratmann, U., Schaarschmidt, K., & Santamaria, P. (1996). Morphometric investigation of condylar cartilage and disc thickness in the human temporomandibular joint: Significance for the definition of osteoarthrotic changes. *Journal of Oral Pathology Medicine, 25,* 200–205.

Syrjanen, S. (1984). Age-related changes in the structure of labial minor salivary glands. *Age and Ageing, 13,* 159–165.

Tomoda, K., Morii, S., Yamashita, T., & Kumazawa, T. (1984). Histology of human eustachian tube muscles: Effect of aging. *Annals of Otology, Rhinology and Laryngology, 93,* 17–24.

Tomonaga, M. (1977). Histochemical and ultrastructural changes in senile human skeletal muscle. *Journal of the American Geriatrics Society, 25,* 125–131.

Tracy, J., Logemann, J., Kahrilas, P., Jacob, P., Kobara, M., & Krugler, C. (1989). Preliminary observations on the effects of age on oropharyngeal deglutition. *Dysphagia, 4,* 90–94.

Truex, R. (1940). Morphological alterations in the Gasserian ganglion cells and their association with senescence in man. *American Journal of Pathology, 16,* 255–268.

Tsuga, K., Carlsson, G., Osterberg, T., & Karlsson, S. (1998). Self-assessed masticatory ability in relation to maximal bite force and dental state in 80-year-old subjects. *Journal of Oral Rehabilitation, 25,* 117–124.

Vaughn, H. (1943). Study of the temporomandibular articulation. *Journal of the American Dental Association, 30,* 1501–1507.

Vissink, A., Panders, A., Gravenmade, E., & Vermey, A. (1988). Causes and consequences of hyposalivation. *Ear, Nose and Throat Journal, 67,* 166–168, 173–176.

Vissink, A., Spijkervet, F., & Van Nieuw Amerongen, A. (1996). Aging and saliva: A review of the literature. *Special Care in Dentistry, 16,* 95–103.

Walter, J., & Soliah, L. (1995). Sweetener preference among non-institutionalized older adults. *Journal of Nutrition for the Elderly, 14,* 1–13.

Weiffenbach, J., Tylenda, C., & Baum, B. (1990). Oral sensory changes in aging. *Journal of Gerontology, 45,* M121–M125.

Weisengreen, H. (1975). Observation of the articular disc. *Oral Surgery, Oral Medicine, Oral Pathology, 40,* 113–121.

Williams, P., Warwick, R., Dyson, M., & Bannister, L. (1989). *Gray's anatomy.* Edinburgh: Churchill Livingstone.

Wohlert, A. (1996a). Perioral muscle activity in young and older adults during speech and nonspeech tasks. *Journal of Speech and Hearing Research, 39,* 761–770.

Wohlert, A. (1996b). Reflex responses of lip muscles in young and older women. *Journal of Speech and Hearing Research, 39,* 578–589.

Wohlert, A. (1996c). Tactile perception of spatial stimuli on the lip surface by young and older adults. *Journal of Speech and Hearing Research, 39,* 1191–1198.

Wohlert, A., & Goffman, L. (1994). Human perioral muscle activation patterns. *Journal of Speech and Hearing Research, 37,* 1032–1040.

Wohlert, A., & Smith, A. (1998). Spatiotemporal stability of lip movements in older adult speakers. *Journal of Speech and Hearing Research, 41,* 41–50.

Yamaguchi, A., Nasu, M., Esaki, Y., Shimada, H., & Yoshiki, S. (1982). Amyloid deposits in the aged tongue: A post mortem study of 107 individuals over 60 years of age. *Journal of Oral Pathology, 11,* 237–244.

Zaino, C., & Benventano, T. (1977). Functional, involutional and degenerative disorders. In C. Zaino & T. Benventano (Eds.), *Radiographic examination of the oropharynx and esophagus* (pp. 141–176). New York: Springer-Verlag.

Zarb, G., & McKay, H. (1988). The partially endentulous patient. 1. The biologic price of prosthetic intervention. *Australian Dental Journal, 25,* 63–68.

5

Neuromuscular Control of Voice and Aging

In several chapters of this book potential effects of age-related changes in the peripheral nervous system on speech and voice production are mentioned. For instance, muscle atrophy with aging has been reported in the respiratory, phonatory, and articulatory systems (see relevant chapters). Such atrophy might be associated with age-related changes in neuromotor function. This chapter discusses changes in the peripheral nervous system with aging and the potential consequences of such changes on speech mechanism functioning. In addition, age-related changes in the central nervous system with implications for speech and voice production by elderly speakers are described.

PERIPHERAL CHANGES

In recent years, much research attention has been focused on the effects of aging on motor functioning. Mechanisms underlying observations of skeletal muscle atrophy in elderly persons have been explored, particularly in extremity muscles. Undoubtedly, factors intrinsic to the muscles, themselves, such as biochemical changes in muscle metabolism and changes in the distribution/size of muscle fibers contribute to the "aging" of skeletal muscles (Carmeli & Reznick, 1994). In addition, external environmental factors such as exercise, disuse, nutrition, and drugs also affect muscle aging (Boreham et al., 1988; McCarter, 1990; McCormick & Thomas, 1992; Rothstein & Rose, 1982; Wilmore, 1991). However, factors related to control of muscle contraction by the motor neural system also have been implicated. Indeed, age-related changes in the peripheral nervous system led to the concept of denervation atrophy of skeletal muscles as a principle mechanism for muscle degeneration in old age. Muscle degeneration has been reported to involve both an overall decline in the number of muscle fibers as well as selective denervation of Type II (fast twitch) muscle fibers. Such changes are particularly marked after age 60 (Carmeli & Reznick, 1994; Doherty, Vandervoort, & Brown, 1993; Doherty, Vandervoort, Taylor, & Brown, 1993; Lexell, 1997; Roos, Rice, & Vandervoort, 1997).

Motor Unit

In Skeletal Muscle

A number of studies have described the age-related changes seen in peripheral nerves as a type of "dying back" neuropathy because changes occur earlier and are more dramatic at the distal end of nerve fibers (Krinke, 1983; Spencer & Ochoa, 1982; Spencer & Schaumburg, 1976). The motor unit is the basic component of the motor system and includes a lower motor neuron (cell body and processes) and all muscle fibers served by the nerve cell. The motor unit has been described as the "final common pathway," because signals from various centers in the central nervous system as well as input from the peripheral nervous system result in all voluntary movement through activation of skeletal muscle. Age-related changes in motor units have been implicated in reductions in contractile strength of muscles even in healthy, active elderly individuals. Such reductions in contractile strength are exhibited similarly by both men and women (Doherty, Vandervoort, & Brown, 1993; Doherty, Vandervoort, Taylor, & Brown, 1993; Frontera, Hughes, Lutz, & Evans, 1991).

One of the neural system changes implicated in muscle degeneration in the elderly involves a decline in the number of motor neurons. Such declines, at least in limb muscle, become apparent after about 60 years of age (Booth, Weeden, & Tseng, 1994; Kawamura, O'Brien, Okazaki, & Dyck, 1977; Tomlinson & Irving, 1977). Estimates place average motor neuron loss from the second to the tenth decade of life at 25%, although losses in some individuals older than 60 years have been reported to exceed 50% (Doherty, Vandervoort, Taylor, & Brown, 1993; Tomlinson & Irving, 1977).

Declines in motor neurons are accompanied by reductions in the number of motor axons, at least in lumbar region. Reductions of 5% in the number of large and intermediate myelinated ventral root fibers (L3–L5) between young adulthood and old age have been reported. No loss in small nerve fibers has been found (Kawamura et al., 1977). Similar losses have been reported in the cervical region, along with reductions in fiber diameter with aging (Mittal & Logmani, 1987).

The neuromuscular junction (NMJ) is crucial for interaction between the muscular and neural systems. Biochemical, morphological, or functional changes at this site will influence the response of a muscle to neural stimulation. Research for several years has indicated that the NMJ is a dynamic structure capable of axonal growth, sprouting, and regeneration capabilities. However, there are many indications that these dynamic processes both in animals and humans decline with aging. With aging, fragmentation of acetylcholine receptors at the endplate of the NMJ has been observed, along with increases in endplate size and reductions in the number of endplates innervated by unbranched axons (Gutmann & Hanzlikova, 1965; Larsson & Ansved, 1995; Oda, 1989). Regressive changes both in the presynaptic region (decreased membrane length) and the postsynaptic region (decreased membrane density) have been identified (Arizono, Koreto, Iwai, Hidaka, & Takeoka, 1984). Interestingly, however, when age-related changes in endplate architecture in various muscles of rats were investigated, extremity muscles of aged animals displayed declines in nerve branch sprouting, whereas the diaphragm of old animals maintained the level of sprouting evident in young animals. However, changes in endplate morphology in the diaphragm of old rats occurred which were similar to age-related morphological changes in rats' extremity muscles, indicating that the diaphragm is not exempt from aging effects (Rosenheimer & Smith, 1985).

Electromyographic (EMG) studies have shown changes both in the duration and amplitude of action potentials of motor units with advancing age. Findings have indicated that the axonal conduction velocity of motor nerve fibers slows with aging (Doherty & Brown, 1993; Doherty, Vandervoot, & Brown, 1993; Hayward, 1977; Howard, McGill, & Dorfman, 1988). It has been suggested that slowing of conduction velocity with aging might be associated with loss of large nerve fibers, segmental demyelination, and reductions in internodal length (Doherty, Vandervoort, & Brown, 1993). However, although aging results in slowing of nerve conduction velocity in peripheral nerves, the degree of this slowing has been characterized as mild (LaFratta & Canestrari, 1966).

Motor unit declines with aging are significant. However, there is evidence from studies with animals and humans that at least some surviving motor units are able to partially compensate for declining motor unit numbers through an increase in average motor unit size with age (increased force output), along with slowing of contractile speed. These alterations result in motor units in elderly muscles that are fewer in number, but larger and slower and capable of partially maintaining the contractile strength of affected muscles. However, increased force output in elderly motor units may occur at the expense of fine motor control, and slower contractile speeds might limit an individual's ability to produce large forces rapidly, such as would be needed to avoid a potential fall. In addition, a progressive reduction in muscle mass and contractile strength would occur once a substantial number of motor units were lost (Doherty & Brown, 1997; Doherty, Vandervoort, & Brown, 1993; Vandervoort & Hayes, 1989; Vandervoort & McComas, 1986).

The extent to which changes in the motor unit occur with aging varies from muscle to muscle. Indeed, some muscles do not seem to be affected by age. Studies with animals suggest that non–weight-bearing muscles are less susceptible to aging effects than are weight-bearing muscles (Carmeli & Reznick, 1994). Differences in aging patterns for various muscle groups may be related to differences in motor unit activity patterns and the corresponding biochemical and ultrastructural characteristics of muscle fibers and motor neurons comprising the different motor units. Environmental effects also may differ among muscle groups (Malmgren & Ringwood, 1988).

In Laryngeal Muscles

Intrinsic laryngeal muscles have use patterns that differ from extremity muscles and even the diaphragm. Laryngeal muscles also differ from most other skeletal muscles in histochemical and ultrastructural characteristics (Malmgren & Ringwood, 1988).

Several studies have reported that intrinsic laryngeal muscles undergo regressive changes with aging (Chapter 3). Some investigators suggest that age-related changes are most dramatic in the posterior cricoarytenoid (PCA), although there is no consensus on this issue (Bach, Lederer, & Dinolt, 1941; Ferreri, 1959; Malmgren & Gacek, 1981). Among laryngeal muscles, the PCA is unique in that it is the only abductor muscle. As such, it is activated during each inspiratory cycle of breathing and also is involved in regulating expiratory airflow during speech production (Bartlett, Remmers, & Gautier, 1973; Gautier, Remmers, & Bartlett, 1973; Hiroto, Hirano, Toyozumi, & Shin, 1967). PCA also is unique ultrastructurally and histochemically in that its muscle fibers are well suited for oxidative metabolism and resistance to fatigue (Gambino, Malmgren, & Gacek, 1990). It has been suggested in several studies that the PCA undergoes early aging (Malmgren & Gacek, 1981; Sherrey & Megirian, 1975; Teig, Dahl, & Thorkelsen, 1978). Indeed, PCA has been reported to display some degree of muscle fiber atrophy by age 46 (Guindi, Michaels, Bannister, & Gibson, 1981).

Aging of PCA may well be associated with changes in the motor unit, although evidence is conflicting. PCA shows indications of partial denervation followed by reinnervation at a relatively early age (Teig et al., 1978). Distal axonal degeneration with aging also has been documented (Perie, St. Guily, Callard, & Sebille, 1997). These findings suggest that degenerative changes in nerve supply begin early in adulthood. In contrast, Gambino et al. (1990) examined NMJ length and axonal terminal branching of PCA in adults of varying ages and observed no age-related differences. These authors argue that PCA may tend to retain neuromotor integrity with aging as a consequence of more constant use over the lifespan in comparison with limb muscles, which incur more variable activity levels.

Other intrinsic laryngeal muscles also display age-related changes in motor units. The thyroarytenoid (TA), interarytenoid (IA), and cricothyroid (CT) are reported to display distal axonal degeneration with aging that is linked to declines in the number of muscle fibers (Perie et al., 1997).

Laryngeal Innervation

Only limited research has been conducted on aging of the laryngeal nerve supply. Malmgren & Ringwood (1988) investigated aging changes in the recurrent laryngeal nerve (RLN) in rats. Although there appears to be no decrease in the total myelinated fiber count in the aging RLN, at least in rats, there is an age-related increase in the size of myelinated fibers. There also is evidence of an age-related increase in regenerated nerve fibers and pathological fibers. It appears, as well, that regulation of the microenvironment of RLN fibers undergoes disruption with advanced old age. Such disruption has been linked to pathological changes in nerve fibers (Watanabe & Ohnishi, 1979).

The superior laryngeal nerve (SLN) also has been shown to undergo age-related changes. In older rats, fibers of the internal branch of the SLN show signs of demyelination and axonal degeneration, although total nerve fiber counts, fiber size (myelinated and unmyelinated), and relative proportions of large and small fibers do not vary with age (Rosenberg, Malmgren, & Woo, 1989). In humans, a 31%

decrease in myelinated nerve fibers has been observed in the SLN with aging, involving primarily small fibers. Small myelinated fibers also show significant declines in axonal diameter (Mortelliti, Malmgren, & Gacek, 1990).

Impact on Speech, Voice, and Swallowing

Although limited research has been conducted on innervation of the articulatory mechanism, Weismer and Liss (1991) suggest that age-related changes in the structure of the peripheral nervous system might influence speech motor control in elderly speakers, citing reports of slower nerve conduction velocities in elderly persons. Although it has yet to be demonstrated that nerve conduction velocity is associated with articulatory behavior even within a given age group, it has been speculated that slowing of conduction velocity could be responsible for the well-documented slowing of speech rate in the elderly (Smith, Wasowicz, & Preston, 1987). Conduction velocity slowing also could disrupt coordination among articulators in older speakers (Weismer & Liss, 1991).

Reductions in nerve supply to muscles of the speech mechanism also might be behind observations of increased stiffness in muscles of the respiratory, phonatory, and supralaryngeal systems in the elderly (Weismer & Liss, 1991). If neural supply to a muscle is disordered, metabolic activity of that muscle is adversely affected and the muscle becomes stiffer and more fibrotic. Examples of such muscle dysfunction can be found in Parkinsonism (Weismer & Liss, 1991). As these authors note, it is important to consider the potential influence of age-related reductions in neural drive on the physical properties of muscles involved in speech production.

Compromised peripheral nerve supply could have significant implications for voice production, respiratory support, and swallow function in the elderly. An age-related pattern of degeneration of nerve fibers followed by regeneration in RLN could alter the distribution of motor units throughout the laryngeal adductor and abductor muscles, compromise motor function, and lead to voice deterioration (Malmgren & Ringwood, 1988, discussion). Similarly, loss of motor neurons and age-related alterations in NMJ architecture in respiratory muscles (Wokke et al., 1990) could result in muscle weakening and compromise breath support in elderly speakers. Degenerative changes in SLN in the aged could affect motor functioning of the cricothyroid muscle as well as airway sensory function. Specifically, if of sufficient magnitude, such changes could interfere with pitch regulation and control and contribute to swallowing disorders in older persons.

CENTRAL CHANGES

Brain and Brainstem

Gross Changes

Brain weight increases from birth until approximately age 20, when the process reverses and brain weight declines through old age. By age 90, brain weight has decreased approximately 10% in comparison with young adulthood. Declining brain size has been evidenced via computed tomography (CT) scans and magnetic resonance imaging (MRI) by shrinkage of convolutions and widening of gyri and a resulting increase in the space between the brain and its meninges. It appears that between the ages of 20 and 50, the largest decline involves gray matter, whereas after that time more white matter is lost than gray (Brody, 1992). Brain atrophy is more pronounced in men than women, although the effect of gender varies according to the subregion of the brain (Xu et al., 2000).

It has been estimated that nerve cell losses in the cortex of the frontal lobe are approximately 40% between the ages of 45 and 83 (Brody, 1970). Similarly, the superior portion of the temporal lobe, the occipital lobe, and the precentral gyrus demonstrates significant decreases in cell number with aging (Brody, 1955). These cortical areas are associated with affect, awareness, personality, hearing, memory, vision, and motor functions. Interestingly, the postcentral gyrus, associated with sensory functions such as touch discrimination, shows no significant change in cell number with aging (Brody, 1992). In addition to declining cell numbers in certain regions of the cortex, there also is evidence that pyramidal cells of the cerebral cortex undergo progressive age-related changes that eventually interfere with communication between cells (Scheibel & Scheibel, 1975).

Changes in the cortex have been implicated in slowing of motor movements in the elderly. Indeed, it has been suggested that age-related declines in the speed of the central component of motor processing might be a more significant factor in age-related slowing of motor acts than are changes in nerve conduction velocity (Knoefel, 1990; Leonard, Matsumoto, Diedrich, & McMillan, 1997). Leonard et al. (1997) found delays in anticipatory postural responses preceding voluntary movement in elderly individuals in comparison with younger adults. These authors concluded that at least part of the observed changes were the result of altered central programming involving changes in temporal sequencing of distal muscle activation in elderly persons. Knoefel (1990) cites studies in which no difference in reaction time was recorded for muscles in the jaw, finger, or foot despite varying distances of peripheral nerve conduction (Birren & Botwinick, 1955). In addition, tasks of greater complexity that require greater cognitive processing show a greater decline with aging than do simple motor tasks. Specifically, elderly persons demonstrate disproportionately greater reaction times, in comparison with younger persons, if the response involves a choice of motor response to varying stimuli as opposed to a simple motor response (Welford, 1977).

Unlike the brain, the brainstem is a region of the nervous system that, with very few exceptions, does not demonstrate cell number decreases with increasing age. Brody (1992), in discussing the disparity in aging effects among cells of the nervous system, noted that it appears that nerve cell loss with aging tends to occur disproportionately within more highly developed cells. Thus even within the cortex of the brain there appears to be a disproportionate loss of association cells. Association cells serve an integrating function and are recognized as the most highly developed nerve cell type in the human brain. If such a hypothesis were true it would account for the relative preservation of brainstem cells with aging, as these cells are involved in more basic life-sustaining processes as opposed to higher level thought processes. However, one area of the brainstem in which age-related declines in cell numbers have been documented is the locus coeruleus, a group of cells in the pons that are related to neurotransmitter release throughout widespread areas of the central nervous system and also have been linked to rapid eye movement (REM) sleep (Brody, 1992).

Dopaminergic Changes

There is substantial evidence that dopamine levels in the human brain decline up to 50% over the life span (Adolfsson, Gottfries, Roos, & Winblad, 1979; Bertler, 1961; Carlsson & Winblad, 1976; Hornykiewicz, 1983; Morgan & Finch, 1988; Reiderer & Wuketich, 1976; Volkow et al., 2000), although some investigators have found no age-related changes, particularly in neostriatal structures (Bird & Iversen, 1974; MacKay et al., 1982; Robinson et al., 1977). Reportedly, declines are quite variable across individuals (Morgan & Finch, 1988). In addition, responsiveness to dopamine of the postsynaptic system also lessens with aging, as indicated by declines in dopamine-stimulated receptor density (DeBlasi & Mennini, 1982; Memo, Lucchi, Spano, & Trabucchi, 1980; Severson & Finch, 1980). The effect of these age-related changes in the dopaminergic system is a substantial deterioration of muscle tone, which results in impaired motor performance and reductions in sensorimotor integration (Morgan & Finch, 1988). Interestingly, however, the venoconstrictive and brain metabolic properties of dopamine do not appear to be altered as a consequence of age-related declines in levels (Harada, Ohmori, Kito, & Fujimura, 1998; Volkow et al., 2000).

Impact on Speech, Voice, and Swallowing

Progressive degeneration of the dopaminergic system with aging may result in generalized slowing of all sensorimotor processes, including speech production. Specifically, neurotransmitter degeneration in the elderly could slow speech rate in elderly speakers (Chapter 9). However, other degenerative changes in the brain also have been shown to affect brain function (Peach, 1987) and might also affect speech rate. For instance, age-related cortical changes, although impacting most significantly on memory, cognition, and language functions, cannot be separated from speech production behaviors. As noted by Weismer and Liss (1991), slowing of speech rate in the elderly could involve an interaction both of altered language processes (lexical access) and degeneration of the dopaminergic system. Indeed, these authors suggest that speaking rate be assessed in the elderly under conditions in which lexical access demands vary to separate out the contribution of these two elements.

Slowing of swallow function with age also has been reported (Rademaker, Pauloski, Calangelo, & Logemann, 1998; Robbins, Hamilton, Lof, & Kempster, 1992; Sonies, Parent, Morrish, & Baum, 1988; Spiegel, Sataloff, & Selber, 1999). Such slowing involves extended bolus transit time through the oropharynx and prolonged closure and opening of the valves associated with swallowing, namely the velopharynx, larynx, and cricopharyngeus (Rademaker et al., 1998). Although it has yet to be demonstrated that such slowing is linked to age-related alterations in the dopaminergic system, it has been suggested that slowing of neural processing time with aging could be a factor in these changes (Caruso & Max, 1997; Rademaker et al., 1998).

Age-related changes in the central nervous system also might play a role in the clinical expression of essential tremor (Elble, 1995). Essential tremor is the most common form of abnormal tremor characterized by action tremor in the absence of other signs of motor dysfunction. Essential tremor is frequently inherited and occurs most often in elderly persons (Elble & Koller, 1990). Mild essential tremor has been implicated as the probable cause of tremulousness in elderly voices (Elble, 1995).

NORMAL MOTOR BEHAVIOR VERSUS PARKINSON DISEASE

A number of different brain lesions have been identified in Parkinson disease. However, it is widely held that damage to or loss of cells in the substantia nigra pars compacta is the major pathological lesion responsible for the characteristic motor signs of the disease (Bernheimer, Birkmayer, Hornykiewicz, Jellinger, & Seitelberger, 1973; McGeer, & McGeer, 1978; McGeer, McGeer, & Suzuki, 1977; Mortimer, 1988). This nucleus is the source of ascending dopaminergic pathways to the striatum. Clinical signs of the disease have been reported to differ in patients with early onset of symptoms and those with symptoms beginning later in life. When Parkinson disease begins in the 40s or 50s it usually is accompanied by rigidity and/or moderate to severe tremor. In contrast, individuals in whom the condition begins after age 70 typically demonstrate rigidity and tremor less prominently in comparison with marked slowing of motor behavior. These differences in clinical signs have led to speculation that there may be age-related subtypes of Parkinson disease, although such variations have not been distinguished pathologically or biochemically (Mortimer, 1988).

Perceptually, the voice of persons with Parkinson disease has been described as breathy, tremulous, high pitched, monotone, and reduced in loudness (Hanson, Gerratt, & Ward, 1984). Visual examination of the larynx using both telescopic cinelaryngoscopy and videostroboscopy has revealed abnormal findings, including disordered phonatory postures, bowed vocal folds, abnormally large glottic aperture during phonation, vertical laryngeal tremor, abnormal phase closure, and severe phase asymmetry (Hanson et al., 1984; Perez, Ramig, Smith, & Dromey, 1996). Acoustic findings of high perturbation (both frequency and amplitude) in Parkinson patients also indicate that the disease has a measurable effect on phonation. In particular, increased variability of perturbation measures in Parkinson patients compared with normal speakers has been reported (Ramig, Scherer, Titze, & Ringel, 1988; Zwirner, Murry, & Woodson, 1991).

Normal elderly individuals have been shown to demonstrate progressive declines in dopamine levels. Therefore, it is probably not surprising that some investigators have speculated that Parkinson disease may be viewed, in part, as an accelerated form of aging (Mortimer & Webster, 1982; Weismer & Liss, 1991). Reported similarities in normal aging and Parkinson disease are listed in Table 5–1. Knoefel (1990) pointed out that the gait of the aged involves a slightly flexed upright position, slowed forward progress, shortened stride, decreased clearance of the foot and heel from the ground, increased side-to-side sway, and extra steps. An extreme form of this gait resembles that of Parkinson disease, absent the tremor and festination. Mortimer (1988) observed that although rigidity and rest tremor (primary signs of Parkinson disease) are absent in normal elderly individuals, reduced motor speed (bradykinesia) is strongly associated with aging both in normal elderly individuals and those with Parkinson disease. More recently, following an EMG investigation, Baker, Ramig, Luschei, and Smith (1998) concluded that reduced thyroarytenoid muscle

Table 5–1. Reported Similarities in Normal Aging and Parkinson Disease

Normal Aging	Parkinson Disease
Gait	
Slightly flexed upright posture	Extreme normal aging gait,
Slowed forward progress	plus tremor and festination
Shortened stride	
Decreased foot and heel ground clearance	
Increased side-to-side sway	
Extra steps	
Motor Speed	
Reduced (bradykinesia)	Reduced (bradykinesia), plus rigidity and rest tremor
Muscle Activity	
Reduced thyroarytenoid activity	Same as normal aging
Speech Acoustics	
Shortening of laryngeal devoicing gesture (/s/ and /p/ VOT)	Same as normal aging
Shallow formant trajectories	
Spirantization of stops	

Note: Compiled from Baker, Ramig, Lusschei, & Smith (1998); Knoefel (1990); Liss, Weismer, & Rosenbek (1990); Mortimer (1988).

activity may accompany both normal aging and Parkinson disease. Liss, Weismer, and Rosenbek (1990) found similarities in the acoustic characteristics of speech produced by males over the age of 87 and Parkinson patients. Specifically, both groups shared the following acoustic features, in comparison with younger elderly persons and young adults: (1) disproportionate shortening of the laryngeal devoicing gesture in two segments (/s/ and /p/ VOT), (2) shallow formant trajectories, and (3) spirantization of stops. As these features of speech require fine motor control and coordination, the authors hypothesized that generalized slowing of speech production processes with aging due to degeneration in the dopaminergic system could be responsible for "Parkinson-like" findings in very old males.

In comparing normal elderly individuals and Parkinson patients, it is instructive to point out differences in these two groups as well as similarities. In kinematic studies of connected speech, Parkinson patients demonstrated slower lip and jaw movements with smaller displacements than those observed for normal geriatric speakers (Forrest, Weismer, & Turner,

1989). Similarly, following a photoglottographic study, Lin, Jiang, Hone, and Hanson (1999) concluded that normal elderly speakers can be distinguished from Parkinson patients on the basis of higher speed quotients (proportion of time for glottal opening relative to glottal closing). This finding was interpreted as a reflection of greater rigidity of the vocalis muscle in the Parkinson group relative to normal elderly speakers. Finally, higher laryngeal resistance values and greater phonation threshold pressures reportedly distinguish Parkinson patients and normal elderly speakers (Jiang et al., 1999). It is important to note, however, that none of these investigations included very old speakers. Without data on very old speakers, it is not possible to definitively state that these parameters continue to distinguish Parkinson patients in advanced old age (Liss et al., 1990).

In summary, there is considerable evidence that the normal aged brain shares many features in common with brain changes evident in Parkinson disease, particularly in very advanced old age. However, Parkinson patients still can be distinguished clinically by the severity, rapid progression, and age of onset of the brain changes (Mortimer & Webster, 1982). It appears, as well, that vocal fold movement patterns and measures of glottal resistance/phonation threshold pressures also may be useful in differentiating Parkinson patients from normal elderly speakers.

SUMMARY

Considerable research has been conducted on the effects of aging on motor function. Although factors intrinsic to muscles, themselves, as well as external environmental factors contribute to muscle "aging," factors related to control of muscle contraction by the motor neural system are thought by many to be the principle mechanism for muscle degeneration in old age. That is, a type of "dying back" neuropathy, particularly in the distal end of peripheral nerve fibers, has been described as occurring with aging. Specific peripheral system changes observed with aging include declines in motor neurons, reductions in the number of motor axons, and changes in endplate architecture. Functionally, slowing of conduction velocity with aging is well documented, although the degree of slowing has been characterized as mild. Although motor unit declines with aging are significant, there is some evidence that surviving motor units are able to partially compensate for motor unit losses by increasing average motor unit size in the elderly. Hence, motor units in elderly muscles are fewer in number but larger and slower and capable of partially maintaining the contractile strength of affected muscles. However, these alterations may limit an elderly person's ability to produce large forces rapidly, as in the case of a sudden fall. In addition, eventual reduction in muscle mass and contractile strength occurs once a substantial number of motor units are lost.

Several studies on laryngeal muscles also have demonstrated regressive changes with aging. The TA, PCA, IA, and CT are reported to display distal axonal degeneration with aging, which is linked to declines in the number of muscle fibers. Although some investigators suggest that aging effects are most dramatic and occur earlier in PCA, there is no consensus on this issue. Indeed, it also has been suggested that the PCA may tend to retain neuromotor integrity, at least in comparison with limb musculature, as a result of more constant use over the life span.

There is evidence, as well, of age-related changes in the RLN and SLN. In rats, an age-related increase in the size of myelinated fibers has been reported, along with increases in regenerated nerve fibers and pathological fibers. The regulation of the microenvironment of RLN fibers also shows signs of disruption with aging. The internal branch of SLN shows signs of age-related demyelination and axonal degeneration in rats. In humans, small myelinated nerve fibers of the SLN show a 31% decrease in number, along with a decline in axonal diameter.

Changes in the peripheral nervous system with aging could influence speech motor control in elderly speakers. Age-related reductions in nerve conduction velocity might be behind the well-documented slowing of speech rate in the elderly and also might disrupt coordination among the articulators in older speakers. Reductions in nerve supply to muscles of the speech mechanism might increase stiffness in muscles of the respiratory, phonatory, and supralaryngeal systems in the elderly. Compromised peripheral nerve supply also could lead to voice deterioration and breath support difficulties in elderly speakers. In addition, degenerative changes in the SLN, if of sufficient magnitude, might interfere with pitch regulation/control and contribute to swallowing disorders in the elderly.

Changes in the central nervous system include nerve cell losses in the brain, particularly involving the more highly developed cells. Cortical losses include areas associated with affect, awareness, personality, hearing, memory, vision, and motor functions. There is evidence, as well, of age-related changes in pyramidal cells of the cortex that eventually interfere with communication between cells. The brainstem is a region of the central nervous system with relatively few cell number decreases with advanced age.

There is substantial evidence that dopamine levels in the brain decline up to 50% over the life span, although these losses are quite variable across individuals. Responsiveness to dopamine in the system also lessens with aging. The effect of these age-related changes in the dopaminergic system is a substantial deterioration of muscle tone, which impairs motor performance and reduces sensorimotor integration.

A significant factor in the slowing of motor acts in the elderly may involve age-related declines in central motor processing, as opposed to slowing of nerve conduction velocity in peripheral nerves. In comparison to young adults, elderly persons have demonstrated the following behaviors leading researchers to such a conclusion: (1) delays in anticipatory postural responses preceding voluntary movement and (2) disproportionate declines in reaction time for motor tasks requiring greater cognitive processing in comparison with simple motor tasks. However, although motor tasks requiring greater cognitive processing may show greater declines with aging, the speed of even simple motor acts slows to some degree in the elderly.

Central nervous system changes with aging could have a significant impact on speech, voice, and swallowing. Neurotransmitter degeneration in the elderly could slow speech rate in the elderly, although such slowing also could involve altered language processes. Slowed swallow function in elderly persons also might be related to neurotransmitter changes. Age-related changes in the central nervous system could play a role in the clinical expression of essential tremor.

Several investigators have speculated that Parkinson disease may be viewed as an accelerated form of aging. Findings in normal elderly persons that are similar to those in Parkinson patients include similarities in gait and reductions in motor speed. Symptoms of Parkinson disease that are absent in normal elderly persons include rigidity and rest tremor. Interestingly, individuals with Parkinson disease beginning after age 70 typically have less prominent rigidity and tremor than individuals displaying the disease in the 40s or 50s, leading to speculation that there may be age-related subtypes of Parkinson disease.

Similarities have been found in the acoustic characteristics of speech produced by normal elderly persons beyond the age of 87 and Parkinson patients. Since the features of speech showing acoustic changes require fine motor control and coordination, these findings have been taken as support for the hypothesis that advanced old age resembles Parkinsonism.

Parkinson patients can be distinguished from normal elderly speakers on the basis of: (1) slower lip and jaw movements with smaller displacements, (2) higher speed quotient, (3) higher laryngeal resistance, and (4) greater phonation threshold pressure. However, because very old speakers have yet to be compared with Parkinson patients on these measures, it remains possible that the two groups cannot be distinguished once advanced old age is reached.

REFERENCES

Adolfsson, R., Gottfries, C., Roos, B., & Winblad, B. (1979). Changes in brain cate-cholamines in patients with dementia of Alzheimer type. *British Journal of Psychiatry, 135,* 216–223.

Arizono, N., Koreto, O., Iwai, Y., Hidaka, T., & Takeoka, O. (1984). Morphometric analysis of human neuromuscular junction in different ages. *Acta Pathologica Japan, 34,* 1243–1249.

Bach, A., Lederer, F., & Dinolt, R. (1941). Senile changes in the laryngeal musculature. *Archives of Otolaryngology, 34,* 47–56.

Baker, K., Ramig, L., Luschei, F., & Smith, M. (1998). Thyroarytenoid muscle activity associated with hypophonia in Parkinson disease and aging. *Neurology, 51,* 1592–1598.

Bartlett, D., Remmers, J. & Gautier, H. (1973). Laryngeal regulation of respiratory airflow. *Respiratory Physiology, 18,* 194–204.

Bernheimer, H., Birkmayer, W., Hornykiewicz, O., Jellinger, K., & Seitelberger, F. (1973). Brain dopamine and the syndromes of Parkinson and Huntington. Clinical, morphological and neurochemical correlations. *Journal of Neurological Sciences, 20,* 415–455.

Bertler, A. (1961). Occurrence and localization of catecholamines in the human brain. *Acta Physiologica Scandanavia, 51,* 97–107.

Bird, E., & Iversen, L. (1974). Huntington's chorea: Post-mortem measurement of glutamic acid decarboxylase, choline acetyltransferase and dopamine in basal ganglia. *Brain, 97,* 457–472.

Birren, J., & Botwinick, J. (1955). Age differences in finger, jaw and foot reaction time to auditory stimuli. *Journal of Gerontology, 10,* 429–432.

Booth, F., Weeden, S., & Tseng, B. (1994). Effect of aging on human skeletal muscle and motor function. *Medicine & Science in Sports & Exercise, 26,* 556–560.

Boreham, C., Watt, P., Williams, P., Merry, B., Goldspink, G., & Goldspink, D. (1988). Effect of ageing and chronic dietary restriction on the morphology of fast and slow muscles of the rat. *Journal of Anatomy, 157,* 111–125.

Brody, H. (1955). Organization of the cerebral cortex. III. A Study of aging in the human cerebral cortex. *Journal of Comprehensive Neurology, 102,* 511–556.

Brody, H. (1970). Structural changes in the aging nervous system. In H. Blumenthal (Ed.), *Interdisciplinary topics in gerontology* (pp. 9–21). Basel: Karger.

Brody, H. (1992). The aging brain. *Acta Neurologica Scandinavica, (Suppl.), 137,* 40–44.

Carlsson, A., & Winblad, B. (1976). The influence of age and time interval between death and autopsy on dopamine and 3-methoxytyramine levels in human basal ganglia. *Journal of Neural Transmission, 38,* 271–276.

Caruso, A., & Max, L. (1997). Effects of aging on neuromotor processes of swallowing. *Seminars in Speech and Language, 18,* 181–192.

Carmeli, E., & Reznick, A. (1994). The physiology and biochemistry of skeletal muscle atrophy as a function of age. *Proceedings of the Society for Experimental Biology & Medicine, 206,* 103–113.

DeBlasi, A., & Mennini, T. (1982). Selective reduction of one class of dopamine receptor binding sites in the corpus striatum of aged rats. *Brain Research, 242,* 361–364.

Doherty, T., & Brown, W. (1993). The estimated numbers and relative sizes of thenar motor units as selected by multiple point stimulation in young and older adults. *Muscle and Nerve, 16,* 355–366.

Doherty, T., & Brown, W. (1997). Age-related changes in the twitch contractile properties of human thenar motor units. *Journal of Applied Physiology, 82,* 93–101.

Doherty, T., Vandervoort, A., & Brown, W. (1993). Effects of ageing on the motor unit: A brief review. *Canadian Journal of Applied Physiology, 18,* 331–358.

Doherty, T., Vandervoort, A., Taylor, A., & Brown, W. (1993). Effects of motor unit losses on strength in older men and women. *Journal of Applied Physiology, 74,* 868–874.

Elble, R. (1995). The role of aging in the clinical expression of essential tremor. *Experimental Gerontology, 30,* 337–347.

Elble, R., & Koller, W. (1990). *Tremor.* Baltimore: Johns Hopkins University Press.

Ferreri, G. (1959). Senescence of the larynx. *Italian General Review of Oto-Rhino-Laryngology, 1,* 640–709.

Forrest, K., Weismer, G., & Turner, G. (1989). Kinematic, acoustic, and perceptual analyses of connected speech produced by Parkinsonian and normal geriatric adults. *Journal of the Acoustical Society of America, 85,* 2608–2622.

Frontera, W., Hughes, V., Lutz, K., & Evans, W. (1991). A cross-sectional study of muscle strength and mass in 45- to 78-yr-old men and women. *Journal of Applied Physiology, 71,* 664–650.

Gambino, D., Malmgren, L., & Gacek, R. (1990). Age-related changes in the neuro-muscular junctions in the human posterior cricoarytenoid muscles: A quantitative study. *Laryngoscope, 100,* 262–268.

Gautier, H., Remmers, J., & Bartlett, D. (1973). Control of the duration of expiration. *Respiratory Physiology, 18,* 205–221.

Guindi, G., Michaels, L., Bannister, R., & Gibson, W. (1981). Pathology of the intrinsic muscles of the larynx. *Clinics in Otolaryngology, 6,* 101–109.

Gutmann, E., & Hanzlikova, V. (1965). Age changes of motor endplates in muscle fibers of the rat. *Gerontologica, 11,* 12–24.

Hanson, D., Gerratt, B., & Ward, P. (1984). Cinegraphic observations of laryngeal function in Parkinson's disease. *Laryngoscope, 94,* 348–353.

Harada, K., Ohmori, M., Kito, Y., & Fujimura, A. (1998). Effects of dopamine on veins in humans: Comparison with noradrenaline and influence of age. *European Journal of Clinical Pharmacology, 54,* 227–230.

Hayward, M. (1977). Automatic analysis of the electromyogram in healthy subjects of different ages. *Journal of the Neurological Sciences, 33,* 397–413.

Hiroto, I., Hirano, M., Toyozumi, Y., & Shin, T. (1967). Electromyographic investigation of the intrinsic laryngeal muscles related to speech sounds. *Annals of Otology, Rhinology and Laryngology, 76,* 861–872.

Hornykiewicz, O. (1983). Dopamine changes in the aging human brain: Functional considerations. In A. Agnoli et al. (Eds.), *Aging, Vol. 23: Aging brain and ergot alkaloids* (pp. 9–14). New York: Raven Press.

Howard, J., McGill, K., & Dorfman, L. (1988). Age effects in properties of motor unit action potentials: ADEMG analysis. *Annals of Neurology, 24,* 207–213.

Jiang, J., O'Mara, T., Chen, H., Stern, J., Vlagos, D., & Hanson, D. (1999). Aerodynamic measurements of patients with Parkinson's disease. *Journal of Voice, 13,* 583–591.

Kawamura, Y., O'Brien, P., Okazaki, H., & Dyck, P. (1977). Lumbar motorneurons of man, I: Numbers and diameter histograms of alpha and gamma axons of ventral roots. *Journal of Neuropathology and Experimental Neurology, 36,* 853–860.

Knoefel, J. (1990). Neurological aging. In E. Cherow (Ed.), *Proceedings of the Research Symposium on Communication Sciences and Disorders and Aging* (pp. 46–53). No. 19, Rockville, MD: ASHA.

Krinke, G. (1983). Spinal radiculopathy in aging rats: Demyelination secondary to neuronal dwindling? *Acta Neuropathologica (Berlin), 59,* 63–69.

LaFratta, C., & Canestrari, R. (1966). A comparison of sensory and motor nerve conduction velocities as related to age. *Archives of Physical Medicine Rehabilitation, 47,* 286–290.

Larsson, L., & Ansved, T. (1995). Effects of ageing on the motor unit. *Progress in Neurobiology, 45,* 397–458.

Leonard, C., Matsumoto, T., Diedrich, P., & McMillan, J. (1997). Changes in neural modulation and motor control during voluntary movements of older individuals. *Journal of Gerontology. Medical Sciences, 52A,* M320–M325.

Lexell, J. (1997). Evidence for nervous system degeneration with advancing age. *Journal of Nutrition, 127 (Suppl.),* 1011S–1013S.

Lin, E., Jiang, J., Hone, S., & Hanson, D. (1999). Photoglottographic measures in Parkinson's disease. *Journal of Voice, 13,* 25–35.

Liss, J., Weismer, G., & Rosenbek, J. (1990). Selected acoustic characteristics of speech production in very old males. *Journal of* Gerontology: *Psychological Sciences, 45,* P35–P45.

MacKay, A., Iversen, L., Rossor, M., Spokes, E., Bird, E., Arregui, A., Creese, I., & Snyder, S. (1982). Increased brain dopamine and dopamine receptors in schizophrenia. *Archives of General Psychiatry, 39,* 991–997.

Malmgren, L., & Gacek, R. (1981). Histochemical characteristics of muscle fiber types in the posterior cricoarytenoid muscle. *Annals of Otology, Rhinology, and Laryngology, 90,* 423–429.

Malmgren, L., & Ringwood, M. (1988). Aging of the recurrent laryngeal nerve: An ultrastructural morphometric study. In O. Fujimura (Ed.), *Vocal physiology: Voice production, mechanisms, and functions.* New York: Raven Press.

McCarter, R. (1990). Age-related changes in skeletal muscle function. *Aging (Milano), 2,* 27–38.

McCormick, K., & Thomas, D. (1992). Exercise-induced satellite cell activation in senescent soleus muscle. *Journal of Applied Physiology, 72,* 888–893.

McGeer, P., & McGeer, E. (1978). Aging and neurotransmitter systems. In C. Finch, D. Potter, & A. Kenny (Eds.), *Parkinson's disease II. Aging and neuroendocrine relationships* (pp. 42–57). New York: Plenum.

McGeer, P., McGeer, E., & Suzuki, J. (1977). Aging and extrapyramidal function. *Archives of Neurology, 34,* 33–35.

Memo, M., Lucchi, L., Spano, P., & Trabucchi, M. (1980). Aging process affects a single class of dopamine receptors. *Brain Research, 202,* 488–492.

Mittal, K., & Logmani, F. (1987). Age-related reduction in 8th cervical ventral nerve root myelinated fiber diameters and numbers in man. *Journal of Gerontology, 42*, 8–10.

Morgan, D., & Finch, C. (1988). Dopaminergic changes in the basal ganglia: A generalized phenomenon of aging in mammals. In J. Joseph (Ed.), General determinants of age-related declines in motor function. *Annals New York Academy of Sciences. Part III. Central neuronal alterations related to motor behavioral control in normal aging: Basal ganglia, 515*, 145–159.

Mortelliti, A., Malmgren, L., & Gacek, R. (1990). Ultrastructural changes with age in the human superior laryngeal nerve. *Archives of Otolaryngology Head and Neck Surgery, 116*, 1062–1069.

Mortimer, J. (1988). Human motor behavior and aging. In J. Joseph (Ed.), General determinants of age-related declines in motor function. *Annals of the New York Academy of Sciences, 515*, 54–65.

Mortimer, J., & Webster, D. (1982). Comparison of extrapyramidal motor function in normal aging and Parkinson's disease. In J. Mortimer, F. Pirozzollo, & G. Maletto (Eds.), *The aging motor system* (pp. 217–241). New York: Praeger.

Oda, K. (1989). Age changes of motor innervation and acetylcholine receptor distribution on human skeletal muscle fibers. *Journal of the Neurological Sciences, 66*, 327–338.

Peach, R. (1987). Language functioning. In H. Mueller & V. Geoffrey (Eds.), *Communication disorders in aging: Assessment and management* (pp. 238–270). Washington, DC: Gallaudet University Press.

Perez, K., Ramig, L., Smith, M., & Dromey, C. (1996). The Parkinson larynx: Tremor and videostroboscopic findings. *Journal of Voice, 10*, 354–361.

Perie, S., St. Guily, J., Callard, P., & Sebille, A. (1997). Innervation of adult human laryngeal muscle fibers. *Journal of Neurological Sciences, 149*, 81–86.

Rademaker, A., Pauloski, B., Calangelo, L., & Logemann, J. (1998). Age and volume effects on liquid swallowing function in normal women. *Journal of Speech and Hearing Research, 41*, 275–284.

Ramig, L., Scherer, R., Titze, I., & Ringel, S. (1988). Acoustic analysis of voices of patients with neurologic disease: Rationale and preliminary data. *Annals of Otology, Rhinology, & Laryngology, 97*, 164–172.

Reiderer, P., & Wuketich, S. (1976). Time course of nigrostriatal degeneration in Parkinson's Disease. *Journal of Neural Transmission, 38*, 277–301.

Robbins, J., Hamilton, J., Lof, G., & Kempster, G. (1992). Oropharyngeal swallowing in normal adults of different ages. *Gastroenterology, 103*, 823–829.

Robinson, D., Sourkes, T., Nies, A., Harris, L., Spector, S., Bartlett, D. & Kaye, I. (1977). Monoamine metabolism in human brain. *Archives of General Psychiatry, 34*, 89–92.

Roos, M., Rice, C., & Vandervoort, A. (1997). Age-related changes in motor unit function. *Muscle and Nerve, 20*, 679–690.

Rosenberg, S., Malmgren, L., & Woo, P. (1989). Age-related changes in the internal branch of the rat superior laryngeal nerve. *Archives of Otolaryngology Head and Neck Surgery, 115*, 78–86.

Rosenheimer, T., & Smith, D. (1985). Differential changes in the end-plate architecture of functionally diverse muscles during aging. *Journal of Neurophysiology, 53*, 1567–1580.

Rothstein, J. & Rose, S. (1982). Muscle mutability: Part 2. Adaptation to drugs, metabolic factors, and aging. *Physical Therapy, 62,* 1788–1798.

Scheibel, M., & Scheibel, A. (1975). Structural changes in the aging brain. In H. Brody (Ed.), *Clinical, morphological and neurochemical aspects of the aging nervous system.* NewYork: Raven Press.

Severson, J., & Finch, C. (1980). Reduced dopaminergic binding during aging in the rodent striatum. *Brain Research, 192,* 147–162.

Sherrey, J., & Megirian, D. (1975). Analysis of the respiratory role of intrinsic laryngeal motoneurons of cat. *Experimental Neurology, 49,* 456–465.

Smith, B., Wasowicz, J., & Preston, J. (1987). Temporal characteristics of the speech of normal elderly adults. *Journal of Speech and Hearing Research, 30,* 522–529.

Sonies, B., Parent, L., Morrish, K., & Baum, B. (1988). Durational aspects of the oral-pharyngeal phase of swallow in normal adults. *Dysphagia, 3,* 1–10.

Spencer, P., & Ochoa, J. (1982). The mammalian peripheral nervous system in old age. In J. Johnson (Ed.), *Aging and cell structure* (pp. 35–57). NewYork: Plenum Press.

Spencer, P., & Schaumburg, H. (1976). Central peripheral distal axonopathy: The pathogenesis of dying-back polyneuropathies. In H. Zimmerman (Ed.), *Progress in neuropathology* (vol. 3, pp. 253–273). NewYork: Grune & Stratton.

Spiegel, J., Sataloff, R., & Selber, J. (1999). Dysphagia in the elderly. In R. Carrau & T. Murry (Eds.), *Comprehensive management of swallowing disorders* (pp. 369–375). San Diego: Singular Publishing Group.

Teig, E., Dahl, H., & Thorkelsen, H. (1978). Actomyosin ATPase activity of human laryngeal muscles. *Acta Otolaryngologica (Stockholm), 85,* 272–281.

Tomlinson, B., & Irving, D. (1977). The numbers of limb motor neurons in the human lumbosacral cord throughout life. *Journal of the Neurological Sciences, 34,* 213–219.

Vandervoort, A., & Hayes, K. (1989). Plantarflexor muscle function in young and elderly women. *European Journal of Applied Physiology & Occupational Physiology, 58,* 389–394.

Vandervoort, A., & McComas, A. (1986). Contractile changes in opposing muscles of the human ankle joint with aging. *Journal of Applied Physiology, 61,* 361–367.

Volkow, N., Logan, J., Fowler, J., Wang, G., Gur, R., Wong, C., Felder, C., Gately, S., Ding, Y., Hitzemann, R., & Pappas, N. (2000). Association between age-related decline in brain dopamine activity and impairment in frontal and cingulate metabolism. *American Journal of Psychiatry, 157,* 75–80.

Watanabe, S., & Ohnishi, A. (1979). Subperineurial space of the sural nerve in various peripheral nerve diseases. *Acta Neuropathologica (Berlin), 46,* 227–230.

Weismer, G., & Liss, J. (1991). Speech motor control and aging. In D. Ripich (Ed.), *Handbook of geriatric communication disorders* (pp. 205–225), Austin, TX: PRO-ED.

Welford, A. (1977). Motor performance. In J. Birren & K. Schaie (Eds.), *Handbook of the psychology of aging.* NewYork: Van Nostrand Reinhold.

Wilmore, J. (1991). The aging of bone and muscle. *Clinics in Sports Medicine, 10,* 231–244.

Wokke, J., Jennekens, F., Oord, C., Veldman, H., Smit, L., & Leppink, G. (1990). Morphological changes in the human end plate with age. *Journal of the Neurological Sciences, 95,* 291–310.

Xu, J., Kobayashi, S., Yamaguchi, S., Iijima, K., Okada, K., & Yamashita, K. (2000). Gender effects on age-related changes in brain structure. *American Journal of Neuroradiology, 21,* 112–118.

Zwirner, P., Murry, T., & Woodson, G. (1991). Phonatory function of neurologically impaired patients. *Journal of Communication Disorders, 24,* 287–300.

CHAPTER

6

Aging and Speech Breathing

Substantial anatomical changes occur in the respiratory system as a function of normal aging (Chapter 2). Given the subtle, complex muscular adjustments and sophisticated neurologic control required for effective speech breathing (MacLarnon & Hewitt, 1999), it is reasonable to predict that the process of speech breathing in elderly speakers is altered. Indeed, research on speech breathing has revealed significant age-related changes. Understanding those changes enables clinicians to recognize those elderly individuals displaying normal speech breathing behaviors, even if behaviors differ from those typically seen in young adults. In addition, such knowledge is critical for the clinical evaluation and treatment of elderly persons with disordered breathing. In this chapter, changes that occur normally in the process of speech breathing with aging are described. In addition, mechanisms thought to be responsible for observed age-related changes are discussed.

The first comprehensive study examining age-related changes in speech breathing was completed by Hoit and Hixon in 1987. These authors investigated speech breathing in 30 White men from three age groups (25, 50, 75 years) who met the criteria: (1) good general health, (2) good respiratory health, (3) average body type, (4) speakers of American English, (5) no history of professional acting/singing experience, (6) no evidence of speech/voice disorders, and (7) adequate hearing sensitivity. Using surface motion magnetometry and the principles of respiratory kinematics (Hixon, Goldman, & Mead, 1987), they examined aspects of general respiratory function as well as speech breathing behaviors (Rochet, 1991).

Hoit, Hixon, Altman, and Morgan (1989) expanded the work begun in 1987 by examining age-related changes in speech breathing in women. Following the same protocol utilized with men, 30 White women in three age groups (25, 50, 75 years) were studied with respect to general respiratory function and speech breathing. An additional criterion of average breast size was added to the protocol to control for mechanical loading of the rib cage. Subsequently, Sperry and Klich (1992) investigated the frequency of inhalation and air expenditure in unphonated expiration during oral reading in 9 young and 9 elderly women.

CHANGES IN GENERAL RESPIRATORY FUNCTION

Measures of general respiratory function (both static and dynamic) are included in the protocol of speech breathing studies because such measures pertain to the most basic of respiratory behaviors and are used routinely in general respiratory function testing (Hoit & Hixon, 1987; Hoit, Hixon, Altman, & Morgan, 1989; Sperry & Klich, 1992). In addition, many of the biomechanical events of speech breathing are lung volume dependent (Agostoni & Hyatt, 1986; Hixon et al., 1987). Static measurements of general respiratory function involve determination of a number of subdivisions of lung volume ((Table 6–1): total lung capacity (TLC), vital capacity (VC), inspiratory capacity (IC), functional residual capacity (FRC), expiratory reserve volume (ERV), and residual volume (RV). Additional static

Table 6–1. Static Measures of General Respiratory Function

Total lung capacity (TLC)	Total volume of air in the lungs after maximum inspiration
Vital capacity (VC)	Largest volume of air expired after maximum inspiration
Inspiratory capacity (IC)	Largest volume of air inspired from resting expiratory level (REL)
Functional residual capacity (FRC)	Volume of air in lungs and airways at REL
Expiratory reserve volume (ERV)	Largest volume of air that can be expired from REL
Residual Volume (RV)	Volume of air left in lungs and airways following maximum expiration

volume measures are calculated relative to total lung capacity to provide normative values (VC/TLC, IC/TLC, FRC/TLC, ERV/TLC, RV/TLC). Dynamic measurements of general respiratory function are made during resting tidal breathing and include tidal volume, relative tidal volume (%VC), breathing rate, minute volume, relative volume contribution of the rib cage, inhalatory flow rate, and exhalatory flow rate.

General respiratory function measures (both static and dynamic) from studies of speech breathing in the elderly compare favorably with similar measures obtained in studies of age-related differences in lung function (Chapter 2). TLC remains unchanged with advancing age in both men and women. This finding apparently relates to the balancing of alterations in active and passive forces of breathing such that TLC remains fairly constant. Similarly, IC (and IC/TLC) as well as FRC (and FRC/TLC) do not differ with aging in men or women, suggesting that the relative recoil pressures of the pulmonary system and the chest wall are unaltered with aging. Also, dynamic measurements of tidal breathing in men do not differ significantly across age groups. In addition, Hoit and Hixon (1987) observed that most men, regardless of age, were similar to normal, young adult male speakers previously studied (Hixon, Goldman, & Mead, 1973) with regard to: (1) background chest wall configuration assumed at resting expiratory level (REL) and (2) chest wall configurations assumed during tidal inspiration reflecting abdominal and rib cage contributions to intake of tidal volume.

Differences in measures of general respiratory functioning as a function of age are summarized in Table 6–2 (Hoit & Hixon, 1987; Hoit et al., 1989). Some interesting gender-related differences are evident in those findings. First, it appears that general respiratory function in women is more affected by aging than is general respiratory functioning in men. For instance, elderly women show evidence of increasing rib cage contribution to tidal breathing in comparison with young women (larger relative volume contribution), whereas men showed no such age-related effect. According to Hoit et al. (1989), variations in individual women's characteristics, such as height and body type rating, failed to explain findings of increased rib cage contribution with age. Women also demonstrated age-related changes on a larger number of static measures of general respiratory function than did men. In addition to the subdivisions of lung volume found to vary in men as a function of age (RV, VC/TLC, RV/TLC), women also showed age-related changes in ERV (and ERV/VC) and VC. At first glance, it might appear that differences in VC and ERV (measured in liters) in women with aging might be accounted for by differences in physical size between the age groups of women. However, Hoit et al. (1989) matched the three age groups of women for body type, a procedure aimed

Table 6–2. Age-Related Patterns of Change in Measures of General Respiratory Function (Subdivisions of Lung Volume and Resting Tidal Breathing) for Men and Women

Men	Women
SUBDIVISIONS OF LUNG VOLUME	
Residual Volume (RV)	
Greater in elderly than young Greater in middle-aged than young	Greater in elderly than young Greater in middle-aged than young
Expiratory Reserve Volume (ERV)	
NSD[1]	Smaller in elderly than young Smaller in elderly than middle-aged
Vital Capacity (VC)	
NSD	Smaller in elderly than young Smaller in elderly than middle-aged
Vital Capacity/Total Lung Capacity (VC/TLC)	
Smaller in elderly than young Smaller in middle-aged than young	Smaller in elderly than young Smaller in elderly than middle-aged Smaller in middle-aged than young
Expiratory Reserve Volume/Total Lung Capacity (ERV/TLC)	
NSD	Smaller in elderly than young Smaller in elderly than middle-aged
Residual Volume/Total Lung Capacity (RV/TLC)	
Larger in elderly than young Larger in middle-aged than young	Larger in elderly than young Larger in elderly than middle-aged Larger in middle-aged than young
RESTING TIDAL BREATHING	
Relative Volume Contribution (Rib Cage)	
NSD	Larger in elderly than young

[1] No significant difference

Note: Compiled from Hoit & Hixon (1987); Hoit, Hixon, Altman, & Morgan (1989).

at equalizing the variable of physical size among groups. Thus it seems unlikely that differences in physical size among the three age groups of women were responsible for the differences observed. Also, such an explanation fails to account for age-related differences in ERV/VC in women.

It appears as well that the magnitude of the decline in VC in women over their life span is greater than the decline experienced by men from young adulthood to old age (Hoit & Hixon, 1987; Hoit et al., 1989). In men, VC/TLC declined from 79.37 in young men to 67.27 in elderly men whereas those values in women declined from 78.23 in young women to 60.53 in elderly women. Similarly, RV/TLC (the counterpart of VC/TLC) increased from 20.63 in young men to 32.73 in elderly men while increasing from 21.75 in young women to 39.47 in elderly women. Although Hoit et al. (1989) acknowledged that differences in VC/TLC and RV/TLC were significant for elderly men and women, they characterized those differences as "slight," as they accounted for only approximately 6.7% TLC. However, VC is considered the most important static observation of general respiratory function in terms of its impact on speech breathing performance (Hoit & Hixon, 1987). Therefore, gender differences in VC/TLC and RV/TLC, along with differences on other measures of general respiratory function, could help to explain declines in measures of speech breathing also found in elderly women. Speech breathing findings are considered next.

CHANGES IN SPEECH BREATHING

Speech breathing changes as a function of age were assessed both from extemporaneous speech and reading in both men and women (Hoit & Hixon, 1987; Hoit et al., 1989; Sperry & Klich, 1992). The reading passages selected for testing protocols provided for expiratory breath groups of various lengths to maximize the opportunity for age-related differences to appear. Measures obtained both from reading and extemporaneous speech included those related to volume, relative volume contribution, and syllable production.

Results of speech breathing testing from extemporaneous speech and reading samples are summarized in Tables 6–3 and 6–4, respectively. In men, extemporaneous speaking appears to be more sensitive to age-related differences in speech breathing than does oral reading. Significant aging effects appear on four measures of extemporaneous speech: lung volume excursion (LVE), rib cage volume initiation referenced to relaxation rib cage volume (RCVI-R), syllables per breath group, and %VC/syllable. In comparison, only one measure produced significant aging effects from oral reading (%VC/syllable). These findings apparently reflect the fact that speakers are more free to make necessary linguistic and respiratory adjustments during extemporaneous speaking, which is a less structured speaking task (Hoit & Hixon, 1987; Rochet, 1991). Hence, adjustments that compensate for age-related limitations in respiratory, laryngeal, or articulatory functioning tend to be more apparent during

Table 6–3. Age-Related Patterns of Change in Measures of Speech Breathing for Men and Women From Extemporaneous Speaking.

Men	Women
Lung Volume Excursion (LVE)	
Larger in elderly than young	Larger in elderly than young
	Larger in middle-aged than young
Rib Cage Volume Excursion (RCVE)	
NSD[1]	NSD
Rib Cage Volume Initiation Referenced to Relaxation Rib Cage Volume (RCVI-R)	
Larger in elderly than young	Larger in elderly than young
Larger in middle-aged than young	
Lung Volume Initiation Referenced to Relaxation Lung Volume (LVI-R)	
NSD	Larger in elderly than young
	Larger in elderly than middle-aged
Syllables/Breath Group	
Fewer in elderly than young	NSD
%Vital Capacity/Syllable (%VC/Syllable)	
Greater in elderly than young	Greater in elderly than young
Frequency of Inhalation	
NT[2]	NT
Air Expenditure: Unphonated Expiration	
NT	NT

[1]No significant difference
[2]Not tested
Note: Compiled from Hoit & Hixon (1987); Hoit, Hixon, Altman, & Morgan (1989).

extemporaneous speaking. Interestingly, recent research on young women has suggested that syllables/breath group decrease and lung volume expenditures per syllable increase under conditions in which cognitive-linguistic demands during speaking are greater. These findings lend support to the notion that some aspects of speech breathing behavior are sensitive to cognitive-linguistic demands imposed by the speaking task (Mitchell, Hoit, & Watson, 1996).

Table 6–4. Age-Related Patterns of Change in Measures of Speech Breathing for Men and Women From Reading.

Men	Women
Lung Volume Excursion (LVE)	
NSD[1]	Larger in elderly than young
	Larger in middle-aged than young
Rib Cage Volume Excursion (RCVE)	
NSD	Larger in elderly than young
	Larger in middle-aged than young
Rib Cage Volume Initiation Referenced to Relaxation Rib Cage Volume (RCVI-R)	
NSD	Larger in elderly than young
Lung Volume Initiation Referenced to Relaxation Lung Volume (LVI-R)	
NSD	NSD
Syllables /Breath Group	
NSD	NSD
%Vital Capacity/Syllable (%VC/Syllable)	
Greater in elderly than young	Greater in elderly than young
Greater in middle-aged than young	Greater in elderly than middle-aged
Frequency of Inhalation	
NT[2]	Greater in elderly than young[3]
Air Expenditure: Unphonated Expiration	
NT	Greater in elderly than young

[1] No significant difference

[2] Not tested

[3] This effect was more marked in continuous passages than in isolated sentences.

Note: Compiled from Hoit & Hixon (1987); Hoit, Hixon, Altman, & Morgan (1989); Sperry & Klich (1992).

In contrast to men, women demonstrated highly similar results (Tables 6–3 and 6–4) during extemporaneous speaking and reading (Hoit et al., 1989). During both activities, elderly women differed significantly from young women on three identical measures: LVE, RCVI-R, and %VC/syllable. In addition, elderly women used larger lung volume initiations (LVI-R) during extemporaneous speech and used larger rib cage volume excursions (RCVE) during reading than did young women. If breathing during reading is more resistant to the effects of aging than breathing during extemporaneous speech (Hoit & Hixon, 1987; Rochet, 1991), then one might conclude that women experience more significant aging effects to speech breathing than do men. This conclusion is further supported by findings of a greater number of age-related changes on measures related to speech breathing in women than in men. Specifically, of the 12 speech breathing measures made on both men and women, and showing age-related changes in either group (Tables 6–3, 6–4), women demonstrated age-related differences on a total of 8 measures, whereas men showed differences on only 5. Of course, it also must be noted that the two groups show marked similarities in age-related speech breathing changes. Both groups utilize greater lung volume and rib cage volume initiations with aging and also expend greater lung volume per syllable during speech tasks. These similarities must not be trivialized.

MECHANISMS OF SPEECH BREATHING CHANGES

Hoit and Hixon (1987) concluded that a number of phenomena may have interacted to account for age-related differences they observed in men's speech breathing patterns. First, they hypothesized that elderly men might have changed their linguistic output during extemporaneous speech to accommodate their need for fewer syllables per breath group. Although Hoit and Hixon (1987) reported that elderly men did not differ from young men in the length of the sentences they produced, they believed that elderly men may have manipulated the phrasing of their utterances by reducing the average number of syllables per breath group. Of course, these authors later reported that the elderly men also demonstrated slower reading rates than did the young men (Hoit et al., 1989), which may have accounted for observed age-related reductions in syllables per breath group (Weismer & Liss, 1991).

Second, Hoit and Hixon (1987) hypothesized that elderly men were faced with inefficient laryngeal and/or upper airway valving, which would explain larger lung volume excursions and a higher %VC/syllable. Although not reaching statistical significance, the authors noted a tendency for elderly men to demonstrate higher cc/syllable values than young men, a trend that further supports the notion that inefficient valving accompanies the aging process in men. Findings of stroboscopic studies (Chapter 7) support the notion of a loss of laryngeal valving capability with aging, as elderly men demonstrate a higher incidence of glottal gaps than do young men (Bless, Biever, & Shaik, 1986; Honjo & Isshiki, 1980).

Women also show age-related increase in air expenditure per sylla-ble. Indeed, perhaps the most intriguing comparison of speech breathing changes with aging in men and women has to do with this issue. Hoit et al. (1989) initially hypothesized that findings of increased %VC/syllable in elderly women arise from the same mechanism hypothesized to explain similar findings in elderly male speakers: an age-related reduction in downstream valving economy, most likely occurring at the larynx. Such an explanation seems unlikely for women, however, given reports of increased vocal fold contact and increased time of vocal fold contact in elderly women in comparison with younger women in stroboscopic and air flow/EGG waveform studies (Biever & Bless, 1989; Higgins & Saxman, 1991; Linville, 1992) (Chapter 7). Indeed, Hoit and Hixon (1992) later con-cluded that elderly women did not evidence reduced laryngeal valving economy in comparison with young women, after finding no significant differences on measures of laryngeal airway resistance (RLAW) among women ranging in age from 25 to 85 years (Hoit & Hixon, 1992). Similarly, Holmes, Leeper, and Nicholson (1994) found no evidence of loss of laryn-geal valving economy in elderly women when RLAW was investigated in women ranging in age from 55 to 75+ under conditions in which vocal sound pressure level was controlled. Indeed, Holmes et al. (1994) reported higher laryngeal airway resistance values at each of four vocal sound pres-sure levels for women in the 75+ age group than for women in the two younger age groups, suggesting that laryngeal valving economy improves in women between middle age and old age. In addition, researchers have observed that although elderly women use a greater volume of air during speech than do young women *relative to their vital capacity,* the two groups do not differ in their exhalatory airflow rates during phonation (Sapienza & Dutka, 1996; Sperry & Klich, 1992).

If increases in %VC/syllable in elderly women cannot be explained on the basis of compromised laryngeal valving, what mechanism might explain such a finding? Hoit and Hixon (1992) reasoned that larger air expenditures in elderly women might be related to changes in other valv-ing structures upstream of the respiratory system, such as the velopharynx, tongue, or lips. If one of these structures loses valving efficiency with aging, then elderly speakers might expend greater airflow per syllable. They also speculated that the larynx in elderly women might be less agile than a youthful larynx and, hence, slower in moving in and out of the air-way during speech production. They hypothesized that such a loss of agility might result in wasted air during nonphonatory intervals. The basis for this hypothesis lies in reports of neuromuscular changes with aging (Chapter 5) including reductions in the number of motor units and an increase in average motor unit size (Cooper, 1990). Additional support for the notion of air wastage in elderly women during nonphonatory intervals

comes from Sperry and Klich (1992). These researchers observed that elderly women expend two to three times more air than do young women
during unphonated expirations immediately following inhalation, but preceding phonation. Although the precise mechanism for this finding
remains unclear (movement patterns of the larynx, variations in consonant
articulation), the speech pattern of older women appears to involve inefficient aerodynamic valving during periods of time when the vocal folds are
not vibrating. Similar studies of air wastage during unphonated intervals
during speech production have yet to be conducted on men. Additional
insight into this issue might come from a recent study of fundamental frequency (F_0) before voice offset and after voice onset in young and aged
speakers producing intervocalic voiceless obstruents (Watson, 1998).
Young speakers increased F_0 slightly during devoicing suggesting that the
process is mediated by vocal fold tensing. In contrast, aged speakers
decreased F_0 during devoicing, suggesting a greater reliance on vocal fold
abduction to achieve devoicing. Presumably, an increased incidence of
vocal fold abduction by elderly speakers during the production of voiceless
phonemes in running speech would increase air expenditure.

Finally, Hoit and Hixon (1987) hypothesized that elderly men may
anticipate the need for more air during speech production by utilizing
higher lung volume initiation levels. Higher initiation levels would be necessary to compensate for larger lung volume excursions that result from
inefficient valving upstream. Hoit and Hixon (1987) viewed the elderly men
in their study as accomplishing this inspiratory volume change primarily
with the rib cage, as opposed to the abdomen. Such a maneuver optimizes
the mechanical advantage of the rib cage for producing high airflow
(Watson & Hixon, 1985) and increases the effectiveness of the respiratory
mechanism in compensating for insufficient valving upstream. However, as
noted by Rochet (1991), higher lung volume initiation levels in elderly men
also might be related to increased closing volume in elderly speakers (see
Chapter 2). That is, elderly speakers may initiate speech at higher lung volume levels to avoid closing volume limitations. Along these lines, Sperry
and Klich (1992) concluded that higher rib cage elevation in elderly women
helped provide sufficient static recoil pressures in conjunction with respiratory muscle forces to support subglottal pressure and airflow.

Weismer and Liss (1991) view the finding of higher starting lung volumes for older speakers as counterintuitive given anatomical changes
with aging that increase the stiffness of the elderly respiratory system
(Chapter 2). They note that elderly speakers would have to work harder
even to match, let alone exceed, the lung volume utilized by younger
speakers (60% of vital capacity). In addition, older speakers might
encounter alveolar relaxation pressures even at 60% of vital capacity that
are in excess of the desired subglottal pressure for speech (Weismer &

Liss, 1991). Weismer and Liss (1991) offer an alternative explanation for findings of higher starting lung volumes in older speakers. They hypothesize that decreased elasticity of lung tissue in elderly speakers may decrease the sensitivity of lung stretch receptors and reduce the efficiency of sensory feedback for lung volume. Speakers then would utilize higher starting lung volumes during speech to augment sensory feedback, using stretch receptors in the chest wall. Proving this hypothesis, however, requires empirical testing, which has not yet been undertaken.

Sperry and Klich (1992) offered some additional information that relates to this question of higher starting lung volumes in elderly women. They observed, not surprisingly perhaps, that elderly women inhaled more deeply and more often than did young women when reading both isolated sentences and continuous passages. However, they also reported that elderly women inhaled more deeply and more often when they read passages than when they read isolated sentences. In contrast, young women did not vary the depth or frequency of their inhalations in these two contexts. The authors hypothesized that the interval of tidal breathing between isolated sentence readings allowed the elderly women to "rest" and inhale for the following isolated sentence in a relatively undemanding manner. However, if required to read continuously without breaks for tidal breathing, elderly women apparently found that the task demanded more respiratory support and hence became more taxing. Because recoil pressures occur at higher lung volumes as age increases as a result of age-related tissue changes (Gibson & Pride, 1976), older speakers may have been forced to inhale more deeply to attain requisite recoil pressures. In addition, more frequent inhalation might have been necessary to maintain high lung volumes in the face of increased air expenditure (Sperry & Klich, 1992).

It also is interesting to consider the issue of age-related changes in starting lung volumes from the perspective of laryngeal functioning. Recently, high lung volume was associated with a lower vertical larynx position (Iwarsson & Sundberg, 1998). As noted by these authors, lowering of laryngeal position has been recommended as a therapeutic strategy to counteract laryngeal hyperfunction in cases of disordered voice (Aronson, 1990). Similarly, teaching lower laryngeal position has been promoted as a mechanism to prevent laryngeal injury in singers through avoidance of overloading/overstretching of the vocalis muscle and the vocal ligament (Sonninen, 1968). Use of high lung volumes by elderly speakers, then, may have the beneficial effect of lowering vertical laryngeal position and producing more relaxed phonatory adjustments in vocal fold tissue. Of course, there is no evidence at present that elderly speakers employ higher lung volumes to improve laryngeal tension adjustments. Indeed, improved laryngeal adjustments could simply be a beneficial side effect of lung volume increases resulting from other age-related changes.

Weismer and Liss (1991) pointed out that findings of higher starting lung volumes and greater volume per syllable in elderly speakers also might be explained on the basis of age-related differences in phonatory intensity (Dromey & Ramig, 1998), a variable that has not been controlled in studies of age-related changes in speech breathing (Hoit & Hixon, 1987, Hoit et al., 1989; Sperry & Klich, 1992). Although recent research would indicate that intensity levels used by elderly and young women during both conversational speech and reading are not significantly different (Morris & Brown, 1994), there is still some controversy as to differences in phonatory intensity with aging, particularly among male speakers (Hollien, 1987). In addition, recent studies of differences in speech breathing in normal, young women suggest that considerable variability exists in lung volume levels both during spontaneous speech and reading (Winkworth, Davis, Adams, & Ellis, 1995; Winkworth, Davis, Ellis, & Adams, 1994). Further, even controlling intensity does not assure that young speakers will utilize the same lung volume strategies when a given intensity level is produced (Stathopolous & Sapienza, 1993; Winkworth & Davis, 1997). Also, controlling intensity runs the risk of introducing a variable of differential energy expenditure in young and elderly speakers, which could impact results (Russell, Cerny, & Stathopoulos, 1998).

Additional investigations examining starting lung volumes in elderly speakers under conditions in which intensity is controlled would be valuable in further elucidating mechanisms controlling lung volume levels in this population. In addition, further investigation is needed to identify the mechanism(s) responsible for observed age-related increases in air expenditures. Carefully controlled studies with elderly speakers in which simultaneous measurement is made of respiratory, laryngeal, and articulatory parameters during speaking tasks would be helpful in clarifying these issues.

TIMING OF SPEECH BREATHING CHANGES

It is of interest, also, to consider when age-related effects begin to appear in speech breathing. Both men and women show some evidence of age-related changes beginning during middle age, a finding that is consistent with reports that changes in general pulmonary functioning with aging begin to become measurable after approximately age 40 (Rochet, 1991). The pattern and extent of those changes appear to vary across gender, however. Men, for instance, begin to demonstrate increases in % VC/syllable during middle age, whereas women show no evidence of increased air expenditure until old age. This finding suggests that declines in aerodynamic valving occur at an earlier age in men, possibly reflecting differences in the mechanism of the valving difficulties.

A second gender-related difference in the onset and extent of speech breathing changes pertains to lung volumes. During middle age in men, increases in rib cage volume initiation (RCVI-R) begin. However, lung volume excursion (LVE) increases in men do not occur in middle age but only appear with advanced age. In addition, rib cage volume excursion (RCVE) remains unaffected by aging in men. In contrast, women show increases in both lung and rib cage volume excursions (LVE, RCVE) beginning during middle age. Rib cage volume initiation (RCVI-R) increases also appear, but only with advanced age in women. These findings suggest that although both men and women begin to show aging effects in terms of lung volumes during middle age, the pattern varies across gender. In addition, women may show aging effects on lung volumes during speech breathing to a greater extent than do men.

CLINICAL IMPLICATIONS: SPEECH BREATHING CHANGES

It is clear that age is a critical factor to consider in assessing speech breathing behavior in healthy adults. Clinicians should expect different speech breathing behavior from an elderly client than from a young adult client. Specifically, both elderly men and women would be expected to demonstrate larger rib cage volume initiations, larger lung volume excursions, and larger lung volume expenditures per syllable than would their young counterparts, particularly during extemporaneous speaking. Additional differences in speech breathing which might be evidenced in elderly women in comparison with young women include: (1) larger rib cage volume excursions during reading, (2) increased frequency of inhalation during reading, (3) increased air expenditure during unphonated intervals during reading, and (4) larger lung volume initiations during extemporaneous speaking. Elderly men might show reductions in the number of syllables produced per breath group in comparison with young men during extemporaneous speaking. These findings mean that clinicians need to develop new norms for speech breathing measures in adults that account for normal changes in speech breathing that occur with aging. A clinician cannot assume that an elderly client presenting with difficulties in respiratory support for speech is displaying a sign of disease. This behavior may be a manifestation of age, disease, or both.

Clinicians also should be alert to potential differences in aerodynamic valving in elderly men and elderly women and consider how these might impact on speech breathing behaviors they are observing. In elderly men, high airflow rates may be related to air wastage at the glottis during phonation resulting from glottal gaps. Similar findings in elderly women would be less likely to result from laryngeal valving deficits during phonation and more likely to result from air wastage during nonphonatory intervals or age-related articulatory variations. Intervention strategies should be directed at minimizing the effects of these deficits through differential treatment plans for elderly men and women.

There is evidence that extemporaneous speech might be more effective in revealing age-related changes in speech breathing than would a reading task. In developing formats to test speech breathing in elderly clients, clinicians would be well advised to include both a reading passage and a sample of extemporaneous speech in the protocol. Of course, in selection of reading passages attention must be paid to ensuring that sentence lengths are varied and that the context is phonetically balanced. Speech intensity also needs to be controlled during all speaking tasks.

SUMMARY

Research into speech breathing changes with aging was undertaken relatively recently and involves examination of measures related to general respiratory function (lung volumes and resting tidal breathing) along with measures obtained from extemporaneous speaking and reading. Trends in general respiratory function changes with aging revealed in speech breathing studies generally are compatible with the general literature on changes in lung function with age (Chapter 2). However, from speech breathing studies there is some suggestion that general respiratory function is more affected by aging in women than in men. Elderly women display: (1) increased rib cage contribution to tidal breathing not seen in elderly men, (2) a larger number of changes in lung volumes than elderly men, and (3) a greater magnitude of decline in vital capacity in comparison with elderly men.

Speech breathing in men has been found to involve fewer age-related changes during oral reading than during extemporaneous speaking. This finding has been interpreted as an indication that speakers are less free to make linguistic and respiratory adjustments during the more structured reading task. Therefore, adjustments that compensate for age-related limitations in respiratory, laryngeal, or articulatory functioning are most apparent during extemporaneous speaking. In contrast, women demonstrate highly similar results during the two speaking tasks, and exhibit age-related changes on a greater number of speech breathing measures than do men, suggesting that the effects of aging on speech breathing may be more marked in women than men.

A number of mechanisms may be operating to account for speech breathing changes with aging. It is possible that men change their linguistic output during extemporaneous speech to accommodate a need for fewer syllables per breath group. Of course, findings of fewer syllables per breath group in elderly men also might be accounted for simply by well-documented slowing of speech rates in the elderly.

Larger lung volume excursions and higher %VC/syllable in elderly men and women appear to arise from different mechanisms. In men, such findings may be tied to inefficient laryngeal valving resulting from glottal gaps that develop with aging. In women, inefficient laryngeal valving does not explain such findings. It has been speculated that age-related changes in valving structures such as the velopharynx, tongue, or lips might be responsible for findings of increased lung volume excursions and air expenditure in elderly women. It also has been hypothesized that laryngeal agility might lessen with aging in women resulting in slowing of the larynx as it moves in and out of the airway during speech production. Findings that elderly women expend two to three times more air than do young women during unphonated portions of expiration lend support to the notion that air wastage in elderly women may involve changes in the speed of laryngeal movements. Studies of air wastage during unphonated portions of expiration have yet to be conducted on men.

Hypotheses explaining higher lung volume initiation levels in elderly speakers include: (1) compensation for larger lung volume excursions resulting from inefficient valving upstream, (2) avoidance of closing volume limitations, or (3) reductions in efficiency of sensory feedback pertaining to lung volume. Interestingly, use of high lung volumes by elderly speakers may have a beneficial effect of lowering vertical laryngeal position and producing more relaxed phonatory adjustments in vocal fold tissue.

Findings of higher starting lung volumes and greater volume per syllable in elderly speakers also might be explained by age-related differences in phonatory intensity, a variable that has not been controlled in studies of age-related differences in speech breathing. A definitive conclusion as to the source of observed changes in lung volume excursions and air expenditure with aging awaits additional research in which phonatory intensity is controlled.

Both men and women show evidence of age-related changes in speech breathing beginning during middle age, although the pattern and extent of those changes varies across gender. In addition, it is possible that women show the effects of aging on lung volumes during speech breathing to a greater extent than do men.

REFERENCES

Agostoni, E., & Hyatt, R. (1986). Static behavior of the respiratory system. In A. Fishman, P. Macklem, J. Mead, & S. Geiger (Eds.), *Handbook of physiology: Vol. 3, section 3. The respiratory system* (pp. 113–130). Bethesda, MD: American Physiological Society.

Aronson, A. (1990). *Clinical voice disorders: An interdisciplinary approach* (3rd ed.). New York: Thieme Inc.

Biever, D., & Bless, D. (1989). Vibratory characteristics of the vocal folds in young adult and geriatric women. *Journal of Voice, 3,* 120–131.

Bless, D., Biever, D., & Shaik, A. (1986). Comparisons of vibratory characteristics of young adult males and females. In J. Hibi, M. Hirano, & D. Bless (Eds.), *Proceedings of the International Conference on Voice* (pp. 46–54). Kurume, Japan.

Cooper, D. (1990, October). *Maturation, characteristics, and aging of laryngeal muscles.* Paper presented at the Pacific Voice Conference, San Francisco.

Dromey, C., & Ramig, L. (1998). The effect of lung volume on selected phonatory and articulatory variables. *Journal of Speech, Language, and Hearing Research, 41,* 491–502.

Gibson, G., & Pride, N. (1976). Lung distensibility, the static pressure-volume curve of the lungs and its use in clinical assessment. *British Journal of Diseases of the Chest, 70,* 143–150.

Higgins, M., & Saxman, J. (1991). A comparison of selected phonatory behaviors of healthy aged and young adults. *Journal of Speech and Hearing Research, 34,* 1000–1010.

Hixon, T., Goldman, M., & Mead, J. (1973). Kinematics of the chest wall during speech production: Volume displacements of the rib cage, abdomen and lung. *Journal of Speech and Hearing Research, 16,* 78–115.

Hixon, T., Goldman, M., & Mead, J. (1987). Kinematics of the chest wall during speech production: volume displacements of the rib cage, abdomen, and lung. In T. J. Hixon & collaborators (Eds.), *Respiratory function in speech and song* (pp. 93–133). San Diego: College-Hill Press.

Hoit, J., & Hixon, T. (1987). Age and speech breathing. *Journal of Speech and Hearing Research, 30,* 351–366.

Hoit, J., & Hixon, T. (1992). Age and laryngeal airway resistance during vowel production in women. *Journal of Speech and Hearing Research, 35,* 309–313.

Hoit, J., Hixon, T., Altman, M., & Morgan, W. (1989). Speech breathing in women. *Journal of Speech and Hearing Research, 32,* 353–365.

Hollien, H. (1987). "Old voices": What do we really know about them? *Journal of Voice, 1,* 2–17.

Holmes, L., Leeper, H., & Nicholson, I. (1994). Laryngeal airway resistance of older men and women as a function of vocal sound pressure level. *Journal of Speech and Hearing Research, 37,* 789–799.

Honjo, I., & Isshiki, N. (1980). Laryngoscopic and voice characteristics of aged persons. *Archives of Otolaryngology, 106,* 149–150.

Iwarsson, J., & Sundberg, J. (1998). Effects of lung volume on vertical larynx position during phonation. *Journal of Voice, 12,* 159–165.

Linville, S. E. (1992). Glottal gap configurations in two age groups of women. *Journal of Speech and Hearing Research, 35,* 1209–1215.

MacLarnon, A., & Hewitt, G. (1999). The evolution of human speech: The role of enhanced breathing control. *American Journal of Physical Anthropology, 109,* 341–363.

Mitchell, H., Hoit, J., & Watson, P. (1996). Cognitive-linguistic demands and speech breathing. *Journal of Speech and Hearing Research, 39,* 93–104.

Morris, R., & Brown, W. (1994). Age-related differences in speech intensity among adult females. *Folia Phoniatrica et Logopaedica, 46,* 64–69.

Rochet, A. (1991). Aging and the respiratory system. In D. Ripich (Ed.), *Handbook of geriatric communication disorders* (pp. 145–163). Austin, TX: PRO-ED.

Russell, B. Cerny, F., & Stathopoulos, E. (1998). Effects of varied vocal intensity on ventilation and energy expenditure in women and men. *Journal of Speech, Language, & Hearing Research, 41,* 239–248.

Sapienza, C., & Dutka, J. (1996). Glottal airflow characteristics of women's voice production along an aging continuum. *Journal of Speech and Hearing Research, 39,* 322–328.

Sonninen, A. (1968). The external frame function in the control of pitch in the human voice. *Annals of the New York Academy of Science, 155,* 68–90.

Sperry, E., & Klich, R. (1992). Speech breathing in senescent and younger women during oral reading. *Journal of Speech and Hearing Research, 35,* 1246–1255.

Stathopoulos, E., & Sapienza, C. (1993). Respiratory and laryngeal function of women and men during vocal intensity variation. *Journal of Speech and Hearing Research, 36,* 64–75.

Watson, B. (1998). Fundamental frequency during phonetically governed devoicing in normal young and aged speakers. *Journal of the Acoustical Society of America, 103,* 3642–3647.

Watson, P., & Hixon, T. (1985). Respiratory kinematics in classical (opera) singers. *Journal of Speech and Hearing Research, 28,* 104–122.

Weismer, G., & Liss, J. (1991). Speech motor control and aging. In D. Ripich (Ed.), *Handbook of geriatric communication disorders* (pp. 205–225). Austin, TX: PRO-ED.

Winkworth, A., & Davis, P. (1997). Speech breathing and the Lombard effect. *Journal of Speech and Hearing Research, 40,* 159–169.

Winkworth, A., Davis, P., Adams, R., & Ellis, E. (1995). Breathing patterns during spontaneous speech. *Journal of Speech and Hearing Research, 38,* 124–144.

Winkworth, A., Davis, P., Ellis, E., & Adams, R. (1994). Variability and consistency in speech breathing during reading: Lung volumes, speech intensity, and linguistic factors. *Journal of Speech and Hearing Research, 37,* 535–556.

Aging and Vocal Fold Function

Age-related anatomical and physiological changes in the vocal folds (Chapter 3) can be expected to alter the functioning of this finely tuned sound generator. Atrophy of muscles and connective tissue, edema, alterations in cartilage composition, erosion of joints, declines in hydration, and disruption of nerve supply result in loss of precision of vibratory motion and incomplete glottal closure patterns. In this chapter, changes in functioning of the vocal folds in men and women with aging are described.

GLOTTAL GAP

Assessed From Visual Examination

Glottal gap refers to imperfect closure of the glottis during phonation. The configuration of various glottal gaps is illustrated in Figure 7–1. An anterior gap (a) is an opening in the glottis in the region of the anterior commissure. An anterior gap combined with a posterior opening in the region between the arytenoid cartilages (posterior chink) is an anterior-posterior

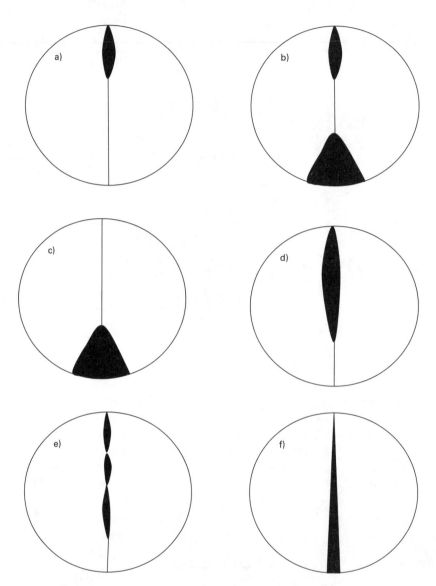

Figure 7–1. Possible glottal configurations, (a) anterior gap, (b) anterior-posterior gap, (c) posterior chink, (d) spindle, (e) irregular gap, and (f) incomplete closure.

gap (b). Posterior chink also may occur alone (c). A larger anterior gap, or spindle (d), involves incomplete closure from the anterior commissure to the vocal processes of the arytenoids. Irregular gaps (e) are identified in instances in which there are several contact points along the length of the glottis, with gaps in between. These often reflect nonlinear vocal fold edges resulting from a variety of vocal fold lesions or inflammatory conditions. Failure of the vocal folds to come into contact along the length of the glottis is incomplete closure (f).

Before considering changes in vocal fold closure that occur with aging (Linville, 1996, 2000) it is instructive to consider glottal closure in normal young adult speakers. Historically, complete glottal closure has been regarded as a characteristic of normal phonation in the young. However, considerable recent research has indicated that some forms of glottal gap also must be considered a normal laryngeal adjustment in young adults, at least under certain phonatory conditions and in certain populations. For instance, posterior chink has been observed commonly in both young and middle-aged women across phonatory conditions (Biever & Bless, 1989; Koike & Hirano, 1973; Linville, 1992; Södersten, 1994; Södersten, Hertegård, & Hammarberg, 1995; Södersten & Lindestad, 1990). In comparison, posterior chink is an unusual finding in young men, at least within the speaking pitch range (Södersten & Lindestad, 1990). The reason for this gender disparity is unclear, although it has been suggested that men may have an anatomical advantage related to the smaller angle between the vocal folds in the resting position (Sulter, Schutte, & Miller, 1996). At high pitch, both males and females demonstrate glottal gaps of varying configurations (Murry, Xu, & Woodson, 1998; Pausewang Gelfer & Bultemeyer, 1990). Similarly, an increase in glottal gaps in both sexes has been correlated with decreased loudness (Rammage, Peppard, & Bless, 1992; Södersten & Lindestad, 1990).

Presumably, atrophic changes in the vocal folds with aging (Chapter 3) increase glottal closure deficits. That is, elderly speakers experiencing such changes either would have a tendency to demonstrate glottal gaps and irregularities along the medial edge of the vocal fold for the first time, or any gaps already in existence would tend to be exacerbated (Lundy, Silva, Casiano, Lu, & Xue, 1998; Tanaka, Hirano, & Chijiwa, 1994). Weakening of the thyroarytenoid and/or alterations in the lamina propria would produce (or exacerbate) an anterior gap. Similarly, age-related weakening of the interarytenoid muscles and/or structural changes in the cricoarytenoid joint would create posterior chink or increase the size of a preexisting chink.

Glottal gap incidence figures from a number of studies of normal young and elderly speakers are plotted in Figure 7–2 (Biever & Bless, 1989; Bless, Biever, & Shaik, 1986; Honjo & Isshiki, 1980; Linville, 1992; Peppard, Bless, & Milenkovic, 1988; Södersten & Lindestad, 1990). In men, visual inspection of the larynx using either indirect laryngoscopy or videostroboscopy reveals the predicted aging pattern in terms of the incidence of glottal gap. That is, glottal gap increases in frequency with advancing age.

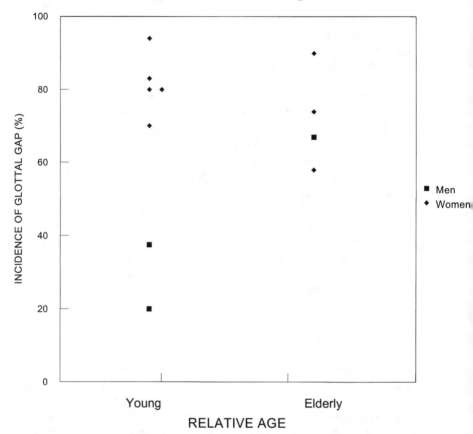

Figure 7–2. Incidence of glottal gap in men and women at different age levels. *Note:* From "The Sound of Senescence" by S. E. Linville, 1996, *Journal of Voice*, 10, p. 194. Copyright 1996 by Lippincott Raven Publishers. Reprinted with permission.

Young men demonstrate an estimated incidence of glottal gap ranging from 20% to 38%, whereas elderly men show an incidence of approximately 67%.

In women, the pattern in terms of the incidence of glottal gap with aging is more interesting. Both young and elderly women display a high incidence of glottal gap. Indeed, the overall incidence of gap in these two groups does not differ significantly. In young women, glottal gap incidence estimates range from 70% to 95% of observations while estimates in elderly women range from 58% to 90%. Young and elderly women differ, however, in the configuration of glottal gaps observed. In Figure 7–3 data are presented from a study of 10 young and 10 elderly women (Linville, 1992). Both anterior gap and spindle occur significantly more frequently in elderly women than in young women. Indeed, anterior gap and spindle configurations are rarely observed in young women. Posterior chink occurs significantly more frequently in young women, along with incomplete closure. Studies of middle-aged women also show a high incidence of posterior chink, suggesting that glottal configurations typical of young adult women carry over into middle age (Södersten et al., 1995).

It is surprising that young women display posterior chink more frequently than elderly women, given anatomical changes in the larynx with aging (Chapter 3). Age-related anatomical changes, such as erosion of the cricoarytenoid joint, muscle atrophy, and connective tissue changes, all work against closure of the posterior glottis, rather than for it. Of course, these anatomical changes in the larynx have been reported less frequently and to a lesser extent in women than men. In contrast, edema has been reported in the superficial layer of the lamina propria in elderly women, although the extent to which edema is present with aging varies considerably among individuals (Hirano, Kurita, & Nakashima, 1983; Hirano, Kurita, & Sakaguchi, 1989). Although edema facilitates closure of the posterior glottis, medical examination of videostroboscopic images showed no evidence of edema in elderly women studied by Linville (1992).

If edema does not account for the lower incidence of posterior chink in elderly women, what phenomenon explains the apparent decline in posterior chink with aging? One possibility is that young women fail to close the posterior glottis for functional reasons. Less forceful contraction of the interarytenoid muscles may be adopted by young women as an economy measure or as a means to accomplish a voice quality aim such as a slightly breathy voice. Young women have been reported to display a significantly greater degree of perceived breathiness than do young men (Södersten & Lindestad, 1990). In elderly women, then, posterior chink might be abandoned as gaps begin to appear in the anterior glottis and closure of the posterior glottis becomes necessary to achieve adequate laryngeal valving. Interestingly, there is some suggestion that the incidence of posterior chink in young women varies across cultures. In a study of Australian women (mean age 29 years) the incidence of posterior chink was only 29% (Pemberton et al., 1993). Of course, in the Australian study a flexible fiberscope, as opposed to a rigid endoscope, was used to assess glottal closure. Flexible fiberscopes have been found to reveal lesser degrees of incomplete

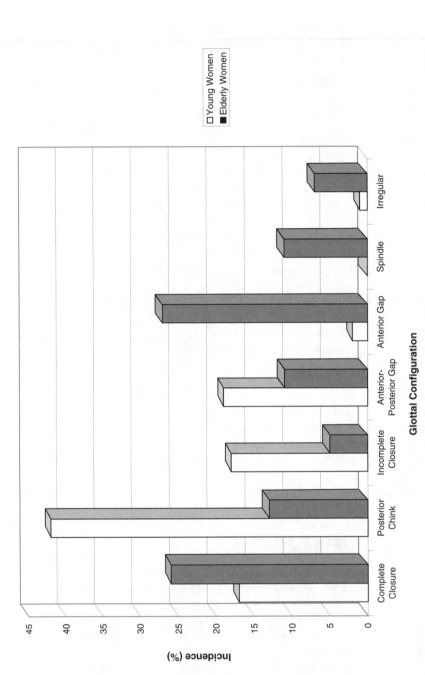

Figure 7–3. Incidence of various glottal configurations (%) in young and elderly women across nine pitch and loudness conditions. *Note:* Data are from Linville (1992). Previously published in "The Aging Voice" by S. E. Linville, in *Voice Quality Measurement*, edited by R. D. Kent & M. J. Ball, 2000, p. 368. San Diego: Singular Publishing Group. Copyright 2000 by Singular Publishing Group. Reprinted with permission.

vocal fold closure in comparison with rigid endoscopes, a factor that could have affected the incidence figures reported (Södersten & Lindestad, 1992). It is interesting, as well, that young adult women with vocal fold atrophy have been found to nearly always demonstrate complete closure of the posterior glottis (Lindestad & Hertegård, 1994). This finding lends support to a model in which posterior chink in young women is a functional adjustment that can be abandoned, if necessary.

A second possibility is that the superior view of the posterior larynx in elderly women is affected by some as yet undetected age-related alteration in the larynx supraglottally. If there are supraglottic laryngeal changes, elderly women may simply appear to achieve closure of the posterior glottis more frequently than young women. However, currently there is no anatomical data supporting such a suggestion. There is evidence, however, that a portion of the posterior glottis remains unclosed normally during vocal fold adduction in both men and women. Investigators have described a conic-shaped space in the posterior glottis that is closed supraglottally along a diagonal path running posterosuperiorly from the base of the vocal processes to the top of the arytenoid apex (Hirano, 1985; Hirano, Kurita, Kiyokawa, & Sato, 1986). In addition, it has been reported that posterior chink occurs even in young adult female professional singers (Hertegård, Gauffin, & Karlsson, 1992; Peppard et al., 1988; Södersten, 1994). If one presumes that professionally trained singers work to maximize glottal efficiency, then findings of posterior chink in young female professional singers argue against a functional adjustment, since posterior chink reduces glottal efficiency. However, that presumption may be faulty, particularly for speaking voice. There is some indication that professional singers do not necessarily apply the same standards to speaking voice applied to singing voice (Chapter 13).

Young and elderly women differ also in the extent to which variations in loudness affect the incidence of posterior chink (Figure 7–4). Although young women demonstrate posterior chink fairly frequently in all loudness conditions, elderly women have a particularly low incidence of posterior chink when phonating loudly. Elderly women may find it problematic to phonate loudly while keeping the posterior glottis open, because they have begun to experience age-related gaps more anteriorly in the glottis. In other words, the appearance of age-related anterior gaps in elderly women may necessitate closing the posterior glottis to achieve adequate loudness. In contrast, young women have the advantage of full muscular capability anteriorly and may have no difficulty achieving adequate loudness, even with the posterior glottis open. This explanation also is speculative. However, a correlation has been reported between maximum intensity of phonation and bowing of the vocal folds (Linville, Skarin, & Fornatto, 1989).

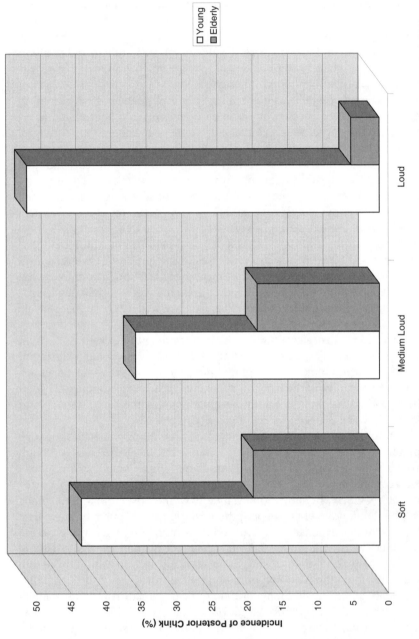

Figure 7–4. Incidence of posterior chink in young and elderly women at various loudness levels. *Note:* Data are from Linville (1992).

Inferred From Aerodynamic and Electroglottographic (EGG) Measures

It is possible to obtain an estimate of the pattern of airflow through the glottis during consecutive cycles of vocal fold vibration from inverse-filtered airflow waveforms (Rothenberg, 1973, 1977). Subsequently, airflow duty cycle can be derived from inverse-filtered airflow waveforms. Airflow duty cycle is defined as the ratio of the time above a set baseline divided by the glottal period. Similarly, EGG duty cycle, which is derived from the EGG waveform, represents the ratio of the time above a set baseline to the glottal period (Higgins & Saxman, 1991). Duty cycle measures are inversely proportional to extent and duration of vocal fold contact. That is, higher duty cycle measures indicate less vocal fold contact for a shorter period of time (Childers & Krishnamurthy, 1985; Fourcin & Abberton, 1971; Lecluse, Brocaar, & Verschuure, 1975; Rothenberg & Mahshie, 1988).

Higgins and Saxman (1991) observed interesting age-related patterns, particularly in women, when airflow duty cycle and EGG duty cycle measures were obtained for speakers of varying ages. As shown in Figure 7–5, elderly men displayed the predicted pattern of longer duty cycles than young men, indicating less complete vocal fold closure with aging. Women, however, showed the reverse pattern of slightly shorter duty cycle measures with advanced age. The pattern observed in women suggested slightly increased vocal fold contact and increased time of contact in elderly women. Although these results for women run counter to what might be predicted given age-related changes in the larynx, such a pattern is consistent with results of stroboscopic studies. Additional evidence that women do not lose laryngeal valving capability with aging comes from Sapienza and Dutka (1996) who found no differences on measures of glottal airflow among women ranging in age from 20 to 73+ years.

In summary, airflow and duty cycle studies indicate that elderly women do not display more glottal gaps than young women. Indeed, elderly women appear to close the glottis more completely than young women. Perhaps these results reflect an age-related shift in women from a larger posterior chink in young adulthood to a smaller anterior gap during geriatric years.

In considering gender differences in vocal aging, it is interesting to examine age-related changes in duty cycle measures with reference to the male-female coalescence model of aging (Chapter 1) proposed by Hollien (1987). According to the coalescence model, hormonal changes at menopause negate some of the gender differences in laryngeal behaviors that appear as a result of hormonal shifts at puberty. Hollien (1987) applied this model to age-related patterns of fundamental frequency

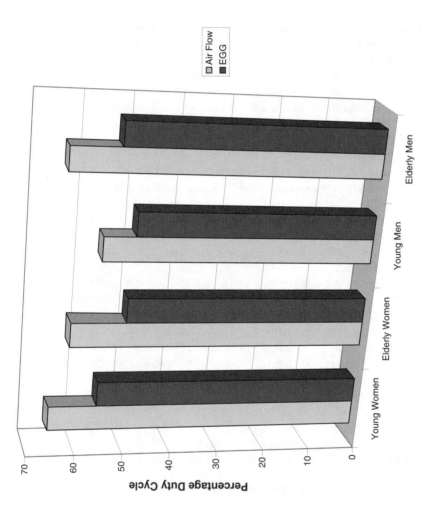

Figure 7–5. Mean air flow duty cycle and electroglottographic duty cycle measures (%) for men and women in two age groups averaged across four pitch and loudness conditions. *Note:* Data are from Higgins & Saxman (1991). Adapted from "The Aging Voice" by S. E. Linville, in *Voice Quality Measurement*, edited by R. D. Kent & M. J. Ball, 2000, p. 370. San Diego: Singular Publishing Group. Copyright 2000 by Singular Publishing Group. Reprinted with permission.

change, noting that the lowering of fundamental frequency experienced by women in midlife contrasts with a rising fundamental frequency pattern in men after middle age. The result of these divergent patterns is that men and women demonstrate greater similarity in fundamental frequency in old age than at any other time in adult life (Chapter 10). As noted by Higgins and Saxman (1991), it appears that the male-female coalescence model also fits duty cycle data related to life span changes in vocal fold contact in men and women.

VOCAL FOLD MOVEMENT PATTERNS

In addition to assessing vocal fold closure patterns, videostroboscopy is useful in making visual-perceptual judgments of symmetry, amplitude, and periodicity of vocal fold motion as well as drawing inferences about the functioning of the vocal fold cover in relation to underlying muscle tissue. Age-related differences in such measures would be predicted as a consequence of anatomic and physiologic changes in the larynx with aging. Therefore, observing and recording such differences makes sense as a strategy for examining age-related differences in vocal fold functioning.

Specific measures commonly assessed from videostroboscopy include symmetry, amplitude, and periodicity of vocal fold motion as well as mucosal wave and stiffness. Symmetry is defined as the extent to which the two vocal folds mirror each other in timing of closure and extent of lateral excursion during vibration. Periodicity refers to the apparent regularity of successive cycles of vocal fold vibration, while amplitude pertains to the extent of horizontal excursion of the vocal fold during vibration. Mucosal wave refers to the presence or absence of an observable wave emanating from the free edge of the vocal fold and moving laterally. Stiffness is observed by the presence of immobility along any part of the vocal fold during vibration (Hirano & Bless, 1993).

Using videostroboscopy, Biever and Bless (1989) assessed vocal fold movement patterns in 40 women ranging in age from 22 to 77 years. Results indicated that elderly women exhibited greater aperiodicity, reduced mucosal wave, and reduced amplitude of vibration in comparison with younger women. Findings of greater aperiodicity in vocal fold movement in elderly women support acoustic findings (Chapter 10) of higher jitter/shimmer levels and higher fundamental frequency standard deviation levels in elderly speakers (Linville & Fisher, 1985; Orlikoff, 1990). Reductions of mucosal wave in elderly women, as noted by the authors, could result from: (1) hormonally-related edema associated with menopause, or (2) drying and thinning of the mucosa related to postmenopausal endocrine changes.

Interestingly, only one elderly woman examined by Biever and Bless (1989) demonstrated increased mucosal wave. Because increased mucosal wave reflects degeneration of the connective tissue between the mucosa the underlying muscle (Hirano et al., 1983), this finding supports reports that age-related changes in the lamina propria (Chapter 3) are not particularly common in females (Kahane, 1990). Reductions of vocal fold amplitude in elderly women correlated with an observation of midmembranous glottal gaps. This correlation suggests that tissue atrophy may have affected the force and degree of vocal fold movement in elderly women. However, as the authors noted, amplitude of vocal fold motion also varies with vocal intensity and vocal intensity was controlled only informally in the study.

IMPLICATIONS OF VOCAL FOLD FUNCTION CHANGES

Glottal Gap

There is evidence that the size of a glottal gap influences measures of vocal function (Hertegård & Gauffin, 1995). Rammage et al. (1992) found a strong relationship between posterior chink size and airflow in 70 young adult women. Omori et al. (1997) reported a correlation between mean airflow rate and the extent of visible bowing in a group of 41 patients diagnosed with vocal fold atrophy. Later, Omori, Slavit, Kacker, and Blaugrund (1998) obtained measures of vocal function (pitch/amplitude perturbation, harmonics-to-noise ratio, high-frequency power ratio, mean airflow rate, AC/DC ratio, and maximum phonation time) in 42 patients with glottic incompetence dysphonia. They concluded that these measures mainly were influenced by glottal gap size as opposed to the etiology of the glottic incompetence (vocal fold paralysis, vocal fold atrophy, sulcus vocalis). Taken together, these studies suggest that an increase in the incidence and/or size of glottal closure deficits with aging would alter acoustic and aerodynamic measures of vocal function. However, the usefulness of this information in detecting the presence of normal age-related glottal gaps in the elderly may be limited. Because young adults (particularly women) frequently have glottal gaps, it could prove a challenge to distinguish purely age-related glottic incompetence using such measures.

A higher incidence of glottal gaps in elderly speakers (presumably men) in comparison with their younger counterparts also may produce perceptual voice changes, including increased breathiness. Interestingly, however, documented glottic incompetence does not always result in an increase in perceived breathiness. Omori et al. (1997) found that 39% of patients diagnosed with vocal fold atrophy had normal (nonbreathy) voice quality. Similarly, Rammage et al. (1992) reported that posterior glottal chink size did not explain perceived breathiness in a group of 70 women. Rammage et al. (1992) proposed three possible explanations for this finding: (1) differences among listeners in the perceptual definition of breathiness, (2) the interaction of several glottic and supraglottic factors that influence perceptual judgments of breathiness (Klatt & Klatt, 1990), and (3) difficulty in defining a perceptual boundary between "normal" and "abnormal" breathiness (Rammage et al., 1992).

A second perceptual voice change resulting from age-related glottal gaps is possible. If elderly speakers increase laryngeal adductory force to compensate for a closure deficit (Remacle, Lawson, & Watelet, 1999; Slavit, 1999), the resulting voice quality may be strained. Indeed, listeners have listed increased strain as a perceptual characteristic of voices judged to be old (Chapter 11). Furthermore, elderly male speakers are reported to demonstrate higher estimated subglottal pressure values than young men, a finding that may reflect vocal fold stiffening (Higgins & Saxman, 1991). In addition, Chan and Titze (1999) found that the viscoelastic shear properties of the superficial layer of the lamina propria increase with aging, particularly in males. This change is thought to reflect increased stiffness of the vocal fold mucosa (Chapter 3).

An additional consequence of vocal fold closure deficits in elderly individuals is a reduction in syllables produced per breath group due to air wastage with phonation (Till, Crumley, Jafari, & Law-Till, 1994). Both men and women decline in maximum phonation time (MPT) with aging. Hence, elderly speakers require a greater number of intrasentence breaths in comparison with young adult speakers (Hoit & Hixon, 1987; Kreul, 1972; Ptacek, Sander, Maloney, & Jackson, 1966). Age-related declines in MPT in women are difficult to explain in terms of laryngeal function, because their incidence of glottal closure deficits does not increase with aging. Therefore, the most likely contributor to declines in MPT may be altered speech breathing (Chapter 6). However, correlations have been reported between MPT and measures of vocal intensity and pitch range in elderly women (Linville, Skarin, & Fornatto, 1989), suggesting that laryngeal factors contribute in some way to age-related shortening of phonation time in this group.

Vocal Fold Movement Patterns

Findings related to vocal fold movement patterns (reduced mucosal wave/amplitude of vibration, greater aperiodicity in older women) have implications for assessment of normalcy of vocal fold functioning in elderly speakers. Clearly, a separate database on stroboscopic characteristics of elderly vocal folds is needed to avoid errors in determining normal vocal fold function in this group (Biever & Bless, 1989). Further, separate norms are needed for elderly men and women to account for gender differences. Finally, given the variability among elderly speakers across all parameters related to vocal functioning, a larger stroboscopic database on this population is necessary prior to definitively assessing the effects of aging on vocal fold vibratory characteristics.

SUMMARY

Imperfect glottal closure must be considered a normal adjustment in young adults, at least under certain phonatory conditions and in certain populations. When young, both sexes demonstrate gaps at high pitch and when phonating softly. In elderly men, vocal fold atrophy increases the overall incidence of glottal gaps. Young and elderly women do not differ in the incidence of glottal gaps although they do differ in gap configurations. Elderly women tend to have more anteriorly placed gaps, with young and middle-aged women demonstrating posterior chink.

It is unclear why younger women demonstrate posterior chink more frequently than elderly women. One possibility is that younger women fail to close the posterior glottis for functional reasons. Alternatively, the superior laryngeal view of the posterior larynx in elderly women may be altered anatomically, although such changes have yet to be detected. A third possibility is that elderly women close the posterior glottis to compensate for age-related gaps more anteriorly in the glottis. Findings of aerodynamic and EGG studies are consistent with stroboscopic findings of more complete glottal closure in elderly women in comparison with young women.

Stroboscopic studies of vocal fold movement patterns in elderly women indicate that aging results in greater aperiodicity, reductions in mucosal wave, and reduced amplitude of vibration. Reductions in mucosal wave could be related to age-related edema or mucosal drying.

It is conceivable that measures of vocal function might be used in the future to assist in the diagnosis of age-related vocal fold atrophy. However, getting to that point will prove a challenge given the frequent occurrence of glottal gaps in normal young adult persons. To further complicate the situation, documented glottic incompetence does not always result in an increase in perceived breathiness. However, perceptual indices of strain and/or measures of vocal function related to vocal fold stiffening may prove useful in detecting age-related vocal fold changes.

REFERENCES

Biever, D., & Bless, D. (1989). Vibratory characteristics of the vocal folds in young adult and geriatric women. *Journal of Voice, 3,* 120–131.

Bless, D., Biever, D., & Shaik, A. (1986). Comparisons of vibratory characteristics of young adult males and females. In J. Hibi, M. Hirano, & D. Bless (Eds.), *Proceedings of International Conference on Voice* (pp. 46–54). Kurume, Japan.

Chan, R., & Titze, I. (1999). Viscoelastic shear properties of human vocal fold mucosa: Measurement methodology and empirical results. *Journal of the Acoustical Society of America, 106,* 2008–2021.

Childers, D., & Krishnamurthy, A. (1985). A critical review of electroglottography. *Critical Review of Biomedical Engineering, 12,* 131–161.

Fourcin, A., & Abberton, E. (1971). First applications of a new laryngograph. *Medical and Biological Illustration, 21,* 172–182.

Hertegård, S., & Gauffin, J. (1995). Glottal area and vibratory patterns studied with simultaneous stroboscopy, flow glottography, and electroglottography. *Journal of Speech and Hearing Research, 38,* 85–100.

Hertegård, S., Gauffin, J., & Karlsson, I. (1992). Physiological correlates of the inverse filtered flow waveform. *Journal of Voice, 6,* 224–234.

Higgins, M., & Saxman, J. (1991). A comparison of selected phonatory behaviors of healthy aged and young adults. *Journal of Speech and Hearing Research, 34,* 1000–1010.

Hirano, M. (1985). Physiology of the posterior glottis. In E. Myers (Ed.), *New dimensions in otorhinolaryngology: Head and neck surgery 1* (pp. 379–382). New York: Excerpta Medica.

Hirano, M., & Bless, D. (1993). *Videostroboscopic examination of the larynx.* San Diego: Singular Publishing Group.

Hirano, M., Kurita, S., Kiyokawa, K., & Sato, K. (1986). Posterior glottis: A morphological study in excised human larynges. *Annals of Otology, Rhinology and Laryngology, 95,* 576–581.

Hirano, M., Kurita, S., & Nakashima, T. (1983). Growth, development and aging of the human vocal folds. In D. Bless & J. Abbs (Eds.), *Vocal fold physiology: Contemporary research and clinical issues* (pp. 22–43). San Diego: College-Hill Press.

Hirano, M., Kurita, S., & Sakaguchi, S. (1989). Aging of the vibratory tissue of human vocal folds. *Acta Otolaryngologica (Stockholm), 107,* 428–433.

Hoit, J., & Hixon, T. (1987). Age and speech breathing. *Journal of Speech and Hearing Research, 30,* 351–366.

Hollien, H. (1987). "Old voices": What do we really know about them? *Journal of Voice, 1,* 2–17.

Honjo, I., & Isshiki, N. (1980). Laryngoscopic and voice characteristics of aged persons. *Archives of Otolaryngology, 106,* 149–150.

Kahane, J. (1990). Age-related changes in the peripheral speech mechanism: Structural and physiological changes. *Proceedings of the research symposium on communicative sciences and disorders and aging. ASHA Reports, No. 19* (pp. 75–87). Rockville, MD: American Speech-Language-Hearing Association.

Klatt, D., & Klatt, L. (1990). Analysis, synthesis, and perception of voice quality variations among female and male talkers. *Journal of the Acoustical Society of America, 87,* 820–857.

Koike,Y., & Hirano, M. (1973). Glottal-area time function and subglottal-pressure variation. *Journal of the Acoustical Society of America, 54,* 1618–1627.

Kreul, E. (1972). Neuromuscular control examination (NMC) for Parkinsonism: Vocal prolongations and diadochokinetic and reading rates. *Journal of Speech and Hearing Research, 15,* 73–83.

Lecluse, F., Brocaar, M., &Verschuure, J. (1975). Electroglottography and its relation to glottal activity. *Folia Phoniatrica (Basel), 27,* 215–224.

Lindestad, P., & Hertegård, S. (1994). Spindle-shaped glottal insufficiency with and without sulcus vocalis: A retrospective study. *Annals of Otology, Rhinology, & Laryngology, 103,* 547–553.

Linville, S. E. (1992). Glottal gap configurations in two age groups of women. *Journal of Speech and Hearing Research, 35,* 1209–1215.

Linville, S. E. (1996).The sound of senescence. *Journal of Voice, 10,* 190–200.

Linville, S. E. (2000).The aging voice. In R. D. Kent & M. J. Ball (Eds.), *Voice quality measurement* (pp. 359–376). San Diego: Singular Publishing Group.

Linville, S. E., & Fisher, H. (1985). Acoustic characteristics of perceived versus actual vocal age in controlled phonation by adult females. *Journal of the Acoustical Society of America, 78,* 40–48.

Linville, S. E., Skarin, B., & Fornatto, E. (1989). The interrelationship of measures related to vocal function, speech rate, and laryngeal appearance in elderly women. *Journal of Speech and Hearing Research, 32,* 323–330.

Lundy, D., Silva, C., Casiano, R., Lu, F., & Xue, J. (1998). Causes of hoarseness in elderly patients. *Otolaryngology Head & Neck Surgery, 118,* 481–485.

Murry,T., Xu, J., & Woodson, G. (1998). Glottal configuration associated with fundamental frequency and vocal register. *Journal of Voice, 12,* 44–49.

Omori, K., Slavit, D., Kacker, A., & Blaugrund, S. (1998). Influence of size and etiology of glottal gap in glottic incompetence dysphonia. *Laryngoscope, 108,* 514–518.

Omori, K., Slavit, D., Matos, C., Kojima, H., Kacker, A., & Blaugrund, S. (1997). Vocal fold atrophy: Quantitative glottic measurement and vocal function. *Annals of Otology, Rhinology, & Laryngology, 106,* 544–551.

Orlikoff, R. (1990). The relationship of age and cardiovascular health to certain acoustic characteristics of male voices. *Journal of Speech and Hearing Research, 33,* 450–457.

Pausewang Gelfer, M., & Bultemeyer, D. (1990). Evaluation of vocal fold vibratory patterns in normal voices. *Journal of Voice, 4,* 335–345.

Pemberton, C., Russell, A., Priestley, J., Havas, T., Hooper, J., & Clark, P. (1993). Characteristics of normal larynges under flexible fiberscopic and stroboscopic examination: An Australian perspective. *Journal of Voice, 7,* 382–389.

Peppard, R., Bless, D., & Milenkovic, P. (1988). Comparison of young adult singers and nonsingers with vocal nodules. *Journal of Voice, 2,* 250–260.

Ptacek, P., Sander, E., Maloney, W., & Jackson, C. (1966). Phonatory and related changes with advanced age. *Journal of Speech and Hearing Research, 9,* 353–360.

Rammage, L., Peppard, R., & Bless, D. (1992). Aerodynamic, laryngoscopic, and perceptual-acoustic characteristics in dysphonic females with posterior glottal chinks: A retrospective study. *Journal of Voice, 6,* 64–78.

Remacle, M., Lawson, G., & Watelet, J. (1999). Carbon dioxide laser microsurgery of benign vocal fold lesions: Indications, techniques, and results in 251 patients. *Annals of Otology, Rhinology, & Laryngology, 108,* 156–164.

Rothenberg, M. (1973). A new inverse-filtering technique for deriving the glottal air flow waveform during voicing. *Journal of the Acoustical Society of America, 53,* 1632–1645.

Rothenberg, M. (1977). Measurement of airflow in speech. *Journal of Speech and Hearing Research, 20,* 155–176.

Rothenberg, M., & Mahshie, J. (1988). Monitoring and vocal fold abduction through vocal fold contact area. *Journal of Speech and Hearing Research, 31,* 338–351.

Sapienza, C., & Dutka, J. (1996). Glottal airflow characteristics of women's voice production along and aging continuum. *Journal of Speech and Hearing Research, 39,* 322–328.

Slavit, D. (1999). Phonosurgery in the elderly: A review. *Ear, Nose, & Throat Journal, 78,* 505–512.

Södersten, M. (1994). Vocal fold closure during phonation: Physiological, perceptual, and acoustic studies. *Studies in Logopedics and Phoniatrics (No. 3).* Stockholm: Department of Logopedics and Phoniatrics, Huddinge University Hospital.

Södersten, M., Hertegård, S., & Hammarberg, B. (1995). Glottal closure, transglottal airflow, and voice quality in healthy, middle-aged women. *Journal of Voice, 9,* 182–197.

Södersten, M., & Lindestad, P. (1990). Glottal closure and perceived breathiness during phonation in normally speaking subjects. *Journal of Speech and Hearing Research, 33,* 601–611.

Södersten, M., & Lindestad, P. (1992). A comparison of vocal fold closure in rigid telescopic and flexible fiberoptic laryngostroboscopy. *Acta Otolaryngologica (Stockholm), 112,* 144–150.

Sulter, A., Schutte, H., & Miller, D. (1996). Standardized videostroboscopic rating: Differences between untrained and trained male and female subjects, and effects of varying sound intensity, fundamental frequency, and age. *Journal of Voice, 10,* 175–189.

Tanaka, S., Hirano, M., & Chijiwa, K. (1994). Some aspects of vocal fold bowing. *Annals of Otology, Rhinology and Laryngology, 103,* 357–362.

Till, J., Crumley, R., Jafari, M., & Law-Till, C. (1994). Aerodynamic and temporal disruptions of speech in laryngeal insufficiency. *Archives of Otolaryngology Head & Neck Surgery, 120,* 317–325.

CHAPTER

8

Aging and Articulation

With changes in the speech production mechanism with aging, it is not surprising that elderly persons experience altered articulation. Age-related loss of neuromuscular control (Chapter 5) accompanied by anatomical changes in the structures of speech production affect oral motor precision, the speed of articulatory gestures, and alter both segmental and suprasegmental aspects of speech. Changes in articulation with aging are tied to changes in vocalization in that certain aspects of speech production (such as intonation and the devoicing gesture) are controlled by laryngeal adjustments that modify with aging. Also, age-related articulatory adjustments affect the resonance characteristics of voice (Chapter 10).

In perceptual studies, listeners have reported with some consistency that elderly speakers use less precise articulation than young adult speakers (Hartman, 1979). As early as 1974, it was suggested that elderly speakers might be considered mildly dysarthric (Ryan & Burk, 1974). More recently, perceptual ratings of normal geriatric speakers by speech-language pathologists on speech characteristics related to articulatory imprecision reveal similarities to patterns characteristic of dysarthric speakers (Amerman & Parnell, 1990; Parnell & Amerman, 1987). Also, when 40 normally aging individuals were assessed on the Frenchay Dysarthria Scale, 80% showed performance characteristics of dysarthria, particularly on the tongue and laryngeal subtests (Wallace, 1991).

Interestingly, however, there also is some suggestion that an elderly speaker's dialect may be a factor in judgments of age-related changes in articulatory precision (Benjamin, 1997). Differences in African-American English articulatory and/or suprasegmental features could explain findings in which normal elderly African-Americans were disproportionately judged as displaying articulatory imprecision, even among African-American judges (Amerman & Parnell, 1990). Benjamin felt that such variations are best considered a cultural difference as opposed to an indicator of advanced age or a speech disorder.

In this chapter changes in both segmental and suprasegmental speech parameters with aging, as currently understood, are discussed. Where appropriate, such changes are presented within the framework of specific articulators involved in production.

SEGMENTAL ARTICULATION

Because the perception of precise speech may be linked to any number of physiological gestures by many different structures in the speech mechanism, the source of perceived imprecision in elderly speech is not easily determined. However, some possible sources have been considered in the literature. A summary of the evidence supporting loss of articulatory precision in elderly males and females is presented in Table 8–1. A detailed discussion of that evidence follows.

Tongue Movement

As noted by Weismer and Liss (1991), information on age-related changes in tongue movement during speech production can be obtained using kinematics (measures of displacement, acceleration, and velocity) as well as acoustic analysis techniques. Kinematic techniques provide the most direct evaluation of lingual behavior during speech production and are especially useful in evaluating compound lingual movements (Kent, 1986). However, kinematic analysis techniques have yet to be employed in the analysis of age-related differences in lingual motion.

Acoustic measurement techniques can provide indirect information on the rate at which articulatory gestures of the tongue are completed. At faster articulatory rates, with accompanying increases in speed of articulatory changes within the vocal tract, vowel formant transitions show a faster rate of frequency change. Liss, Weismer, and Rosenbek (1990) showed that very old male speakers (87–93 years) had slower transition rates than did young adult males and younger geriatric males. These

Table 8–1. Evidence of Articulatory Imprecision in Elderly Male and Female Speakers

Acoustic Evidence		
Males	**Females**
Smaller rate of frequency change along formant transitions suggesting slower tongue movements	No Data
Evidence of longer stop closure intervals suggesting deterioration of muscle control and strength of articulators (lips, tongue)[1]	Evidence of longer stop closure intervals but declines in muscle control/strength *may* be less than in males
Noisy stop closure intervals suggesting inefficient constriction: stop consonant production (spirantization). Suggests less extensive lip and tongue movements	No Data
Shorter voiceless interval for voiceless fricatives/stops. Suggests loss of posterior cricoarytenoid effectiveness/ range of motion in cricoarytenoid joint. (Reduced maximum opening of vocal folds during devoicing)[2]	Voiceless interval unchanged suggesting that the female larynx is affected less by aging than is the male larynx
VOT findings conflicting. Some indication VOT distinction is compressed slightly in producing voiced/voiceless stops primarily due to shorter VOT values for voiceless stops.[3]	Same as male
Ultrasound Evidence	
Subtle differences in tongue movement and position during isolated phoneme production. Suggests *possible* decline in oral motor precision	Same as male

(continued on next page)

141

Table 8–1. (continued from previous page)

Acoustic Evidence	
Males	**Females**
	EMG Evidence
No Data	Reduced average peak EMG activity/increased variability (lips) suggesting decline in lip muscle activity with aging
	Higher correlation of EMG activity among sites surrounding the lips. Increased lip muscle coupling: speech production. Possibly reflects reduced flexibility of fine motor control
	Kinematic Evidence
Higher STI: reduced spatiotemporal stability (lips)[4]	Same as male

[1] Stop closure interval is the period of time between cessation of formants for the preceding vowel and the burst.

[2] Voiceless interval is the interval from the last glottal pulse preceding to the first glottal pulse following a period of voicelessness associated with either voiceless fricatives or stops (Weismer & Fromm, 1983).

[3] VOT is the time interval between the burst and the initiation of glottal pulsing for the vowel that follows.

[4] STI is the sum of standard deviations of kinematic waveforms from multiple utterance repetitions.

slower transition rates were interpreted to reflect, at least in part, slower tongue movements among very old speakers. However, as noted by Weismer and Liss (1991), these acoustic findings need confirmation by direct kinematic measures of lingual performance. Formant transition rates in elderly women have yet to be investigated.

Slowing of articulatory gestures with aging also can be evidenced acoustically in the stop closure interval accompanying production of stop consonants. The stop closure interval is the period of time between the cessation of formants for the preceding vowel and the burst. Benjamin (1982) reported longer stop closure intervals in elderly speakers (10 males, 10 females) in comparison with young adult speakers (10 males, 10 females), regardless of gender. She attributed this phenomenon to slowing of articulatory gestures accompanying closure of the vocal tract. Such a slowing might be observed as a consequence of deterioration of muscle control and strength. For stops in which vocal tract closure involves a constriction created by the tongue, such as /k/, loss of muscle control and strength specifically involves the tongue. Interestingly, however, although both males and females showed the same pattern of increasingly long closure intervals with advancing age, the magnitude of change with aging (averaged across 18 stop consonants) in males was greater (15 msec) than in females (11.1 msec), suggesting that males demonstrated greater relative deterioration of muscle function than did females. Further evidence that males show greater age-related tongue function loss than females comes from perceptual studies in which listeners perceived elderly males as showing greater articulatory imprecision overall than elderly females (Benjamin, 1986).

Conflicting data have been reported by Weismer and Fromm (1983), who observed no difference in stop closure intervals of 6 elderly men compared with young adults. These disparate findings might reflect the variability inherent in measuring the performance of elderly individuals on any number of variables (Chapter 12). That is, because elderly speakers differ widely from individual to individual in their performance on speech production variables, a larger sample of subjects might be needed to observe age-related differences. Although data on stop closure intervals suggest that elderly males experience greater declines in tongue muscle control and strength than do elderly females, definitive resolution of this issue awaits additional research involving even larger samples of elderly speakers.

There is acoustic evidence, as well, of decreases in the extent of tongue movement in elderly speakers, at least elderly men. Spirantization refers to inefficient constriction during the closure interval for stop consonant production. Such a leaky constriction is evidenced acoustically by noise during the normally silent closure interval. This time interval is associated with the ability of the speaker to interrupt the air stream by closing the vocal tract. In the case of velar/palatal stops, such closure is accomplished by the tongue. Presumably, acoustic evidence of spirantization implies less extensive tongue movements during the production of stop and fricative consonants. It has been shown that males over the age of 87 demonstrate spirantization at rates higher than young adult males and younger geriatric males. Interestingly, very old males demonstrate even higher rates of spirantization than rates observed in males with Parkinson disease (Liss et al., 1990; Weismer, 1984). Elderly women have yet to be studied for evidence of spirantization during stop consonant production.

Ultrasound technology also has been employed in an attempt to obtain preliminary information on tongue motion patterns during speech in elderly persons (Sonies & Caruso, 1990). Ultrasound technology has the advantage of having no known negative bioeffects. Sonies, Baum, and Shawker (1984) applied this technology with a small number of elderly speakers (males = 8; females = 6) and reported subtle differences in tongue movement and position during the production of isolated phonemes (/i/, /a/, /k/). Specifically, elderly speakers tended to minimize tongue retraction on /a/ in comparison with younger adults. Although the investigators noted that the elderly speakers had normal-sounding speech, the extent to which subtle, systematic differences existed in the acoustic signal of the elderly productions is unknown. In addition, the extent to which findings of differences in tongue movement/position patterns would persist in speech gestures during conversational speech is unknown. Finally, the extent to which these results would hold up on a large sample of elderly speakers awaits additional research.

Lip and Jaw Movements

As noted by Weismer and Liss (1991), lip gestures necessary for speech production are somewhat coarse and, therefore, potentially less affected by the aging process than are movements of the tongue. Nonetheless, there is acoustic evidence that very old males spirantize bilabial stops to a greater extent than do younger elderly and young adult males. This suggests that lip movements become less extensive with very advanced age, at least in male speakers (Liss et al., 1990). In addition, evidence that the closure interval for bilabial stop consonants is longer in elderly speakers than young adult speakers suggests that the speed of lip movements is negatively affected by aging (Benjamin, 1982).

Changes in lip muscle activity during speech production with aging have been examined more directly using electromyographic (EMG) data.

Average peak EMG activity in orbicularis oris superior and orbicularis oris inferior during the production of consonant-vowel tokens (p ae) by a small group (n = 3) of elderly women was found to be reduced by approximately 50% in comparison with such activity in a small group (n = 8) of young adults (gender unspecified). In addition, elderly women showed greater variability in peak EMG activity of those muscles during the rapid syllable production than did the young adults (Rastatter, McGuire, Bushong, & Loposky, 1987). However, given the small number of elderly women studied and variability in EMG activity demonstrated by those women, it is difficult to draw any conclusions as to differences in lip muscle activity with aging. Additional investigations on larger numbers of elderly speakers are needed to confirm these findings.

EMG data have been used, as well, to examine the functional relationships among the perioral muscles during speech production, as opposed to activation patterns for individual muscles. The advantage of this procedure is that information is gained on the coordination of muscles in producing speech. Because speech production requires intricate coordination of the articulators to produce an acceptable acoustic output, information on relationships among muscle activation patterns during speech production may reveal subtle effects of aging that are not evident from studies of muscles individually (Weismer & Liss, 1991). Wohlert (1996) examined correlations of EMG activity among paired sites surrounding the lips in 22 young adult and 22 elderly women during both conversational speech and reading. She found lower correlations among the lip sites during speech produced by young women in comparison with elderly women. These results imply that aging increases muscle coupling during speech production, possibly as a consequence of reduced flexibility of fine oral motor control in the elderly.

Kinematic techniques also have been applied to the evaluation of lip motion during speech production by elderly speakers. Wohlert and Smith (1998) evaluated lip movement variability during production of short phrases at three speech rates (habitual, slow, fast) using the spatiotemporal index (STI). The STI is the sum of standard deviations of kinematic waveforms across multiple repetitions of a given utterance (Smith, Goffman, Zelaznik, Ying, & McGillem, 1995). Despite completely intelligible and error-free speech in the elderly adults, their STI values at habitual rate were significantly higher (more variable) than STI values observed for young adults. These findings suggest that spatiotemporal stability of lip movement at habitual speech rate is reduced in elderly speakers. Findings of greater variability in elderly speakers' lip movements may reflect increased accommodation in the elderly mechanism to the progressive physiological changes of old age. The fact that the speech of elderly subjects was effective despite increased variability of lip motion probably reflects the limited requirements of speech for refined lip gestures and/or the subtlety of age-related changes in lip movements.

Aging changes in jaw movements during speech production have not been investigated to date. Significant anatomical changes occur in the temporomandibular joint (TMJ) with aging, along with measurable change in muscles servicing the jaw region. These changes have been shown to affect nonspeech movements of the mandible, such as biting and chewing (Chapter 4). Opinion is divided as to whether speech production is likely to be affected to a significant degree by age-changes in jaw function. Although some investigators believe that speech production is not likely to be affected to a significant degree (Kahane, 1990), others suggest that mandibular function may play a more significant role in changes in articulatory behavior in the elderly (Weismer & Liss, 1991). Resolution of this issue requires direct investigation.

Pharyngeal Adjustment

Alterations in adjustment of the pharynx during speech production affect the resonance quality of voice as well as consonant and vowel articulation. Changes in voice quality with aging are discussed at some length in Chapters 10 and 11. From the viewpoint of articulation, alterations in the cross-sectional area of the pharyngeal lumen have been shown to vary as a function of vowel height (Minifie, Hixon, Kelsey, & Woodhouse, 1970). To date, no studies have been conducted to determine if age-related changes in pharyngeal anatomy and physiology (Chapter 4) produce measurable changes in the precision of vowel articulation, although such effects are possible. It has been suggested that an ultrasound investigation of lateral pharyngeal wall movement during vowel production by young and elderly speakers, accompanied by measurement of vowel formant frequencies, would be an appropriate methodology to employ in answering this question (Weismer & Liss, 1991). Weismer and Liss (1991) also suggest conducting a study in which the duration of vocal fold vibration during the closure interval for voiced stops for young and elderly speakers is investigated. They hypothesize that muscle weakness and atrophy in the pharynx may inhibit the ability of elderly speakers to perform the rapid muscular changes necessary to expand the pharynx during voiced stop production and maintain airflow through the glottis with accompanying vibration of the vocal folds. Failure to perform the expansion maneuver rapidly could result in shorter duration of vocal fold vibration during a closure interval in elderly speakers compared with young adult speakers. Studies such as these would add considerably to current knowledge regarding the effects of aging on articulatory precision.

Laryngeal Gestures

Laryngeal gestures play a role in articulatory precision both through the laryngeal devoicing gesture (devoicing of voiceless obstruents) and through laryngealization that can be used to mark the onset of a phrase initiated by a vowel (Umeda, 1982). Weismer and Liss (1991) hypothesized that increased stiffness of laryngeal structures associated with aging, along with age-related declines in laryngeal innervation (Chapter 3), could result in loss of compression in the larynx sufficient to prevent the laryngeal gestures necessary to accomplish laryngealization. They speculated that laryngealization might be a less frequent occurrence in casual speech produced by elderly persons in comparison with young persons. A study investigating this issue could provide additional insight into potential differences in the articulatory behaviors of speakers with aging.

Examination of the laryngeal devoicing gesture during the production of voiceless obstruents in young and elderly speakers has revealed significant age-related differences. The laryngeal devoicing gesture refers to opening and closing adjustments of the vocal folds during the production of voiceless obstruents (Weismer, 1980). According to Hirose (1976), production of the laryngeal devoicing gesture involves both the posterior cricoarytenoid muscle during the opening portion of the gesture and the interarytenoid muscles during the closing portion. The voiceless interval, which is an index of the duration of the laryngeal devoicing gesture, has been defined as the interval extending from the last glottal pulse preceding, to the first glottal pulse following, a period of voicelessness associated with either voiceless fricatives or stops (Weismer & Fromm, 1983). Acoustic evidence suggests that aging compromises the fine motor coordination required to open and close the vocal folds during the production of voiceless obstruents, at least in male speakers. Elderly male speakers produce shorter voiceless intervals than do young adult males (Weismer & Fromm, 1983). A likely explanation for this finding involves loss of muscle effectiveness and reduced range of motion at the cricoarytenoid joint (Weismer & Liss, 1991). Such changes would decrease the maximum opening of the vocal folds during devoicing resulting in a shorter voiceless interval. Interestingly, elderly males also produce shorter voiceless intervals than do elderly females, with elderly females performing similarly to young adult speakers. This finding supports those of anatomical studies indicating that the male larynx shows the effects of aging more dramatically than does the female larynx (Chapter 3). Interestingly, when Shanks (1970) examined rapid repetition of a glottal fricative-vowel syllable in 120 women (20–80 years), she found no significant difference in rate of syllable repetitions. This finding provides additional articulatory evidence that female laryngeal structures are relatively unaffected by aging.

The devoicing gesture also may be accomplished by differing mechanisms in young and elderly speakers. Watson (1998) found that young speakers show a small increase in fundamental frequency (F_0) during devoicing of an intervocalic voiceless obstruent (10 cycles before voice offset and after voice onset), whereas aged speakers showed a decrease. This difference was interpreted as evidence that the aged larynx may limit the role of increased vocal fold stiffness in the devoicing gesture, whereas the younger larynx allows for such a mechanism. Elderly speakers, therefore, may rely more on vocal fold abduction to accomplish devoicing.

Laryngeal gestures are important, as well, in the fine motor coordination necessary to maintain adjustments of the articulatory and laryngeal systems represented by voice onset time (VOT). VOT is the time interval between the release of the oral constriction for production of a plosive and the initiation of glottal pulsing for the vowel that follows. Given changes in the neural system as well as the respiratory, phonatory, and articulatory structures with aging, several investigators have hypothesized that VOT would be altered in elderly speakers and have conducted studies aimed at uncovering such changes. Results of studies on VOT and aging have yielded conflicting results. Some investigators have reported shorter VOT measures for elderly speakers in comparison with young speakers (Benjamin, 1982; Liss et al., 1990). Others, however, report that VOT does not differ across age groups (Petrosino, Colcord, Kurcz, & Yonker, 1993; Smith, Wasowicz, & Preston, 1987; Sweeting & Baken, 1982) or differs only in certain phonetic contexts (Neiman, Klich, & Shuey, 1983; Decoster & Debruyne, 1997).

As noted by Weismer and Fromm (1983), differences in VOT in young adult and elderly speakers appear to be subtle. Indeed, Sweeting and Baken (1982) concluded that although mean VOT does not differ across age groups, variability increases with aging both within and between groups. Further, when minimal separation of VOTs for individual subjects is examined (difference between longest VOT for /b/ and shortest for /p/), the average of these minimal separations diminishes with advanced age, regardless of speaker gender (Sweeting & Baken, 1982). Compression of VOT distinctions in elderly speakers is evidenced primarily as shortening of VOT values for voiceless stops. Interpreting findings of compressed VOT values in elderly speakers accurately is facilitated if VOT is considered along with information on voiceless interval duration and stop closure duration (Weismer & Fromm, 1983). In elderly females, shorter VOT values for voiceless stops are accompanied by longer stop closure intervals (Benjamin, 1982) and unchanged voiceless intervals (Weismer & Fromm, 1983). It appears, therefore, that the timing of supraglottic/glottic events in voiceless stops produced by elderly women is affected primarily by deterioration of muscle control and strength in supraglottic articulators (lips, tongue), as opposed to aging of laryngeal tissues. In elderly males, however, shorter VOT values are accompanied by shorter voiceless intervals as well as reports of longer stop closure intervals. Although elderly men appear to demonstrate deterioration of muscle control and strength in supraglottic articulators, those changes with aging may be less significant in the production of voiceless stops than are age-related laryngeal changes. Of course, this interpretation must be considered speculative given conflicting findings regarding VOT changes with aging, as well as reports of markedly high variability in VOT measures for elderly speakers. A definitive conclusion as to aging effects on VOT awaits a carefully controlled study on a large number of elderly speakers in which physiological variables are directly assessed in conjunction with VOT.

Phoneme Duration

Several studies have resulted in findings of vowel and consonant durations that are longer in elderly speakers than those observed in young speakers (Amerman & Parnell, 1992; Benjamin, 1982; Forrest, Weismer, & Turner, 1989; Morris & Brown, 1987, 1994; Smith et al., 1987). Segment durations in elderly speakers have been reported to be 20%-25% longer at both normal and fast speaking rates (Smith et al., 1987). In addition, vowel and consonant durations produced by elderly speakers tend to be proportionately longer than those produced by young adult speakers when placed in stressed contexts (Benjamin, 1982; Morris & Brown, 1987). Elderly speakers show some flexibility in segment durations, however. For example, when faced with a speaking situation requiring longer utterances, elderly speakers frequently will reduce phoneme segment durations to maintain the physiological support necessary to produce the utterances successfully (Amerman & Parnell, 1992). Hence, elderly speakers appear to be sensitive to age-related declines in their abilities (Benjamin, 1997).

Investigators have speculated that segment duration increases in elderly speakers could be related to findings of decreases in nerve conduction velocities in regions of the body unrelated to speech production. Nerve supply in the forearm, for example, has been reported to decline in conduction velocity by approximately 16% (Kenney, 1982). Smith and his associates (1987) hypothesized that similar declines in conduction velocity in nerves servicing the speech production mechanism might explain longer segment durations in elderly speakers. It has been noted, however, that there is no evidence that nerve conduction velocities are correlated with articulatory behavior (Weismer & Liss, 1991). Resolution of this question awaits a study in which conduction velocities and speech timing are measured and compared across age groups (Weismer & Liss, 1991).

It has been hypothesized, as well, that longer segment durations in elderly speakers might involve age-related changes in central neurotransmitters that result in slowing of all sensorimotor processes (Weismer & Liss, 1991). Evidence supporting this hypothesis includes findings of progressive degeneration of the dopaminergic system with advanced age (Morgan & Finch, 1988), as well as behavioral findings that appear to be consistent with such deterioration (McNeill, Koek, Brown, & Rafols, 1988; Mortimer, 1988). Similarities between normal aging and Parkinson disease (Chapter 5) have been pointed out by several investigators (Liss et al., 1990; Mortimer, 1988; Weismer & Liss, 1991).

Syllable Repetition (Oral Diadochokinesis)

Some investigators have examined articulatory functioning with aging through measurement of oral diadochokinesis (Amerman & Parnell, 1982; Ptacek, Sander, Maloney, & Jackson, 1966). That is, investigators have measured the maximum speed of alternating articulatory movements involving the lips, tongue, and jaw (oral consonant + vowel syllables). Although acceptably rapid and precise movements reflect intact neuromotor functioning, excessively slow or irregular performance would suggest deterioration of neuromotor functioning (Darley, Aronson, & Brown, 1975). When maximum speed of alternating articulatory movements have been compared in elderly speakers and young adult speakers, older adults produce fewer syllables in a specified time, indicating some decline in neuromotor functioning with aging. In addition, both the amplitude and duration of such productions by elderly speakers are more variable than productions by young speakers. Increased variability in the duration of individual syllables during sequences produced by elderly speakers is an indication of reduced motor precision with age. Increased variability in the amplitude of adjacent syllables suggests age-related reductions in biomechanical competency related to controlling air pressure/flow during rapid, repetitive speech movements. Of course, the extent to which such deficits translate into similar findings during conversational speech production can only be determined with additional research in which conversational utterances are directly examined.

SUPRASEGMENTAL ARTICULATION

Just as aging of structures of the speech mechanism may affect the precision of segmental articulation, aging also may affect changes in suprasegmental aspects of speech production. In addition, elderly speakers might alter suprasegmental aspects of speech production functionally in association with a"sociolect of age"that involves a learned pattern of speech production consistent with societal expectations for elderly speakers (Ramig, 1986). Although the existence of an elderly speech pattern arising from dialectical adjustments remains speculative, evidence of age-related changes in suprasegmental parameters of speech might support such a notion. In addition, such findings might help explain reports from listeners that elderly speakers (at least male speakers) read with"more authority" than do younger male speakers (Ryan & Capadano, 1978).

Intonation

Benjamin (1986) investigated intonational variation in male and female speakers who were young (approximately 29 years) and elderly (approximately 74 years) during a reading task. Specifically, maximum inflections (semitones) and number of inflections were compared. Elderly speakers, regardless of gender, used a greater number of inflections and demonstrated a wider range of semitones in their inflections than did young adult speakers. Noting that listeners did not perceive excessive pitch variability in passages read by elderly speakers, Benjamin concluded that social factors, as opposed to physiological changes with aging, may have accounted for the findings. Indeed, listeners commented on the"dramatic style" employed by some elderly speakers. Also, some elderly speakers commented that they had been taught as children to"read with feeling,"a factor that could have accounted for observed age-related differences.

Age-related differences in intonation also have been investigated on a limited basis in French (Ryalls, Le Dorze, Lever, Ouellet, & Larfeuil, 1994). These authors asked middle-aged (m = 52 years) and older (m = 67 years) speakers to read a list of statements and questions and calculated the difference in F_0 between the final syllable productions of the two utterance types. Although no significant age-related differences were found, it is difficult to draw conclusions from this study, given the fairly restricted age range studied and the limited nature of the intonational measurements that were calculated.

There are suggestions, as well, that elderly speakers are more variable in their intonational patterns than are young adult speakers, particularly if speech rate is varied. In a study involving only a very small number of speakers, Weismer and Fromm (1983) reported little or no influence of fast speaking rate on F_0 contours in two young adult speakers. In contrast, one elderly speaker showed much greater contour variability at a faster speaking rate. The second elderly speaker demonstrated markedly variable F_0 contours even at conversational speaking rates making it impossible to judge the effect of increased speaking rate. If findings of increased variability in F_0 contours at fast speaking rates could be replicated on a larger number of subjects, it might be possible to draw inferences as to the role of speaking rate as a performance stress variable to elderly speakers.

Stress

Contrastive stress is the level of prominence of a syllable or word within an utterance. A limited number of studies have examined age-related differences in this aspect of speech production. Scukanec, Petrosino, and Colcord (1996) reported that elderly women consistently produced a greater extent of F_0 change than did young women when producing stressed words in statements read aloud. Elderly women also were more variable in F_0 when producing stressed words than young women. In contrast, although both age groups also increased intensity and lengthened duration during stressed words, young and elderly women did not differ significantly in the relative intensity of durational change observed during this task.

These findings for contrastive stress are similar to those of Benjamin (1986) for intonation reported in the previous section. That is, elderly speakers used a wider F_0 range during connected speech than did young speakers. Elderly speakers may mark stress more heavily than do young speakers, either because of functional alterations in their use of the speaking mechanism (age-related differences in speech style) or because of age-related changes in the mechanism that result in declines in phonatory control/compensatory adjustments by elderly speakers.

Interestingly, Wingfield, Lahar, and Stine (1989) concluded that elderly adults derive greater benefit from prosody in terms of speech recall than do younger adults. They hypothesized that use of exaggerated intonation and stress by young speakers when talking to elderly listeners ("elderspeak"; Cohen & Faulkner, 1986) facilitates communication. Others, however, have cautioned that "elderspeak" may amount to overaccommodation and, as such, could be viewed as patronizing (Wingfield et al., 1989). More recently, Kemper and Harden (1999) concluded that providing semantic elaborations and reducing the use of subordinate and embedded clauses when talking to the elderly facilitated communication, whereas simply reducing sentence length, using high pitch, and slowing speech rate did not. In any case, elderly speakers' use of more marked changes in F_0 when producing suprasegmental parameters of speech parallels reported age-related changes in perception. That is, although contradictory evidence has been reported, elderly speakers may produce those contrasts in their own speech that facilitate maximum recall of speech if they are the listener.

SUMMARY

Evidence of articulatory imprecision in the speech of elderly adults has been gathered from several sources. Although acoustic evidence supports loss of articulatory precision in both males and females with aging, males appear to show more dramatic declines, particularly in measures reflecting laryngeal functioning (voiceless interval). Both aging males and females show acoustic evidence of deterioration in muscle control and strength in the lips and tongue, although there is some suggestion that such deterioration may be more marked in males.

Ultrasound evidence is scarce, although limited data that are available suggest that elderly speakers of both genders experience declines in oral motor precision. EMG and kinematic studies involving the lips have suggested that lip muscle activity declines with aging and is accompanied by reductions in flexibility of fine motor control and spatiotemporal instability.

Although longer phoneme durations have been observed in both men and women with aging, elderly speakers also demonstrate flexibility in phoneme durations when attempting to maintain physiological support and successfully produce an utterance. Longer segment durations in elderly speakers have been speculated to result from: (1) decreases in nerve conduction velocity, or (2) changes in central neurotransmitters. Elderly speakers have also been reported to experience declines in maximum speed of alternating articulatory movements (oral diadochokinesis), as well as increased variability in these movements.

Suprasegmental parameters also change with aging. Specifically, elderly speakers demonstrate a wider range of semitones in their inflections, as well as a greater number of inflections in comparison with young speakers. The extent to which these differences stem from physiological changes in the mechanism with aging as opposed to social factors is open to some question. Findings with regard to age-related changes in contrastive stress are similar to those for intonation. Namely, elderly speakers, at least elderly women, appear to use a wider F_0 range when producing stressed words than do young women. Of course, elderly women also appear to be more variable in F_0 on stressed words than are their younger counterparts. It is interesting that elderly speakers' production of more marked changes in F_0 in suprasegmental parameters of speech reportedly parallels age-related changes in perception, although opinion on this issue is divided. That is, there is some suggestion that elderly speakers produce contrasts in their own speech (wider F_0 range) that also may facilitate maximum recall of speech, if they function as the listener.

REFERENCES

Amerman, J., & Parnell, M. (1982). Oral motor precision in older adults. *Journal of the National Student Speech Language Hearing Association, 10,* 55–66.

Amerman, J., & Parnell, M. (1990). Auditory impressions of the speech of normal elderly adults. *British Journal of Communication Disorders, 25,* 35–43.

Amerman, J., & Parnell, M. (1992). Speech timing strategies in elderly adults. *Journal of Phonetics, 20,* 65–76.

Benjamin, B. (1982). Phonological performance in gerontological speech, *Journal of Psycholinguistic Research, 11,* 159–167.

Benjamin, B. (1986). Dimensions of the older female voice. *Language and Communication, 6,* 35–45.

Benjamin, B. (1997). Speech production of normally aging adults. *Seminars in Speech and Language, 18,* 135–141.

Cohen, G., & Faulkner, D. (1986). Does 'elderspeak' work? The effect of intonation and stress on comprehension and recall of spoken discourse in old age. *Language and Communication, 6,* 91–98.

Darley, F., Aronson, A., & Brown, J. (1975). *Motor speech disorders.* Philadelphia: W. B. Saunders.

Decoster, W., & Debruyne, F. (1997). Changes in spectral measures and voice-onset time with age: A cross-sectional and a longitudinal study. *Folia Phoniatrica et Logopaedica, 49,* 269–280.

Forrest, K., Weismer, G., & Turner, G. (1989). Kinematic, acoustic, and perceptual analyses of connected speech produced by Parkinsonian and normal geriatric patients. *Journal of the Acoustical Society of America, 85,* 2608–2622.

Hartman, D. (1979). The perceptual identity and characteristics of aging in normal male adult speakers. *Journal of Communication Disorders, 12,* 53–61.

Hirose, H. (1976). Posterior cricoarytenoid as a speech muscle. *Annals of Otology, Rhinology, and Laryngology, 85,* 335–342.

Kahane, J. (1990). Age-related changes in the peripheral speech mechanism. Structural and physiological changes. In E. Cherow (Ed.), *Proceedings of the research symposium on communication sciences and disorders and aging* (pp. 75–87). *ASHA Reports, No. 19.* Rockville, MD: American Speech-Language-Hearing Association.

Kemper, S., & Harden, T. (1999). Experimentally disentangling what's beneficial about elderspeak from what's not. *Psychology & Aging, 14,* 656–670.

Kenney, R. (1982). *Physiology of aging: A synopsis.* Chicago: Year Book Medical Publishers.

Kent, R. (1986). The iceberg hypothesis: The temporal assembly of speech movements. In J. Perkell & D. Klatt (Eds.), *Invariance and variability in speech processes* (pp. 234–242). Hillsdale, NJ: Lawrence Erlbaum.

Liss, J., Weismer, G., & Rosenbek, J. (1990). Selected acoustic characteristics of speech production in very old males. *Journal of Gerontology Psychological Sciences, 45,* P35–P45.

McNeill, T., Koek, L., Brown, S., & Rafols, J. (1988). Age-related changes in the nigrostriatal system. In J. Joseph (Ed.), General determinants of age-related declines in motor function. *Annals of the New York Academy of Sciences, 515,* 239–248.

Minifie, F., Hixon, T., Kelsey, C., & Woodhouse, R. (1970). Lateral pharyngeal wall movement during speech production. *Journal of Speech and Hearing Research, 13,* 584–595.

Morgan, D., & Finch, C. (1988). Dopaminergic changes in the basal ganglia: A generalized phenomenon of aging in mammals. In J. Joseph (Ed.), General determinants of age-related declines in motor function. *Annals New York Academy of Sciences. Part III. Central neuronal alterations related to motor behavioral control in normal aging: Basal ganglia, 515,* 145–159.

Morris, R., & Brown, W. (1987). Age-related voice measures among adult women. *Journal of Voice, 1,* 38-43.

Morris, R., & Brown, W. (1994). Age-related differences in speech variability among women. *Journal of Communication Disorders, 27,* 49–64.

Mortimer, J. (1988). Human motor behavior and aging. In J. Joseph (Ed.), General determinants of age-related declines in motor function. *Annals of the New York Academy of Sciences, 515,* 54–65.

Neiman, G., Klich, R., & Shuey, E. (1983). Voice onset time in young and 70-year-old women. *Journal of Speech and Hearing Research, 26,* 118–123.

Parnell, M., & Amerman, J. (1987). Perception of oral diadochokinetic performances in elderly adults. *Journal of Communication Disorders, 20,* 339–351.

Petrosino, L., Colcord, R., Kurcz, K., & Yonker, R. (1993). Voice onset time of velar stop productions in aged speakers. *Perceptual and Motor Skills, 76,* 83–88.

Ptacek, P., Sander, E., Maloney, W., & Jackson, C. (1966). Phonatory and related changes with advanced age. *Journal of Speech and Hearing Research, 9,* 353–360.

Ramig, L. (1986). Aging speech: Physiological and sociological aspects. *Language and Communication, 6,* 25–34.

Rastatter, M., McGuire, R., Bushong, L., & Loposky, M. (1987). Speech-motor equivalence in aging subjects. *Perceptual and Motor Skills, 64,* 635–638.

Ryalls, J., Le Dorze, G., Lever, N., Ouellet, L., & Larfeuil, C. (1994). The effects of age and sex on speech intonation and duration for matched statements and questions in French. *Journal of the Acoustical Society of America, 95,* 2274–2276.

Ryan, E., & Capadano, H. (1978). Age perceptions and evaluative reactions toward adult speakers. *Journal of Gerontology, 33,* 98–102.

Ryan, W., & Burk, K. (1974). Perceptual and acoustic correlates of aging in the speech of males. *Journal of Communication Disorders, 7,* 181–192.

Scukanec, G., Petrosino, L., & Colcord, R. (1996). Age-related differences in acoustical aspects of contrastive stress in women. *Folia Phoniatrica et Logopaedica, 48,* 231–239.

Shanks, S. (1970). Effect of aging upon rapid syllable repetition. *Perceptual and Motor Skills, 30,* 687–690.

Smith, A., Goffman, L., Zelaznik, H., Ying, G., & McGillem, C. (1995). Spatiotemporal stability and patterning of speech movement sequences. *Experimental Brain Research, 104,* 493–501.

Smith, B., Wasowicz, J., & Preston, J. (1987). Temporal characteristics of the speech of normal elderly adults. *Journal of Speech and Hearing Research, 30,* 522–529.

Sonies, B., Baum, B., & Shawker, T. (1984). Tongue motion in elderly adults: Initial in situ observations. *Journal of Gerontology, 39,* 279–283.

Sonies, B., & Caruso, A. (1990). The aging process and its potential impact on measures of oral sensorimotor function. In E. Cherow (Ed.), *Proceedings of the research symposium on communication sciences and disorders and aging, ASHA Reports, No. 19* (pp. 114–124). Rockville, MD: American Speech-Language-Hearing Association.

Sweeting, P., & Baken, R. (1982). Voice onset time in a normal-aged population. *Journal of Speech and Hearing Research, 25,* 129–134.

Umeda, N. (1982). Boundary: Perceptual and acoustic properties and syntactic and statistical determinants. In N. Lass (Ed.), *Speech and language: Advances in basic research and practice* (Vol. 7, pp. 333–371). New York: Academic Press.

Wallace, G. (1991). Assessment of oral peripheral structure and function in normal aging individuals with the Frenchay. *Journal of Communication Disorders, 24,* 101–109.

Watson, B. (1998). Fundamental frequency during phonetically governed devoicing in normal young and aged speakers. *Journal of the Acoustical Society of America, 103,* 3642–3647.

Weismer, G. (1980). Control of the voicing distinction for intervocalic stops and fricatives: Some data and theoretical considerations. *Journal of Phonetics, 8,* 417–428.

Weismer, G. (1984). Articulatory characteristics of Parkinsonian dysarthria: Segmental and phrase-level timing, spirantization, and glottal-supraglottal coordination. In M. McNeil, J. Rosenbek, & A. Aronson (Eds.), *The dysarthrias* (pp. 101–130). San Diego: College-Hill Press.

Weismer, G., & Fromm, D. (1983). Acoustic analysis of geriatric utterances. In D. Bless and J. Abbs (Eds.), *Vocal fold physiology: Contemporary research and clinical issues* (pp. 317–332). San Diego CA: College-Hill Press.

Weismer, G., & Liss, J. (1991). Speech motor control and aging. In D. Ripich (Ed.), *Handbook of geriatric communication disorders* (pp. 205–225). Austin, TX: PRO-ED.

Wingfield, A., Lahar, C., & Stine, E. (1989). Age and decision strategies in running memory for speech: Effects of prosody and linguistic structure. *Journal of Gerontology Psychological Sciences, 44,* P106–P113.

Wohlert, A. (1996). Perioral muscle activity in young and older adults during speech and nonspeech tasks. *Journal of Speech and Hearing Research, 39,* 761–770.

Wohlert, A., & Smith, A. (1998). Spatiotemporal stability of lip movements in older adult speakers. *Journal of Speech, Language, and Hearing Research, 41,* 41–50.

9

Aging and Speaking Rate

In Chapter 8, a number of temporal variations at the segmental level were discussed that appear to distinguish the speech of young adults and elderly speakers. A question remains, however, as to the influence of temporal variation in elderly speech patterns on overall speaking rate. As noted by Benjamin (1988), subtle differences in articulatory timing may be a factor in listeners' perceptions of imprecise articulation as a characteristic of elderly speech (Chapter 11). In terms of laryngeal function, alterations in speaking rate with aging can be linked to pause time. If elderly speakers are forced to pause more frequently to inhale because of inadequate laryngeal valving (Chapter 7), or respiratory limitations (Chapter 6), speech rate will slow.

In this chapter substantial evidence is reviewed indicating that speaking rate in elderly persons is slower than younger adults. Potential explanations for slowing of speech are explored, along with evidence tying speaking rate to speech recall in elderly individuals. In addition, research concerning dysfluent speech behavior in elderly persons is discussed.

SLOWING OF SPEECH RATE

Numerous studies have demonstrated that elderly persons speak at a slower rate than do younger adults (Amerman & Parnell, 1992; Brown, Morris, & Michel, 1989; Duchin & Mysak, 1987; Hartmann & Danhauer,

1976; Mysak, 1959; Mysak & Hanley, 1959; Oyer & Deal, 1985; Ramig, 1983; Ryan, 1972; Shipp, Qi, Huntley, & Hollien, 1992; Smith, Wasowicz, & Preston, 1987). Slower rates have been reported in elderly speakers in comparison with young adult speakers during both oral reading and spontaneous speech, although the two groups do not differ in the relative rate of speech used under various speaking conditions. That is, both young adult and elderly speakers use slower speaking rates when cognitive processing demands increase, such as during picture description, in comparison to more automatic speaking tasks, such as oral reading (Duchin & Mysak, 1987).

Elderly speakers are 20%–25% slower than young adults when speaking at their normal speaking rate. In addition, elderly speakers are 55% more variable than young speakers when allowed to speak at their habitual rate. Interestingly, evidence suggests that elderly speakers are capable of increasing their speech rate so that they are speaking as rapidly as young adults talking at their normal rate. However, elderly speakers typically do not utilize such a rapid rate. When both groups are asked to talk rapidly, elderly speakers are unable to match the rate used by young speakers; they are 20%–25% slower (Benjamin, 1997).

It is interesting, as well, that older adults consistently produce longer durations in their speech than young adults, both at typical and fast speaking rates (Chapter 8). This finding holds true for sentence durations, syllable durations, and consonant/vowel durations (Smith et al., 1987). Also, elderly men pause more frequently to breathe than do young men (Shipp et al., 1992), and elderly men in poor physiological condition use more pause time during connected speech than do their counterparts in good condition (Ramig, 1986). Further, elderly speakers are not as effective as are young adult speakers at reducing pause length to further increase speaking rate when speaking at fast rates (Benjamin, 1987).

The bulk of studies examining speaking rate have focused on male speakers. Although some studies have reported that women also demonstrate slowing of speech rate with aging (Brown et al., 1989; Oyer & Deal, 1985; Smith et al., 1987), findings of similar speaking rates in young and elderly women also have been reported (Hoit, Hixon, Altman, & Morgan, 1989). It is possible that women demonstrate slowing of speech rate with aging to a lesser extent than do men. Findings of differences in aging effects in women compared to men certainly are not unprecedented. Indeed, gender disparity has been reported for a number of aging biological systems including the larynx and the respiratory system. In general, the disparity appears to be in the direction of relative preservation of function in females with aging (Chapter 12).

WHY SPEECH RATE SLOWS

Slowing of speech rate in the elderly is not unexpected if one considers the general slowing of performance that occurs with aging. Slowing of performance has been characterized as one of the most widespread changes in old age, affecting both motor output and sensory input, as well as higher level cognitive processes (Birren, Woods, & Williams, 1980; Salthouse, 1993a, 1993b, 1994). There is evidence of age-related declines both in sensory-motor speed (the speed with which an individual registers a stimuli and produces simple responses) and perceptual-cognitive speed (the speed with which a person can perform basic cognitive tasks). Relatively little is known about the source of the relationship between age and speed, although recent reports suggest that overall health status, at least among relatively healthy elderly adults, is only related to a minor degree with declining speed (Earles & Salthouse, 1995).

Although several hypotheses have been put forth to explain speech rate slowing in elderly speakers (Table 9–1), the phenomenon is perhaps most commonly attributed to alterations in the nervous system with aging. Specifically, generalized neuromuscular slowing associated with advanced chronological age often is mentioned as a potential cause (Ramig, 1983; Smith et al., 1987). It is hypothesized that the well-documented slowing of nerve conduction velocities in the elderly (Chapter 5) slows phonemic rates (Smith et al., 1987) and disrupts coordination among the articulators (Weismer & Liss, 1991). In addition, alterations in nerve supply in the elderly could be the reason for respiratory limitations observed in this population. As noted by Weismer and Liss (1991), disordered nerve supply affects muscle metabolic activity and results in stiffer, more fibrotic muscles. Increased stiffness in respiratory musculature would increase muscle resistance and ultimately slow the breathing process in elderly speakers (Chapter 6) and increase pause time during speech production.

Table 9–1. Possible Explanations for Speech Rate Slowing in the Elderly

Nervous System Aging
  Neuromuscular Slowing
  Altered Nerve Supply
Increased Cautiousness
Compensatory Adjustment to Maintain/Enhance Fluency
Declines in Speed of Information Processing

A second hypothesis put forth to explain speech rate slowing in the elderly is increased cautiousness associated with aging. It has been suggested that elderly adults speak more slowly because they monitor their output more carefully than do young adults (Kent & Burkard, 1981). Although more careful monitoring by elderly speakers certainly could be a factor in slower speech rate, particularly for spontaneous speech production, elderly subjects also speak more slowly than young adults when required to produce single, memorized sentences very rapidly (Smith et al., 1987). This finding suggests that a mechanism other than monitoring differences in the two groups is responsible, at least in part, for age-related speech slowing. In addition, speech rate differences in elderly and young speakers have been found to be comparable at both slow and fast rates under conditions in which no creative linguistic processing is occurring, such as the production of memorized sentences (Smith et al., 1987). This finding suggests that a more "low level" process is responsible for the slowing phenomenon.

Although it appears unlikely that increased cautiousness accounts entirely for slowing of speech rate in the elderly, this phenomenon can not be ruled out as a contributing factor. As noted by Birren et al. (1980), cautiousness is related to reluctance to make a mistake. When considering cautiousness in the elderly, Botwinick (1978) concluded that older persons show some tendency to react slowly to avoid the risk of being wrong. Presumably, this pattern of behavior would have developed over time as a consequence of learning that precipitous action (or statements) can have negative consequences (Birren et al., 1980). Amerman and Parnell (1992) also considered increased cautiousness as one of several possible explanations for observed slowing of speech rate in elderly persons. These authors observed that elderly speakers maintain the same adjustments in consonant duration observed in young adults when utterance length and consonant/vowel spatial relationships are varied, while still demonstrating an overall decline in speech rate.

Perhaps an interaction of neuromuscular and sociolinguistic factors is responsible for slowing of speech rate with aging. The notion that neuromuscular and sociolinguistic factors interact in the slowing of speech rate in the elderly is not incompatible with evidence recently gathered on speech rate in young adult speakers. In an investigation involving a large sample of normal young adult speakers, Tsao and Weismer (1997) concluded that neuromuscular constraints play a role in establishing a speaker's habitual speaking rate. This conclusion was based on evidence that some young speakers were capable of talking more rapidly than other young speakers. Also, habitual speaking rate was associated with maximum speaking rate in all speakers. In addition, regardless of whether young speakers habitually spoke "slow" or "fast," both groups showed a similar magnitude of change as they shifted from their habitual speaking rate to maximum rate. However, neuromuscular factors did not account entirely for speaking rates used by young speakers. A small number of subjects were able to speak at very fast maximum rate despite habitual speaking rates that were considered somewhat slow.

It has been speculated, as well, that slowing of speech rate in the elderly may be a compensatory adjustment adopted by older speakers to maintain or enhance speech fluency (Duchin & Mysak, 1987). Noting that reduction of speech rate has been an effective strategy for reducing dysfluencies in young speakers, Caruso, McClowry, and Max (1997) speculated that elderly speakers could adopt slower speaking rates in an effort to avoid dysfluent speech. However, evidence gathered by Leeper and Culatta (1995) might suggest otherwise. These authors considered the relationship between fluency, speaking rate, and age. They found that although speech rate decreased with advancing age, dysfluencies did not decrease with decreasing speech rate.

Interesting data from the field of psychology related to word recall in the elderly could bear on the issue of speech rate in the aged population. As an indicator of brain pathology, psychologists frequently employ tests of verbal fluency. During these tests individuals are asked to recall as many words as possible meeting particular criteria within a set time limit, such as words beginning with a particular letter of the alphabet, words belonging to a certain category, or words *not* containing a particular letter. In considering age-related changes in performance on these tests in normal individuals, it is interesting that elderly persons perform as well as young persons when generating words beginning with a particular letter (Bolla, Lindgren, Bonaccorsy, & Bleecker, 1990; Bryan, Luszcz, & Crawford, 1997; Heller & Dobbs, 1993; Tomer & Levin, 1993; Troyer, Moscovitch, & Winocur, 1997). However, elderly persons demonstrate small but significant declines in performance in comparison with young persons if asked to generate words belonging within a particular category (such as animals) or to produce words in which certain letters are absent (Bryan et al., 1997; Heller & Dobbs, 1993; Kempler, Teng, Dick, Taussig, & Davis, 1998; Tomer & Levin, 1993). From such findings, Bryan et al. (1997) concluded that elderly persons are able to retain their ability to recall words with the same initial letter because this task, to a large extent, relies on an individual's word knowledge base. The elderly show small declines in performance when producing words in which a letter is absent because this task relies to a greater extent on speed of information processing. If elderly persons have declines in speed of information processing, and word retrieval is slowed as a consequence, such delays could cause speech rate to slow. In particular, pause length would be extended as the retrieval process is extended.

Some recent psychoacoustic data supports the notion that elderly individuals show delays in information processing in comparison with young adults, particularly under conditions of increased speech rate (Wingfield & Ducharme, 1999). While conflicting data has been reported (Gordon-Salant & Fitzgibbons, 1997; Taylor et al., 1994), some researchers have found that asking elderly listeners to recall spoken discourse presented at rapid speech rates produces special difficulty for elderly listeners in comparison with young adult listeners (Riggs, Wingfield, & Tun, 1993; Wingfield & Lindfield, 1995). If there are proportionally large speech processing deficits in the elderly under conditions in which speech is presented rapidly, it might make sense for elderly speakers to adjust their own speaking rate downward. Such an adjustment could allow for consistency in processing and production aspects of speech. Of course, any such explanation is speculative and does not rule out the involvement of other systems (such as neuromuscular slowing) in age-related slowing of speech rate. Indeed, it seems likely that slowing of speech rate in the elderly is a multidimensional adjustment related both to age-related changes in speech processing and speech production.

DYSFLUENCY AND AGING

A relatively modest amount of research has been conducted to date on age-related changes in speech fluency among normal, nonstuttering adult speakers. A review of research is provided by Caruso et al. (1997), who note that findings are somewhat conflicting. Early findings by Yairi and Clifton (1972) suggest that "normal" dysfluencies (incomplete phrases, interjections, revisions) increase in elderly speakers. That is, older speakers produced these types of dysfluencies more frequently than did high school seniors. Indeed, Manning and Shirkey (1981) proposed a model of age-related changes in speech fluency in which the incidence of dysfluent speech increased in old age. However, this model was revised by Manning and Monte (1981) after examining spontaneous speech fluency in 40 non-stutterers ranging in age from 50 to 95 years. These authors noted that the incidence of "formulative" fluency breaks (revisions of words/phrases, interjections, fillers, and repetitions of words/phrases), which constitute the majority of any normal speaker's dysfluencies, increased from age 50 to age 70, but then decreased in frequency after age 70. "Motoric" speech breaks (repetitions of sounds/syllables, sound prolongations, dysrhythmic phonations, cessation of voicing/airflow), which are considered more pathological, occurred only rarely across all age groups studied and the incidence was unchanged with aging. Manning and Monte (1981) concluded that motoric fluency breaks are unaffected by aging and that formulative fluency breaks decrease during late adulthood (after age 70).

This conclusion has not been supported in subsequent research, however. Duchin and Mysak (1987) reported that, although speech rate slowed significantly with advanced age in men, the incidence of dysfluent speech did not differ significantly among young, middle-aged, and elderly speakers, even those beyond age 70. More recently, Leeper and Culatta (1995) measured speech fluency as a function of speaking rate in 98 speakers (49 males, 49 females) ranging in age from 55 to 92 years on a variety of speaking tasks (oral reading, picture descriptions, spontaneous speech). No age-related differences in speech fluency were observed for picture descriptions or spontaneous speech. Although dysfluencies increased with aging during oral reading, the incidence of dysfluent words was low for all age groups while reading (less than 2%), minimizing the practical significance of this finding. Overall, results of Leeper and Culatta (1995) indicate that elderly individuals do not differ from young adult speakers in dysfluent speech production. Interestingly, however, although not reaching statistical significance, a tendency toward greater dysfluency was noticed for males in comparison with females, regardless of age.

One reason for disparate findings in studies of dysfluency in the elderly may be increased variability among aged speakers. Many of the investigators examining age-related fluency changes have commented that elderly speakers show a wider range of fluency performance than do younger speakers, a finding that parallels results comparing young adults and elderly persons across a broad spectrum of performance variables. Greater variability among elderly speakers indicates that some elderly individuals are relatively immune from changes in speech fluency, whereas others show age-related deterioration. It has been speculated that heterogeneity among elderly speakers might be accounted for on the basis of propensity for dysfluent speech production. That is, perhaps nonstuttering elderly speakers falling at the "lower limits" of normal in terms of fluency are at greater risk of demonstrating age-related increases in dysfluency than are nonstuttering elderly at the "upper limits" of the normal range (Caruso et al., 1997). Longitudinal studies on speech fluency in adults would provide valuable additional information on this issue.

Based on research to date, it appears reasonable to conclude that speech fluency does not change appreciably with aging, at least under normal speaking conditions. It is possible, however, that elderly speakers have greater difficulty maintaining fluent speech under circumstances of greater cognitive stress. For instance, there is some suggestion that elderly speakers find it more difficult than younger speakers to maintain fluent speech under conditions in which highly automated word-reading responses must be suppressed, and the color of a presented word must be named instead (Caruso et al., 1997). Findings of a breakdown in fluency in normal elderly speakers under high-stress conditions are consistent with findings of other studies examining motor skills, vocal behavior, and physiological systems in aged individuals (Ramig & Ringel, 1983; Ringel & Chodzko-Zajko, 1990; Welford, 1982).

SUMMARY

There is ample evidence indicating that elderly speakers demonstrate reduced speech rates in comparison with young speakers. Elderly speakers average 20%–25% reductions in speech rate and are substantially more variable in speech rate in comparison with young adult speakers. Sentence durations, syllable durations, and consonant/vowel durations all are longer in elderly speakers, as well as an increase in the number of breath pauses. However, it is conceivable that women experience less slowing of speech rate than do men. Evidence supporting this notion comes from disparate research findings for women in which no age-related differences in speaking rate were observed.

Several hypotheses have been put forth to account for speech rate slowing. Perhaps most frequently this phenomenon is attributed to changes in the nervous system, either in the form of general neuromuscular slowing or altered nerve supply with aging. Increased cautiousness with aging also has been mentioned as a potential cause, possibly in conjunction with alterations in the nervous system. It has been speculated, as well, that elderly speakers adopt slower speech rates to maintain or enhance speech fluency. Finally, evidence that older individuals show small but significant declines in psychological tests of verbal fluency suggests that the elderly experience declines in speed of information processing. Such declines could slow word retrieval and contribute to slower speech rate through longer pause time.

Although early research suggested that the elderly show increases in "normal" dysfluencies, more recent studies have indicated that young and elderly speakers do not differ with regard to dysfluent speech production. Part of the reason for the disparate findings might have to do with increased variability in fluency of speech in elderly speakers. It appears that some elderly individuals are relatively immune from changes in speech fluency, whereas others show greater age-related deterioration. Considering the entire body of evidence currently available, it appears that speech fluency does not change appreciably with aging, at least under normal speaking conditions.

REFERENCES

Amerman, J., & Parnell, M. (1992). Speech timing strategies in elderly adults. *Journal of Phonetics, 20,* 65–76.

Benjamin, B. (1987). *Temporal alteration strategies in older speakers.* Paper presented at the annual convention of the Speech Communication Association, Boston, MA.

Benjamin, B. (1988). Changes in speech production and linguistic behavior with aging. In B. Shadden (Ed.), *Communication behavior and aging: A sourcebook for clinicians* (pp.162–181). Baltimore: Williams and Wilkins.

Benjamin, B. (1997). Speech production of normally aging adults. *Seminars in Speech and Language, 18,* 135–141.

Birren, J., Woods, A., & Williams, M. (1980). Behavioral slowing with age: Causes, organization, and consequences. In L. Poon (Ed.), *Aging in the 1980s: Psychological Issues* (pp. 293–308). Washington, D C: American Psychological Association.

Bolla, K., Lindgren, K., Bonaccorsy, C., & Bleecker, M. (1990). Predictors of verbal fluency (FAS) in the healthy elderly. *Journal of Clinical Psychology, 46,* 623–628.

Botwinick, J. (1978). *Aging and behavior.* New York: Springer.

Brown, W., Morris, R., & Michel, J. (1989). Vocal jitter in young and aged female voices. *Journal of Voice, 3,* 113–119.

Bryan, J., Luszcz, M., & Crawford, J. (1997). Verbal knowledge and speed of information processing as mediators of age differences in verbal fluency performance among older adults. *Psychology and Aging, 12,* 473–478.

Caruso, A., McClowry, M. T., & Max, L. (1997). Age-related effects on speech fluency. *Seminars in Speech and Language, 18,* 171–180.

Duchin, S., & Mysak, E. (1987). Dysfluency and rate characteristics of young adult, middle-aged, and older males. *Journal of Communication Disorders, 20,* 245–257.

Earles, J., & Salthouse, T. (1995). Interrelations of age, health, and speed. *Journal of Gerontology: Psychological Sciences, 50B,* P33–P41.

Gordon-Salant, S., & Fitzgibbons, P. (1997). Selected cognitive factors and speech recognition performance among young and elderly listeners. *Journal of Speech, Language, and Hearing Research, 40,* 423–431.

Hartman, D., & Danhauer, J. (1976). Perceptual features of speech for males in four perceived age decades. *Journal of the Acoustical Society of America, 59,* 713–715.

Heller, R., & Dobbs, A. (1993). Age differences in word finding in discourse and nondiscourse situations. *Psychology and Aging, 8,* 443–450.

Hoit, J., Hixon, T., Altman, M., & Morgan, W. (1989). Speech breathing in women. *Journal of Speech and Hearing Research, 32,* 353–365.

Kempler, D., Teng, E., Dick, M., Taussig, I., & Davis, D. (1998). The effects of age, education, and ethnicity on verbal fluency. *Journal of the International Neuropsychological Society, 4,* 531–538.

Kent, R., & Burkard, R. (1981). Changes in acoustic correlates of speech production. In D. Beasley & G. Davis (Eds.), *Aging: Communication processes and disorders* (pp. 47–62). New York: Grune & Stratton.

Leeper, L., & Culatta, R. (1995). Speech fluency: Effect of age, gender, and context. *Folia Phoniatrica, 47,* 1–14.

Manning, W., & Monte, K. (1981). Fluency breaks in older speakers: Implications for a model of stuttering throughout the life cycle. *Journal of Fluency Disorders, 6,* 35–58.

Manning, W., & Shirkey, E. (1981). Fluency and the aging process. In D. Beasley & G. Davis (Eds.), *Aging: Communication processes and disorders* (pp.175–189). New York: Grune & Stratton.

Mysak, E. (1959). Pitch and duration characteristics of older males. *Journal of Speech and Hearing Research, 2,* 46–54.

Mysak, E., & Hanley, T. (1959) Vocal aging. *Geriatrics, 14,* 652–656.

Oyer, H., & Deal, L. (1985). Temporal aspects of speech and the aging process. *Folia Phoniatrica (Basel), 37,* 109–112.

Ramig, L. (1983). Effects of physiological aging on speaking and reading rates. *Journal of Communication Disorders, 16,* 217–226.

Ramig, L. (1986). Aging speech: Physiological and sociological aspects. *Language and Communication, 6,* 25–34.

Ramig, L., & Ringel, R. (1983). Effect of physiological aging on selected acoustic characteristics of voice. *Journal of Speech and Hearing Research, 26,* 22–30.

Riggs, K., Wingfield, A., & Tun, P. (1993). Passage difficulty, speech rate, and age differences in memory for spoken text: Speech recall and the complexity hypothesis. *Experimental Aging Research, 19,* 111–128.

Ringel, R., & Chodzko-Zaiko, W. (1990). Some implications of current gerontological theory for the study of voice. *Proceedings of the research symposium on communication sciences and disorders and aging, ASHA Reports, 19,* 66–74. Rockville, MD: American Speech-Language-Hearing Association.

Ryan, W. (1972). Acoustic aspects of the aging voice. *Journal of Gerontology, 27,* 265–268.

Salthouse, T. (1993a). Speed and knowledge as determinants of adult age differences in verbal tasks. *Journal of Gerontology: Psychological Sciences, 48,* P29–P36.

Salthouse, T. (1993b). Speed mediation of adult age differences in cognition. *Developmental Psychology, 29,* 722–738.

Salthouse, T. (1994). The nature of the influence of speed on adult age differences in cognition. *Developmental Psychology, 30,* 240–259.

Shipp, T., Qi, Y., Huntley, R., & Hollien, H. (1992). Acoustic and temporal correlates of perceived age. *Journal of Voice, 6,* 211–216.

Smith, B., Wasowicz, T., & Preston, T. (1987). Temporal characteristics in the speech of normal elderly adults. *Journal of Speech and Hearing Research, 30,* 522–528.

Taylor, J., Yesavage, J., Morrow, D., Dolhert, N., Brooks, J., & Poon, L. (1994). The effects of information load and speech rate on younger and older aircraft pilots' ability to execute simulated air-traffic controller instructions. *Journal of Gerontology: Psychological Sciences, 49,* P191–P200.

Tomer, R., & Levin, B. (1993). Differential effects of aging on two verbal fluency tasks. *Perceptual and Motor Skills, 76,* 465–466.

Troyer, A., Moscovitch, M., & Winocur, G. (1997). Clustering and switching as two components of verbal fluency: Evidence from younger and older healthy adults. *Neuropsychology, 11,* 138–146.

Tsao, Y., & Weismer, G. (1997). Interspeaker variation in habitual speaking rate: Evidence for a neuromuscular component. *Journal of Speech and Hearing Research, 40,* 858–866.

Weismer, G., & Liss, J. (1991). Speech motor control and aging. In D. Ripich (Ed.), *Handbook of geriatric communication disorders* (pp. 205–225). Austin, TX: PRO-ED.

Welford, A. (1982). Motor skills and aging. In J. Mortimer, F. Pirozzolo, & G. Maletta (Eds.), *The aging motor system* (pp. 152–187). New York: Praeger.

Wingfield, A., & Ducharme, J. (1999). Effects of age and passage difficulty on listening-rate preferences for time-altered speech. *Journals of Gerontology. Series B. Psychological Sciences & Social Sciences, 54,* P199–P202.

Wingfield, A., & Lindfield, K. (1995). Multiple memory systems in the processing of speech: Evidence from aging. *Experimental Aging Research, 21,* 101–121.

Yairi, E., & Clifton, N. (1972). Dysfluent speech behavior of preschool children, high school seniors, and geriatric persons. *Journal of Speech and Hearing Research, 15,* 714–719.

10

Acoustic Aspects of Aging Voice

The aging process results in anatomical alterations in the mechanism that affect the functioning of structures responsible for speech production. The precise nature of those anatomical and physiological changes has been outlined in some detail in previous chapters. Alterations in function subsequently affect the sound that is created when speech is produced. That is, the acoustic signal leaving the lips of an elderly speaker bears the imprint of having been created by an altered mechanism.

Much research attention of late has been devoted to discovering acoustic changes that occur normally in voice with aging. Voice scientists view such information as important if normal vocal characteristics of elderly speakers are to be differentiated from vocal changes resulting from disease processes. A normative database representing the range of values to be expected from elderly individuals on a variety of acoustic measures of voice would be useful in early diagnosis of various medical problems afflicting older persons. However, development of such a database has proven to be a challenge to researchers.

In this chapter, acoustic characteristics of voice that have been observed to change with aging are reviewed. Because acoustic features of voice are affected both by phonatory and resonance events, the discussion focuses first on acoustic parameters related to respiration and phonation that have been documented to change with aging. Second, acoustic features related to resonance events that vary with aging are discussed.

ACOUSTIC CHANGES RELATED TO RESPIRATION AND PHONATION

In considering acoustic changes in voice with aging, it is often helpful to separate acoustic parameters related to phonatory quality from those related to resonance quality. Phonatory quality relates to changes in the acoustic properties of an individual's voice deriving from events within the larynx or the respiratory system. Specifically, acoustic parameters such as speaking fundamental frequency, fundamental frequency/amplitude stability, intensity of phonation, and spectral noise reflect the functioning of the respiratory and/or phonatory mechanisms.

Changes to the larynx and respiratory system with aging also affect the maximum and minimum performance capabilities of the vocal mechanism. The upper and lower limits of the fundamental frequency and intensity range of the voice are felt to be sensitive to subtle differences in capability. Measurement of these values in young and elderly speakers may well uncover aging effects. What follows is a review of documented changes in voice with aging that have to do with respiratory and phonatory functioning. Some of these changes pertain to performance capabilities of the aged mechanism and some reflect the acoustic properties of speech produced by older speakers.

Speaking Fundamental Frequency (SF$_0$)

In both men and women, SF$_0$ changes as an individual moves from young adulthood into old age. However, the pattern of change is quite different for the two genders.

Females

The pattern of SF$_0$ change observed in women during adulthood is graphed in Figure 10–1. In this figure, data for nonsmokers is plotted separately from data including both smokers and nonsmokers (Brown, Morris, Hollien, & Howell, 1991; Honjo & Isshiki, 1980; Pegoraro Krook, 1988; Saxman & Burk, 1967; Stoicheff, 1981). Speaking fundamental frequency remains fairly constant in women until menopause, when a drop occurs (approximately 10 Hz–15 Hz). This drop in SF$_0$ presumably results from hormonal changes during menopause that produce changes in the

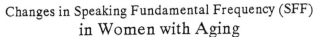

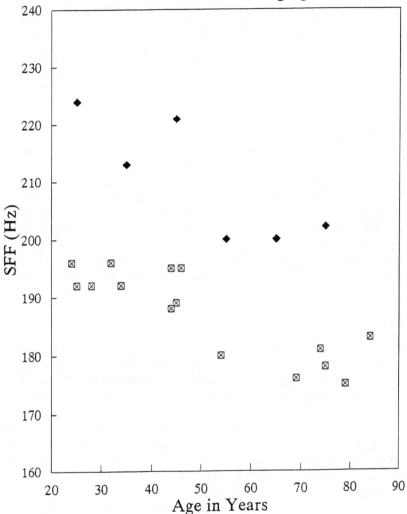

Figure 10–1. Speaking fundamental frequency as a function of age in women. *Note:* From "The Sound of Senescence," by S. E. Linville, 1996, *Journal of Voice, 10,* p. 192. Copyright 1996 by Lippincott-Raven Publishers. Reprinted with permission.

laryngeal mucosa, including thickening and edema (Abitbol, Abitbol, & Abitbol, 1999; Hirano, Kurita, & Nakashima, 1983; Hirano, Kurita, & Sakaguchi, 1989). Both smokers and nonsmokers show the same pattern of SF_0 drop during adulthood; smoking simply lowers SF_0 across age levels. Women maintain a fairly stable SF_0 level into old age. Although there have been reports of increases in SF_0 in women with advanced old age, such increases have not been statistically significant and therefore cannot be considered substantial (Pegoraro Krook, 1988; Max & Mueller, 1996; Mueller, Sweeney, & Baribeau, 1984). It also has been reported that SF_0 in centenarian females lowers in relation to younger elderly women (Awan & Mueller, 1992). However, variability of SF_0 among centenarian females is quite large, indicating that a larger sample of women in this age group must be tested prior to drawing conclusions.

Interestingly, findings from longitudinal studies suggest that lowering of SF_0 in women after middle age may be greater than what is indicated from cross-sectional studies. De Pinto and Hollien (1982) reported a drop of almost 50 Hz for a group of Australian women between young adulthood (18–25 years) and late middle age or early old age (52–60 years). Continued aging of these women did not appreciably alter SF_0 when a portion of the subject pool was re-recorded 12 years later (Russell, Pemberton, & Penny, 1995).

Males

Data on lifespan changes in SF_0 for men, compiled from a large number of sources, are plotted in Figure 10–2 (Brown et al., 1991; Hollien & Jackson, 1973; Hollien & Shipp, 1972; Mysak, 1959; Pegoraro Krook, 1988). In men, SF_0 lowers approximately 10 Hz from young adulthood to middle age. The reason for this drop in SF_0 is unclear. However, Hollien and Shipp (1972) speculated that the decline may be associated with subclinical trauma related to normal vocal use. After middle age, SF_0 in men rises substantially (approximately 35 Hz) into advanced old age. Thus, a man's SF_0 reaches the highest level of his adult life by about age 85 (Decoster & Debruyne, 1997). The rise in SF_0 in men after middle age has been attributed to muscle atrophy or an increase in stiffness of vocal fold tissue with aging (Kahane, 1987; Segre, 1971).

Maximum Phonational Frequency Range (MPFR)

Hollien and his associates defined MPFR as the complete range of frequencies that an individual can produce from the lowest tone sustainable (excluding vocal fry) to the highest falsetto tone, inclusive (Hollien, Dew, & Philips, 1971). The process of aging appears to alter MPFR in both sexes.

Changes in Speaking Fundamental Frequency (SFF)
in Men with Aging

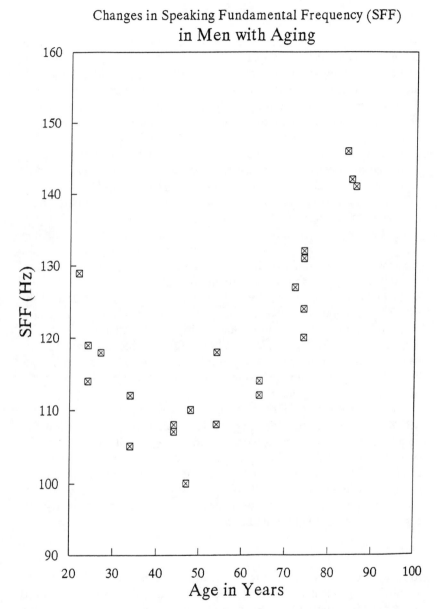

Figure 10–2. Speaking fundamental frequency as a function of age in men. *Note:* From "The Sound of Senescence," by S. E. Linville, 1996, *Journal of Voice, 10,* p. 191. Copyright 1996 by Lippincott-Raven Publishers. Reprinted with permission.

Females

In women, it appears that changes develop at both ends of the MPFR with aging, although such changes occur during different stages of adult life. Menopause changes the low end of the MPFR, with middle-aged post-menopausal women having an ability to produce lower frequencies than both young adult women and elderly women (Linville, 1987). Expansion of low frequency capabilities following menopause presumably is the result of hormonal changes producing an increase in vocal fold mass. It is interesting, however, that expansion of low frequency capability in post-menopausal middle-aged women has not been observed when musically acceptable low pitches were studied (Bohme & Hecker, 1970).

While middle-aged women may be able to produce lower frequencies than women at other ages, this increased capacity for low frequency production is not great enough to significantly expand total MPFR capabilities (Linville, 1987). Changes in pitch production capability that have the greatest impact on total MPFR in women are those that occur at the high end of the MPFR range later in life (Linville, 1987; Ptacek, Sander, Maloney, & Jackson, 1966). Indeed, restriction of the upper end of the MPFR is a phenomenon of aging that may be biologically determined and, as such, occurs even in individuals with professional voice training (Brown, Morris, Hicks, & Howell, 1993). Factors that may account for restriction of high frequency voice production in elderly women include intrinsic muscle weakening, ossification and calcification of laryngeal cartilages, and changes in vocal fold mass.

Elderly women do not maintain the expansion at the low end of the MPFR observed during middle age, tending to revert back to the low frequency capabilities of young women (Linville, 1987). Similarly, the range of musically acceptable low pitches restricts after age 65 (Bohme & Hecker, 1970). It appears that the passage of time between middle age and old age in women is critical both for reversing a drop in the floor of the frequency range that occurs during middle age and, perhaps more significantly, restricting the upper end of the MPFR.

Males

In men, findings with regard to age-related changes in MPFR have been somewhat equivocal. Ptacek et al. (1966) found that elderly men displayed the same MPFR pattern observed in elderly women. That is, elderly men demonstrated restriction of MPFR, accounted for primarily by loss of ability to phonate high pitches. On the other hand, Ramig and Ringel (1983) found no significant differences in phonation range among 48 men ranging in age from 25 to 75 unless physical condition was taken into account.

The authors acknowledged, however, that the design of the study may have affected results with regard to chronological age. That is, factors such as large within group physiological variation may have obscured significant chronological age effects.

Fundamental Frequency (F_0) and Amplitude (Amp) Stability

Measures of F_0 and amp stability have been examined as an aspect of vocal aging because they reflect the regulation and control of voice. The assumption is that a decrement in function accompanies increasing age, resulting in increased instability of vocal fold vibration. Changes in the larynx and the respiratory system with aging might contribute to unstable vocal fold vibration. These changes include degeneration of laryngeal muscle and connective tissue, ossification and calcification of laryngeal cartilages, diminished elastic recoil of lung tissue, and reductions in vital capacity (Bach, Lederer, & Dinolt, 1941; Bode, Dosman, Martin, Ghezzo, & Macklem, 1976; Chebotarev, Korkushko, & Ivanov, 1974; Ferreri, 1959; Frank, Mead, & Ferris, 1957; Gibson, Pride, O'Caine, & Quagliato, 1976; Hirano et al., 1983; Kahane, 1980, 1981b; Lynne-Davies, 1977; Malinowski, 1967; Mittman, Edelman, Norris, & Shock, 1965; Pierce & Ebert, 1958; Roncallo, 1948; Segre, 1971; Turner, Mead, & Wohl, 1968).

Interestingly, reports from listeners regarding vocal cues that they felt marked old speakers suggest that elderly speakers demonstrate greater instability in F_0 than young speakers (Hartman, 1979; Ryan & Burk, 1974). Specifically, reports that elderly speakers display increased hoarseness and harshness suggest higher jitter and shimmer levels. Reports of more vocal tremor in old voices might indicate higher F_0 standard deviation (F_0 SD) or amplitude SD (Amp SD) values in older speakers. Further, reports of more pitch breaks in elderly speakers suggest greater F_0 instability.

Jitter and Shimmer

Measures of stability of vocal fold vibration fall in one of two groups: (a) measures of small, cycle-to-cycle variations in vocal fold vibration and (b) measures reflecting more gross fluctuations over time. Jitter is a measure of cycle-to-cycle fluctuations in the fundamental period of vocal fold vibration. Shimmer reflects cycle-to-cycle variation in waveform amplitude.

Firm conclusions as to the effect of aging on jitter and shimmer levels are not now possible. Numerous factors have been recently uncovered that can interfere with valid and reliable cycle-to-cycle perturbation measurement. Factors such as mean sound pressure level (SPL) of phonation

(Lee, Stemple, & Kizer, 1999; Orlikoff & Kahane, 1991), mean fundamental frequency of phonation (Orlikoff & Baken, 1990), and analysis system differences (Gelfer & Fendel, 1995; Jiang, Lin, & Hanson, 1998; Karnell, Scherer, & Fischer, 1991) have been reported to affect measured jitter and shimmer levels, particularly in female voices. Findings of earlier studies examining age-related differences in jitter and shimmer need to be interpreted cautiously in light of these issues.

Some clue as to age-related differences on these measures might be gleaned from more recent jitter and shimmer data obtained from men's voices, however. As a group, elderly men appear to display higher jitter and shimmer values than young men (Orlikoff, 1990). Elderly men also demonstrate considerably more variability in jitter and shimmer measures than do young men. Findings of increased variability in elderly speakers are not uncommon in studies of age-related differences in both acoustic and physiological measures (Kahane, 1987; Karnell et al., 1991; Linville & Fisher, 1985; Linville, Skarin, & Fornatto, 1898; Max & Mueller, 1996; Orlikoff, 1990; Orlikoff & Baken, 1990; Orlikoff & Kahane, 1991; Ramig & Ringel, 1983). Individual health and fitness variables may be responsible for this increase in variability. In fact, it has been reported that differences in jitter with age tend to be eliminated once health and fitness variables are taken into consideration. Shimmer differences, on the other hand, tend to remain even after accounting for an individual's health and fitness (Orlikoff, 1990; Ramig & Ringel, 1983).

F_0 SD and Amp SD

Measures of F_0 SD and Amp SD reflect more gross fluctuations over time. These measures also tend to increase with increasing age. In fact, F_0 SD measures may be a better discriminator of vocal age than jitter (Linville & Fisher, 1985; Orlikoff, 1990).

In men, substantial differences in F_0 SD have been reported with aging. Levels more than double between young adulthood and old age. Similarly, women also demonstrate increases, with levels jumping 71% over a similar period. It is noteworthy, as well, that F_0 SD ranges for young and elderly speakers, regardless of gender, demonstrate little overlap. That is, some young speakers are able to phonate at F_0 SD stability levels that no elderly speakers can duplicate. On the other hand, jitter measures have been reported to overlap extensively, especially in women (Linville & Fisher, 1985; Orlikoff, 1990).

Measures of Amp SD also differ across age groups, at least for men. Elderly men demonstrated an increase in Amp SD of 54% in comparison with young men (Orlikoff, 1990). Data on Amp SD for women as a function of age are not available.

Speech Intensity

When intensity was examined from samples of connected speech, age-related differences in speech intensity were reported for men, but not for women. Ryan (1972) examined speech intensity in 80 men ranging in age from 40 to 79 years from a sample of conversation as well as a reading passage. Results indicated that men over the age of 70 used higher conversational speech intensity levels than did the younger men during both speaking tasks. More recently, Morris and Brown (1994) examined speech intensity in 50 women ranging in age from 20 to 90 from a reading passage, as well as conversational speech. No age-related differences in intensity were observed in women for either speaking condition. In both investigations participants passed hearing screenings. Ryan (1972) required a pure tone average of at least 30 dB (ISO) in the better ear. Morris and Brown (1994) required levels of 35 dB SPL or better for the frequencies of 500, 1000, and 2000 Hz in the better ear.

Morris and Brown (1994) hypothesized that higher speech intensity in elderly men might be an adaptive mechanism related to findings of decreased laryngeal airway resistance with aging (Melcon, Hoit, & Hixon, 1989). However, it seems more plausible that lower airway resistance values in elderly men result in lower speech intensity rather than the opposite. That is, lower airway resistance (related to incomplete approximation of the vocal folds during phonation) would compromise the valving capability of the laryngeal mechanism, making it more difficult for elderly men to sustain higher intensity levels during conversation. Thus, elderly men would tend to use lower conversational intensity levels. A definitive answer as to the physiological basis of age-related increases in intensity levels of conversational speech in men awaits further study.

Intensity Range

Intensity range has been investigated as a function of age through examination of maximum intensity vowel productions. In both men and women, maximum vowel intensity decreases with advanced age. Ptacek et al. (1966) compared individuals younger than 40 with those older than 65 and determined that maximum vowel intensity was reduced 5.3 dB in elderly men and 7.6 dB in elderly women, in comparison with their younger counterparts. More recently, Morris and Brown (1987) also reported lower maximum vowel intensities for elderly women. In addition, elderly women displayed elevated minimum intensity vowels when compared with younger women. However, young and elderly women used similar intensity levels when producing vowels within a conversational range

(Biever & Bless, 1989; Morris & Brown, 1987, 1994). In men, minimum vowel intensities and conversational range vowel intensities as a function of age have not been examined.

Findings of lower maximum vowel intensities for elderly men and women are likely a reflection of age-related changes in the respiratory and phonatory system. Reductions in vital capacity and loss of elasticity of lung tissues would reduce an elderly speaker's ability to drive air out of the lungs with great force. This reduction in power might not be apparent in conversational speech, but would become a significant factor in a maximum performance task. Similarly, an increased incidence of glottal gaps might account for reductions in maximum vowel intensity, particularly in elderly men in whom a higher incidence of glottal gaps has been reported in comparison with younger men (Honjo & Isshiki, 1980). Elevated minimum intensity levels of phonation in elderly women in comparison with young women might reflect loss of respiratory and/or phonatory control with aging.

Spectral Noise

Spectral noise is the presence of noise components in the spectra of vowels. It has been suggested that spectral noise originates from turbulent airflow resulting from incomplete closure of the vocal folds, or irregular glottal cycles (Yanagihara, 1967). Spectral noise levels might be expected to rise if the vocal folds fail to adduct completely during the vibratory cycle, as would be the case if a glottal gap were present. Spectral noise levels have proven useful clinically as an indicator of the degree of hoarseness in a voice (Deal & Emanuel, 1978; Yumoto, Gould, & Baer, 1982). Specifically, as the level of spectral noise increases, the degree of perceived hoarseness in the voice also increases (Yumoto, Sasaki, & Okamura, 1984).

Ramig (1983) investigated vowel spectral noise in men's voices as a function of aging, with the assumption that age-related changes in laryngeal physiology resulting from anatomical alterations in laryngeal structures are potential sources of elevated spectral noise levels. Vowel spectral noise levels were investigated in sustained phonations of 48 men ranging in age from 25 to 75 years, both as a function of chronological age and physiological condition. Although spectral noise levels were not associated with chronological age in men, noise levels were associated with speakers' physiological condition. These results emphasize the relationship between physiological condition of the general body and acoustic characteristics of voice reflecting laryngeal changes.

ACOUSTIC CHANGES RELATED TO RESONANCE

As a result of the aging process, the supraglottic vocal tract in both men and women undergoes significant changes (Chapter 4). Those changes include growth of the facial skeleton (Israel, 1968, 1973; Lasker, 1953), tooth loss (Adams, 1991), atrophy of pharyngeal musculature (Zaino & Benventano, 1977), atrophy/hypertrophy of tongue musculature (Balogh & Lelkes, 1961, Cohen & Gitman, 1959; Silverman, 1972), and loss of mobility of the temporomandibular joint (Kahane, 1981a). Further, it has been suggested that the larynx lowers in the neck with aging. Vocal tract lengthening in the elderly was reported as early as 1959 by Ferreri. Kahane (1980) brought attention to this early report, noting that Ferreri used the term "laryngeal ptosis" to describe an aging process in which the larynx assumes a position one to three vertebrae lower in the neck than the position observed in young adults. Citing additional anatomic data (Grant, 1940; Macklin & Macklin, 1942), Kahane suggested that weakening of structural support elements in the vertebral column in the elderly produces a series of changes in the lower respiratory tract, including lowering of the larynx, tracheobronchial tree, and lungs. Interestingly, Biever and Bless (1989) observed darker images during stroboscopic examinations on elderly women, in comparison with younger women. They interpreted this observation as indirect evidence of vocal tract lengthening with aging, as darker images suggest greater distance between the camera lens and the vocal folds in elderly women.

Age-related vocal tract lengthening might be expected to affect the resonance characteristics of aged voice. In particular, lowering of formant frequencies in elderly speakers would be predicted. Vocal tract resonance in elderly speakers also might be affected by altered articulatory gestures accompanying age-related loss of joint mobility and muscle weakening.

Formant Frequency Alterations

Formant frequencies of vowels are a measure of the resonance characteristics of the vocal tract. Factors such as vocal tract dimensions and constrictions within the tract (articulatory adjustments) affect formant frequencies. If age-related changes in formant frequencies are systematic and of sufficient magnitude, vocal quality could be altered sufficiently to allow for perceptually meaningful cues to speaker age. That is, a speaker might be perceived as "sounding old" on the basis of the resonance quality of his or her voice (Chapter 11).

There is acoustic evidence from several reports suggesting that elderly speakers tend to centralize tongue position during vowel production.

Benjamin (1982) reported that some elderly speakers (mean age 74) demonstrated formant frequency ratios that were more dispersed through the vowel quadrilateral in comparison with younger adults. This phenomenon was attributed to a loss of articulatory precision resulting in vowel centralization. It is significant, however, that some elderly speakers studied by Benjamin did not display acoustic evidence of centralization. Indeed, she reported a substantial increase in formant frequency variability both within and across elderly speakers, indicating that just as many older speakers showed no indication of centralization (Benjamin, 1982, 1997). Rastatter and Jacques (1990) also reported formant frequency evidence of vowel centralization in elderly speakers during production of isolated vowels. They acknowledged that findings from running speech could yield different results, however, and proceeded to examine vowels in carrier phrases. That investigation indicated that only elderly men showed formant frequency evidence of vowel centralization. Elderly women maintained formant frequency patterns observed in young women (Rastatter, McGuire, Kalinowski, & Stuart, 1997). Interestingly, Liss, Weismer, and Rosenbek (1990) also found consistent evidence of vowel centralization in a group of very old male speakers (over age 87). Those findings led Benjamin (1997) to conclude that a tendency to centralize vowels may become more pervasive with advanced old age, at least in men.

Formant frequencies of elderly speakers also appear to reflect vocal tract lengthening. Endres, Bambach, and Flosser (1971) examined formant frequencies of four male and two female speakers longitudinally over periods of up to 29 years. They reported lowering of the formant frequencies of seven vowels and two diphthongs in content-controlled running speech samples in both men and women. Similarly, in a cross-sectional study of 75 women producing sustained /æ/ vowels, Linville and Fisher (1985) reported significant lowering of F_1 and F_2 with advancing age, although lowering of F_2 was less prominent with increasing age than lowering of F_1. Also, Scukanec, Petrosino, and Squibb (1991) reported lower F_1 frequencies for three elderly women in comparison with six young women on four vowels (/i/, /æ/, /u/, and /a/). Lower F_2 values also were reported for the elderly women, although significant lowering occurred only for /a/ and /u/.

Additional evidence supporting vocal tract lengthening in elderly speakers comes from a recent investigation of long-term average spectra (LTAS) from dynamic speech produced by young and elderly adults (Linville & Rens, in press). LTAS provides an averaged spectra of all voiced sounds across a relatively long speech sample. By including only voiced sounds, the contaminating influence of voiceless phonemes on the resulting spectrum is avoided. The advantage of using LTAS to examine vocal tract resonance changes is that investigators can look across all vowel productions in running speech for consistent acoustic evidence of vocal tract lengthening. LTAS has been used most frequently to draw conclusions as to patterns characteristic of given phonatory vocal qualities, such as breathiness, by comparing acoustic energy levels in various frequency regions (for instance above 1 KHz and below 1 kHz). However, LTAS also has been used to provide spectral information on the relative positioning of the larynx during dynamic speech (Sundberg & Nordstrom, 1976). These authors measured LTAS from a song sung twice by a singer, once with a lowered larynx and once with a raised larynx. They observed lowering of the first three spectral peaks in the lowered larynx condition. In addition, they found good agreement between LTAS findings and lowering of formant frequencies observed to accompany laryngeal lowering in two additional experiments: (a) a study of sustained vowel productions, and (b) a computer simulation study. Sundberg and Nordstom (1976) concluded that the effects on formant frequencies from laryngeal positioning alterations can be identified in LTAS.

Using LTAS, Linville & Rens (in press) investigated the resonance characteristics of dynamic speech in 80 young adult and elderly speakers. They found significant lowering of peak 1 with aging in both men and women. Peaks 2 and 3 also lowered significantly across the adult lifespan in women and showed a tendency to lower in men. Further, the decline in frequency experienced by female speakers with aging for peaks 1, 2, and 3 (29%, 10%, 9%, respectively) was proportionately greater in magnitude than the decline observed in male speakers (11%, 2%, 2%, respectively) suggesting that women may undergo more pronounced age-related lengthening of the vocal tract. Alternatively, it is possible that elderly men tend to alter tongue position systematically during vowel production, while elderly women are less likely to do so.

Considered in total, studies examining the formant frequency characteristics of aged speech suggest a "blended" model of vocal tract resonance changes (Figure 10–3). In such a model, there is an interaction among gender, the resonance effects of vocal tract lengthening, and vowel articulatory patterns. To prove this model, additional studies are needed that directly relate vocal tract configurations to acoustic variables.

Nasal Resonance Changes

The effect of aging on nasal resonance has not been extensively investigated and findings are contradictory. Hutchinson, Robinson, and Nerbonne (1978) obtained measures of nasalance (the quotient of nasal sound pressure level to nasal + oral sound pressure level) from 50- to 80-year-old speakers while reading a passage loaded with orally produced phonemes. These nasalance measures were compared to those obtained by Fletcher (1973) from speakers ranging in age from 18 to 38. Results

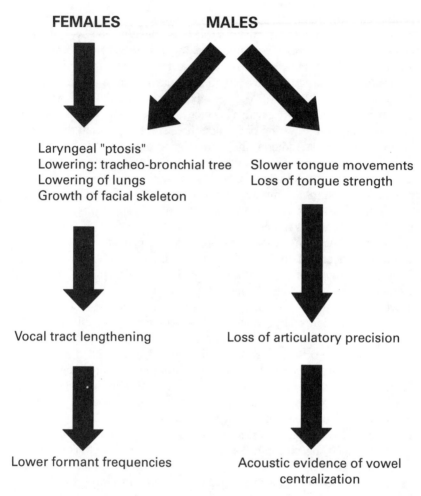

FEMALES   MALES

Laryngeal "ptosis"
Lowering: tracheo-bronchial tree   Slower tongue movements
Lowering of lungs   Loss of tongue strength
Growth of facial skeleton

Vocal tract lengthening   Loss of articulatory precision

Lower formant frequencies   Acoustic evidence of vowel
                                     centralization

Figure 10–3. Flowchart illustrating the blended model of vocal tract resonance changes with aging.

indicated that older speakers had higher nasalance values than younger speakers, leading the authors to conclude that the velopharynx becomes less competent with age.

The conclusions of Hutchinson et al. (1978) were questioned by Hoit and her associates. Hoit, Watson, Hixon, & Johnson (1994) investigated nasal airflow during oral and nasal utterances in 80 men and women ranging in age from 20 to 97 and found no age-related differences in nasal airflow. Indeed, these authors concluded that velopharyngeal function for speech production does not change from young adulthood to senescence. Hoit et al. (1994) speculated that findings of higher nasalance values in elderly speakers by Hutchinson et al. (1978) might have been the result of either: (a) age-related structural modifications in the craniofacial skeleton (such as density reduction), (b) age-related differences in the spectral content of the speech signal that influenced nasalance values, or (c) smaller mouth openings in older speakers in comparison with younger speakers.

Nasalance values in elderly speakers also have been investigated from the perspective of denture use. Scarsellone, Rochet, and Wolfaardt (1999) found lower nasalance values in elderly patients when maxillary dentures were removed for testing, although the magnitude of difference with dentures removed averaged only approximately 2%. This finding led the authors to conclude that normative data for nasalance may safely be applied to elderly speakers regardless of status with regard to maxillary dentition (natural or prosthetic).

SUMMARY

Acoustic characteristics of men's and women's voices are altered as an individual matures. Change occurs both in acoustic characteristics associated with phonatory events and in those related to resonance transfer of voice. In terms of acoustic events related to phonatory function, speaking fundamental frequency in men lowers from young adulthood into middle age and then rises again into old age. In women, SF_0 remains fairly constant into middle age when a slight drop occurs. From middle age to old age in women SF_0 appears to remain relatively unchanged. Elderly women demonstrate restriction of high frequency phonation in comparison with younger women. Middle-aged women may demonstrate expanded capability for low frequency production. In elderly men, high frequency production also appears to be restricted in comparison with younger men, although results of studies have been somewhat equivocal. Fundamental frequency and amplitude instability appear to increase with aging in both men and women. Although definitive conclusions regarding jitter and shimmer changes with aging are not possible at this time, there are suggestions that shimmer, in particular, may be higher in elderly speakers. Increases in F_0 SD and amp SD have been demonstrated in both men and women with aging. Vocal intensity during conversational speech has been reported to increase in men with aging. In women, no changes in intensity of conversational speech with aging have been uncovered. In both men and women, reductions of maximum intensity of vowel productions have been reported. In addition, women have been observed to have elevated minimum vowel intensities in comparison with younger women. Spectral noise levels have been examined in men's voices as a function of aging.

Although noise levels are not associated with chronological aging in men, such levels do vary as a function of physiological condition.

Resonance characteristics of voice vary as a function of aging as well. There is considerable evidence that formant frequencies lower with aging across vowels, suggesting vocal tract lengthening with age. In addition, there is evidence that formant pattern changes with aging are related to centralization of vowels, at least in elderly men. In terms of nasal resonance, although it has been suggested that the velopharynx becomes less competent with aging, those findings have been refuted by researchers who conclude that velopharyngeal function does not change from young adulthood to senescence. Further, recent findings suggest that normative data for nasalance in elderly speakers may safely be applied regardless of maxillary denture status.

REFERENCES

Abitbol, J., Abitbol, P., & Abitbol, B. (1999). Sex hormones and the female voice. *Journal of Voice, 13,* 424-446.

Adams, D. (1991). Age changes in oral structures. *Dental Update, 18,* 14–17.

Awan, S., & Mueller, P. (1992). Speaking fundamental frequency characteristics of centenarian females. *Clinical Linguistics and Phonetics, 6,* 249–254.

Bach, A., Lederer, F., & Dinolt, R. (1941). Senile changes in laryngeal musculature. *Archives of Otolaryngology, 34,* 47–56.

Balogh, K., & Lelkes, K. (1961). The tongue in old age. *Gerontologica Clinica, 3,* 38–54.

Benjamin, B. (1982). Phonological performance in gerontological speech. *Journal of Psycholinguistic Research, 11,* 159–167.

Benjamin, B. (1997). Speech production of normally aging adults. *Seminars in Speech and Language, 18,* 135–141.

Biever, D., & Bless, D. (1989). Vibratory characteristics of the vocal folds in young adult and geriatric women. *Journal of Voice, 3,* 120–131.

Bode, F., Dosman, J., Martin, R., Ghezzo, H., & Macklem, P. (1976). Age and sex differences in lung elasticity and in closing capacity in nonsmokers. *Journal of Applied Physiology, 41,* 129–135.

Bohme, G., & Hecker, G. (1970). Gerontologische Untersuchungen uber Stimmumfang und Sprechstimmlage [Gerontological studies on vocal range and vocal register]. *Folia Phoniatrica (Basel), 22,* 176–184.

Brown, W., Morris, R., Hicks, D., & Howell, E. (1993). Phonational profiles of female professional singers and nonsingers. *Journal of Voice, 7,* 219–226.

Brown, W., Morris, R., Hollien, H., & Howell, E. (1991). Speaking fundamental frequency characteristics as a function of age and professional singing. *Journal of Voice, 5,* 310–315.

Chebotarev, D., Korkushko, O., & Ivanov, L. (1974). Mechanics of hypoxemia in the elderly. *Journal of Gerontology, 29,* 393–400.

Cohen, J., & Gitman, L. (1959). Oral complaints and taste perception in the aged. *Journal of Gerontology, 14,* 294–298.

Deal, R., & Emanuel, F. (1978). Some waveform and spectral features of vowel roughness. *Journal of Speech and Hearing Research, 21,* 250–263.

Decoster, W., & Debruyne, F. (1997). The ageing voice: Changes in fundamental frequency, waveform stability and spectrum. *Acta Oto-Rhino-Laryngologica (Belgium), 51,* 105–112.

de Pinto, O., & Hollien, H. (1982). Speaking fundamental frequency characteristics of Australian women: Then and now. *Journal of Phonetics, 10,* 367–375.

Endres, W., Bambach, W., & Flosser, G. (1971). Voice spectrograms as a function of age, voice disguise, and voice imitation. *Journal of the Acoustical Society of America, 49,* 1842–1847.

Ferreri, G. (1959). Senescence of the larynx. *Italian General Review of Otology-Rhinology-Laryngology, 1,* 640–709.

Fletcher, S. (1973). *Manual for measurement and modification of nasality with TONAR II.* University of Alabama in Birmingham.

Frank, N., Mead, J., & Ferris, B. (1957). The mechanics of the lungs in healthy elderly persons. *Journal of Clinical Investigation, 36,* 1680–1686.

Gelfer, M., & Fendel, D. (1995). Comparisons of jitter, shimmer, and signal-to-noise ratio from directly digitized versus taped voice samples. *Journal of Voice, 9,* 378–382.

Gibson, G., Pride, N., O'Caine, C., & Quagliato, R. (1976). Sex and age differences in pulmonary mechanics in normal non-smoking subjects. *Journal of Applied Physiology, 41,* 20–25.

Grant, J. (1940). *A method of anatomy* (2nd ed.). Baltimore: Williams & Wilkins.

Hartman, D. (1979). The perceptual identity and characteristics of aging in normal male adult speakers. *Journal of Communication Disorders, 12,* 53–61.

Hirano, M., Kurita, S. & Nakashima, T. (1983). Growth, development and aging of the human vocal folds. In D. Bless & J. Abbs (Eds.), *Vocal fold physiology: Contemporary research and clinical issues* (pp. 22–43). San Diego: College-Hill Press.

Hirano, M., Kurita, S., & Sakaguchi, S. (1989). Ageing of the vibratory tissue of human vocal folds. *Acta Otolaryngologica (Stockh.), 107,* 428–433.

Hoit, J., Watson, P., Hixon, K., & Johnson, C. (1994). Age and velopharyngeal function during speech production. *Journal of Speech and Hearing Research, 37,* 295–302.

Hollien, H., Dew, D., & Philips, P. (1971). Phonational frequency ranges of adults. *Journal of Speech and Hearing Research, 14,* 755–760.

Hollien, H., & Jackson, B. (1973). Normative data on the speaking fundamental frequency characteristics of young adult males. *Journal of Phonetics, 1,* 117–120.

Hollien, H., & Shipp, T. (1972). Speaking fundamental frequency and chronologic age in males. *Journal of Speech and Hearing Research, 15,* 155–159.

Honjo, I., & Isshiki, N. (1980). Laryngoscopic and voice characteristics of aged persons. *Archives of Otolaryngology, 106,* 149–150.

Hutchinson, J., Robinson, K., & Nerbonne, M. (1978). Patterns of nasalance in a sample of normal gerontologic speakers. *Journal of Communication Disorders, 11,* 469–481.

Israel, H. (1968). Continuing growth in the human cranial skeleton. *Archives of Oral Biology, 13,* 133–137.

Israel, H. (1973). Age factor and the pattern of change in craniofacial structures. *American Journal of Physical Anthropology, 39,* 111–128.

Jiang, J., Lin, E., & Hanson, D. (1998). Effect of tape recording on perturbation measures. *Journal of Speech, Language, and Hearing Research, 41,* 1031–1041.

Kahane, J. (1980). Age-related histological changes in the human male and female laryngeal cartilages: Biological and functional implications. In V. Lawrence (Ed.), *Transcripts of the Ninth Symposium Care of the Professional Voice* (pp. 11–20). New York: Voice Foundation.

Kahane, J. (1981a). Anatomic and physiologic changes in the aging peripheral speech mechanism. In D. Beasley & G. Davis (Eds.), *Aging communication processes and disorders* (pp. 21–45). New York: Grune & Stratton.

Kahane, J. (1981b). Postnatal development and aging of the human larynx. *Seminars in Speech and Language, 4,* 189–203.

Kahane, J. (1987). Connective tissue changes in the larynx and their effects on voice. *Journal of Voice, 1,* 27–30.

Karnell, M., Scherer, R., & Fischer, L. (1991). Comparison of acoustic voice perturbation measures among three independent voice laboratories. *Journal of Speech and Hearing Research, 34,* 781–790.

Lasker, G. (1953). The aging factor in bodily measurements of adult male and female Mexicans. *Human Biology, 25,* 50–63.

Lee, L., Stemple, J., & Kizer, M. (1999). Consistency of acoustic and aerodynamic measures of voice production over 28 days under various testing conditions. *Journal of Voice, 13,* 477–483.

Linville, S. E. (1987). Maximum phonational frequency range capabilities of women's voices with advancing age. *Folia Phoniatrica (Basel), 39,* 297–301.

Linville, S. E., & Fisher, H. (1985). Acoustic characteristics of perceived versus actual vocal age in controlled phonation by adult females. *Journal of the Acoustical Society of America, 78,* 40–48.

Linville, S. E., & Rens, J. (in press). Vocal tract resonance analysis of aging voice using long-term average spectra. *Journal of Voice.*

Linville, S. E., Skarin, B., & Fornatto, E. (1989). The interrelationship of measures related to vocal function, speech rate, and laryngeal appearance in elderly women. *Journal of Speech and Hearing Research, 32,* 323–330.

Liss, J., Weismer, G., & Rosenbeck, J. (1990). Selected acoustic characteristics of speech production in very old males. *Journal of Gerontology: Psychological Sciences, 45,* P35–P45.

Lynne-Davies, P. (1977). Influence of age on the respiratory system. *Geriatrics, 32,* 57–60.

Macklin, C., & Macklin, M. (1942). Respiratory system. In E. Cowdry (Ed.), *Problems of ageing* (2nd ed., pp. 185–253). Baltimore: Williams & Wilkins.

Malinowski, A. (1967). The shape, dimensions, and process of calcification on the cartilaginous framework of the larynx in relation to age and sex in the Polish population. *Folia Morphologica, 26,* 118–128.

Max, L., & Mueller, P. (1996). Speaking F_0 and cepstral periodicity analysis of conversational speech in a 105-year-old woman: Variability of aging effects. *Journal of Voice, 10,* 245–251.

Melcon, M., Hoit, J., & Hixon, T. (1989). Age and laryngeal airway resistance during vowel production. *Journal of Speech and Hearing Disorders, 54,* 282–286.

Mittman, C., Edelman, N., Norris, A., & Shock, N. (1965). Relationship between chest wall and pulmonary compliance and age. *Journal of Applied Physiology, 20,* 1211–1216.

Morris, R., & Brown, W. (1987). Age-related voice measures among adult women. *Journal of Voice, 1,* 38–43.

Morris, R., & Brown, W. (1994). Age-related differences in speech intensity among adult females. *Folia Phoniatrica (Logop.), 46,* 64–69.

Mueller, P., Sweeney, R., & Baribeau, L. (1984). Acoustic and morphologic study of the senescent voice. *Ear, Nose, and Throat Journal, 63,* 292–295.

Mysak, E. (1959). Pitch and duration characteristics of older males. *Journal of Speech and Hearing Research, 2,* 46–54.

Orlikoff, R. (1990). The relationship of age and cardiovascular health to certain acoustic characteristics of male voices. *Journal of Speech and Hearing Research, 33,* 450–457.

Orlikoff, R., & Baken, R. (1990). Consideration of the relationship between the fundamental frequency of phonation and vocal jitter. *Folia Phoniatrica (Basel), 42,* 31–40.

Orlikoff, R., & Kahane, J. (1991). Influence of mean sound pressure level on jitter and shimmer measures. *Journal of Voice, 5,* 113–119.

Peroraro Krook, M. (1988). Speaking fundamental frequency characteristics of normal Swedish subjects obtained by glottal frequency analysis. *Folia Phoniatrica (Basel), 40,* 82–90.

Pierce, J., & Ebert, R. (1958). The elastic properties of the lungs in the aged. *Journal of Laboratory and Clinical Medicine, 51,* 63–71.

Ptacek, P., Sander, E., Maloney, W., & Jackson, C. (1966). Phonatory and related changes with advanced age. *Journal of Speech and Hearing Research, 9,* 353–360.

Ramig, L. (1983). Effects of physiological aging on vowel spectral noise. *Journal of Gerontology, 38,* 223–225.

Ramig, L., & Ringel, R. (1983). Effects of physiological aging on selected acoustic characteristics of voice. *Journal of Speech and Hearing Research, 26,* 22–30.

Rastatter, M., & Jacques, R. (1990). Formant frequency structure of the aging male and female vocal tract. *Folia Phoniatrica (Basel), 42,* 312–319.

Rastatter, M., McGuire, R., Kalinowski, J., & Stuart, A. (1997). Formant frequency characteristics of elderly speakers in contextual speech. *Folia Phoniatrica et Logopedia, 49,* 1–8.

Roncallo, P. (1948). Researches about ossification and conformation of the thyroid cartilage in men. *Acta Otolaryngologica, 36,* 110–134.

Russell, A., Pemberton, C., & Penny, L. (1995). Speaking fundamental frequency changes in women with age: A longitudinal study. *Journal of Speech and Hearing Research, 38,* 101–109.

Ryan, W. (1972). Acoustic aspects of the aging voice. *Journal of Gerontology, 27,* 265–268.

Ryan, W., & Burk, K. (1974). Perceptual and acoustic correlates in the speech of males. *Journal of Communication Disorders, 7,* 181–192.

Saxman, J., & Burk, K. (1967). Speaking fundamental frequency characteristics of middle-aged females. *Folia Phoniatrica (Basel)*, *19*, 167–172.

Scarsellone, J., Rochet, A., & Wolfaardt, J. (1999). The influence of dentures on nasalance values in speech. *Cleft Palate-Craniofacial Journal*, *36*, 51–56.

Scukanec, G., Petrosino, L., & Squibb, K. (1991). Formant frequency characteristics of children, young adult, and aged female speakers. *Perceptual and Motor Skills*, *73*, 203–208.

Segre, R. (1971). Senescence of the voice. *Eye, Ear, Nose, Throat Monthly*, *50*, 223–227.

Silverman, S. (1972). Degeneration of dental and orofacial structures. In: Orofacial function: Clinical research in dentistry and speech pathology. *ASHA Reports Number 7*. Washington, DC: ASHA.

Stoicheff, M. (1981). Speaking fundamental frequency characteristics of nonsmoking female adults. *Journal of Speech and Hearing Research*, *24*, 437–441.

Sundberg, J., & Nordstrom, P. (1976). Raised and lowered larynx—The effect on vowel formant frequencies. *Speech Transmission Laboratory. Quarterly Progress and Status Report*, *2/3*, 35–39.

Turner, J., Mead, J., & Wohl, M. (1968). Elasticity of human lungs in relation to age. *Journal of Applied Physiology*, *25*, 664–671.

Yanagihara, N. (1967). Significance of harmonic changes and noise components in hoarseness. *Journal of Speech and Hearing Research*, *10*, 531–541.

Yumoto, E., Gould, W., & Baer, T. (1982). Harmonics-to-noise ratio as an index of the degree of hoarseness. *Journal of the Acoustical Society of America*, *71*, 1544–1550.

Yumoto, E., Sasaki, Y., & Okamura, H. (1984). Harmonics-to-noise ratio and psychophysical measurement of the degree of hoarseness. *Journal of Speech and Hearing Research*, *27*, 2–6.

Zaino, C., & Benventano, T. (1977). Functional involutional and degenerative disorders. In C. Zaino & T. Benventano (Eds.), *Radiologic examination of the oropharynx and esophagus*. New York: Springer-Verlag.

11

Listeners' Perceptions of the Aging Voice

An individual's voice quality is affected by a number of factors, including cultural expectations, gender-related expectations, and personality variables. The fact that friends can readily recognize each others' voices over the telephone and that relatives can identify other members of the family from hearing their voices in the next room bears testament to the power of the voice in conveying unique information about a speaker. It is probably not too surprising, therefore, that listeners also demonstrate the ability to identify speaker age with some degree of accuracy simply from hearing a voice sample.

A considerable amount of research has been devoted to the issue of age recognition from voice. Information on the acoustic characteristics of voices perceived as "old" is of interest to speech pathologists as they work with individuals interested in "sounding young." Scientists looking into artificial intelligence systems also would find such information useful as they attempt to develop realistic synthesized voices. Age recognition from voice has implications as well for forensic scientists involved in voice identification in criminal investigations.

In some studies, listeners were asked to estimate speaker age from voice samples and then were questioned afterward about the vocal characteristics they responded to in those speakers unambiguously judged as old (Hartman, 1979; Hartman & Danhauer, 1976; Ryan & Burk, 1974). Vocal characteristics that listeners considered typical of "old" voices (Table 11–1) included lower vocal pitch (regardless of speaker gender), increased hoarseness or harshness, increased strain, vocal tremor, increased breathiness, and reduced loudness. In addition, older speakers were thought to demonstrate slower speech rate, greater hesitancy, less precise articulation, and longer duration of pauses. Although some of these vocal characteristics correspond to actual acoustic changes in voice with chronological aging, others do not. For instance, although listeners reported responding to lower pitch as characteristic of advanced age in men's voices, acoustic analysis on older men's voices consistently has revealed higher fundamental frequency (F_0) levels in elderly men, in comparison with younger men (Chapter 10). Similarly, vocal characteristics mentioned as typical of "old" voice do not always agree with acoustic measures found to actually correlate with perceived age estimates (Horii & Ryan, 1981; Shipp, Qi, Huntley, & Hollien, 1992). Such discrepancies are explored as the chapter progresses.

In this chapter, information on listener accuracy in judging speaker age from voice samples is discussed. In addition, acoustic features of voice that correlate with age estimates (perceptual correlates) are reviewed. Also, instances in which perceived age correlates differ from acoustic changes with chronological aging are noted.

Table 11–1. Vocal characteristics considered by listeners as typical of "old" voices.

Lower vocal pitch (regardless of speaker gender)
Increased hoarseness or harshness
Increased strain
Vocal tremor
Increased breathiness
Reduced loudness
Slower speech rate
Greater hesitancy
Less precise articulation
Longer duration of pauses

Note: Compiled from Hartman, 1979; Hartman & Danhauer, 1976; Ptacek & Sander, 1966; Ryan & Burk, 1974. Previously published in "The Aging Voice" by S. E. Linville, 2000, in R. D. Kent & M. J. Ball (Eds.) *Voice Quality Measurement*, p. 361. San Diego: Singular Publishing Group. Copyright 2000 by Singular Publishing Group. Reprinted with permission.

ACCURACY OF LISTENERS' AGE ESTIMATES

Listeners are reasonably accurate in their estimates of speaker age from taped voice samples. Listeners' accuracy scores in several different studies are presented in Table 11–2. The difficulty of the task varies with the precision of the age estimate required. That is, listeners find it easier deciding if a speaker is young versus old than they do making a direct estimate of the speakers' age. The difficulty of the age estimation task also varies with the nature of the speech sample presented. Listeners are most accurate in judging age from reading samples played forward. Accuracy rates decline progressively when listeners judge age from reading samples played backward, normally phonated vowels, and whispered vowels. In other words, as less acoustic information is present in a sample, the task becomes more difficult for listeners. This result is to be expected. It is interesting, however, that listeners are not reduced to random guessing, even when judging age from samples devoid of voicing information, such as whispered vowels. However, listener accuracy at assessing age from whispered vowels is not particularly good, suggesting that a number of individual speakers would be misperceived under such a condition.

It also is interesting that listeners have been reported to maintain accuracy of speaker age estimation even if speakers attempted to disguise their age during speech production (Lass et al., 1982). That is, relatively small differences in listeners' age estimations ($M = 3.20$ years) resulted when speakers were instructed to read sentences in a manner in which they attempted to sound much younger or much older than they actually

Table 11–2. Accuracy of listeners' age estimates from a variety of speech stimuli.

Listening Task	Relative Age		Direct Age
	Young/Old	Young/Middle-Aged/Old	
Read Forward	99%[a]		.88[b] .93[c] .93[d]
Read Backward	87%		
Phonated Vowels	78%	51%[e]	
Whispered Vowels		43%	

[a]Ptacek & Sander, 1966

[b]Shipp & Hollien, 1969

[c]Ryan & Capadano, 1978

[d]Hartman, 1979

[e]Linville & Fisher, 1985

Source: From "The Sound of Senescence" by S. E. Linville, 1996, *Journal of Voice, 10*, p. 191. Copyright 1996, by Lippincott-Raven Publishers. Adapted by permission.

were. Of course, as the authors pointed out, speakers were not given suggestions as to which vocal parameters they might vary to accomplish the
intended goal.

Although listeners tend to be accurate in their age estimations of
speakers from voice samples, certain factors may affect listener accuracy
(Table 11–3). Linville and Korabic (1986) found that elderly women were
not as accurate as young women in perceiving speaker age from sustained
vowels, although the two groups tended to categorize individual speakers
similarly. Although hearing loss and age-related differences in the auditory system may have accounted in part for the differences observed, such
differences did not entirely explain the poorer performance of elderly
women. The authors concluded that overall listening performance is
adversely affected by advanced age. Interestingly, it appears that young
adulthood and middle age may be the optimum stages of life for judging
age from voice samples. Using a direct age estimation task, Huntley,
Hollien, and Shipp (1987) observed that both adolescent listeners (aged 9
to 15 years) and elderly listeners (aged 60 to 84 years) were less accurate in
their age estimates than were young adults (aged 20 to 30) and middle-
aged adults (aged 40 to 50 years). The authors speculated that poorer performance by adolescent and elderly listeners resulted, in part, from listener
bias from lack of familiarity with the full range of chronological ages represented by the speakers.

Response bias might also explain findings that listeners are more
accurate in their age estimations of young speakers than elderly speakers,
even if the listeners are themselves elderly (Hollien & Tolhurst, 1978;
Jacques & Rastatter, 1990; Neiman & Applegate, 1990). Perhaps listeners
hesitate to assign older age categories to speakers, tending to use the
younger age category more frequently during the course of the listening
experiment. This conclusion is speculative, however, as the authors of
these studies did not report data pertaining to the overall frequency of
"young" and "old" responses. Of course, previous investigators looked for
evidence of response bias in young listeners and found none (Linville &
Fisher, 1985).

Table 11–3. Factors that may influence listeners' age estimates.

Listener age
Response bias among listeners
Variability among old speakers in showing the effects of aging
Speaker race

Findings of "age bias" are not unprecedented, however, at least with respect to studies looking at vocal pleasantness. Deal and Oyer (1991) reported that when young and elderly listeners responded to samples of reading passages, both groups assigned higher "unpleasantness" ratings to older speakers in comparison with younger speakers. The authors suggested that this finding may be related to societal values regarding youth and aging.

If listeners are more accurate in estimating the age of young speakers, the finding might not be related to listener bias at all. It is possible that listeners simply are responding to increased variability among elderly speakers in the extent to which they display acoustic changes in their voices that mark them as "old" speakers. In other words, chronologically old speakers may tend to sound young more often than chronologically young speakers tend to sound old. Support for this hypothesis can be found in results of two studies. Linville and Fisher (1985) found that two of 25 elderly speakers (70–80 years) consistently were perceived by listeners as young (25–35 years) when producing phonated vowels. In contrast, none of the 25 young speakers were perceived as old. Also, Ramig (1986) observed that listeners were more accurate in rating the age of elderly speakers who were in "poor" physiological condition than elderly speakers in "good" physiological condition from sustained vowel productions. Ramig (1986) concluded that the voices of old speakers in "good" condition provided little acoustic information reflecting laryngeal degeneration. In contrast, mechanisms of speakers in "poor" condition demonstrated physiological aging changes reflected in the acoustic characteristics of the voices they produced.

It has been reported that speaker race also might be a variable in accuracy of listener judgments of speaker age. McCloskey and Moran (1988) played tape recorded reading passages from 14 Black and 14 White males between the ages of 65 and 85 to two groups of speech pathology graduate students (10 White, 7 Black). Recordings were played both forward and backward to control for suprasegmental and segmental cues. Regardless of listener race and stimulus type, White male speakers were correctly identified as to age more frequently than were Black male speakers. Black speakers exhibited more within sentence pauses, longer within sentence pauses, and slower reading rates than did the White speakers. Slower speaking rate has been reported consistently as a marker of elderly voices (Hartman & Danhauer, 1976; Mysak, 1959; Mysak & Hanley, 1959; Ryan, 1972; Ryan & Capadano, 1978). This variable, in contrast with vocal quality, may have influenced listeners age estimates, if listeners tended to identify Black speakers as older than White speakers. Data on the frequency of young and old age estimates of Black and White speakers were not reported. It also is interesting to consider these findings relative to findings that elderly African-Americans are disproportionately judged as displaying articulatory imprecision, even among African-American judges (Amerman & Parnell, 1990). As noted earlier in this chapter, articulatory imprecision is one of the vocal characteristics listeners reported as typical of "old" voices. If listeners tend to identify Black speakers as older than White speakers, it is possible that dialectical variations interact with age factors in voice, resulting in perceptual confusion as to correct age estimation. Additional research is necessary to answer this question.

ACOUSTIC CORRELATES OF PERCEIVED AGE

Fundamental Frequency (F_0)

Evidence suggests that F_0 is a very powerful and resilient cue to perceived age. Specifically: (a) listeners are significantly more accurate in their age estimates when judging phonated vowels as opposed to whispered vowels (Jacques & Rastatter, 1990; Linville & Fisher, 1985), (b) listeners perform similarly when judging age from tapes of unaltered phonated vowels and altered tapes in which resonance features of voice are low-pass filtered from the acoustic signal (Jacques & Rastatter, 1990), and (c) mean F_0 correlates significantly with listeners' judgments of age from phonated vowels in the absence of a significant correlation of formant information (Linville & Fisher, 1985). These findings indicate that F_0 dominates resonance information in the perception of speaker age (Table 11–4). However, if F_0 information is unavailable in the signal, as in the case of whispered vowels, formant frequency measures do correlate with age estimates (Linville & Fisher, 1985).

Table 11–4. Acoustic correlates of vocal age in speakers perceived as "old".

Men	Women
Speaking F_0 higher	Speaking F_0 lower
	Jitter uncorrelated
F_0 standard deviation higher	F_0 standard deviation higher
Intensity variability higher	
Spectral noise higher (visual examination)	
	Formant frequencies (æ) lower (whispered vowels only)
Slower speech rate	
More breath pauses	
Longer duration breath pauses	

Note: Blanks indicate unavailable data.

The tendency for F_0 cues to dominate resonance information might be more pronounced in young listeners than elderly listeners. Linville and Korabic (1986) observed that young listeners focused on voicing information (mean F_0 and F_0 standard deviation [F_0 SD] differences) and disregarded resonance information (lower F_1 and F_2 frequencies) when judging age from phonated vowel productions. In contrast, elderly women employed a wider range of acoustic cues.

Correlations of F_0 with perceived age estimates correspond with changes in F_0 that occur with chronological age. That is, women tend to be perceived as older if their F_0 is lower, at least when age is judged from sustained vowel productions (Linville & Fisher, 1985). Men, on the other hand, tend to be perceived as older if their F_0 is higher (Horii & Ryan, 1981; Shipp et al., 1992). However, no significant differences in speaking F_0 have been found between men perceived as young and men perceived as middle aged, suggesting that the categories of "perceived young" and "perceived middle aged" in men are created by listeners employing acoustic information other than just F_0.

It is significant, as well, that correlations of F_0 with perceived age do not agree entirely with listener reports of reactions to F_0 when making age judgments. In both men and women, listeners have reported responding to lower pitch in marking speakers as "old" (Ptacek & Sander, 1966). However, higher speaking F_0 values in male speakers actually correlate with older age estimations (Shipp et al., 1992). This finding indicates that listeners may engage in stereotyping to some degree with regard to F_0 and age.

Stability of F_0 and Amplitude

Measures of stability of vocal fold vibration can be classified as either measures of small, cycle-to-cycle variations in vibration or measures reflecting more gross fluctuations over time. Jitter reflects cycle-to-cycle fluctuations in the fundamental period of vocal fold vibration. Shimmer, on the other hand, is a measure of cycle-to-cycle variations in waveform amplitude.

Perceptually, jitter and shimmer correlate with a voice quality referred to as rough, harsh, or hoarse, at least in pathological voices (Deal & Emanuel, 1978; Lieberman, 1963). That is, voices are perceived by listeners as rough if jitter and/or shimmer levels for those voices are very high. Interestingly, although listeners report feeling that older speakers display hoarse, rough voices (Hartman, 1979), jitter is not associated with perceived age estimates, at least from women's voices (Linville & Fisher, 1985). That is, women's voices with higher levels of jitter do not tend to be perceived as older by listeners, even if their jitter levels are considerably higher than levels considered characteristic of normal voices. If jitter levels reflect perceived roughness, then vocal roughness is not particularly significant as a cue to vocal age in women. However, shimmer may be a more sensitive measure of perceived roughness than jitter. Indeed, there are indications that the perceptual effects of jitter and shimmer are additive (Deal & Emanuel, 1978; Hillenbrand, 1988). Further study is required before a definitive statement can be made regarding the significance of roughness as a perceptual marker of perceived age.

Although the importance of jitter and shimmer as markers of perceived age is open to some question, there is substantial evidence that measures reflecting more gross fluctuations in frequency and amplitude over time are important to age estimations. Higher F_0 SD values in women's voices are associated with older age estimates by listeners (Linville & Fisher, 1985). In men, as well, higher F_0 SD values are reported in individuals perceived as old, in comparison with men perceived as young (Shipp et al., 1992). In addition, Ramig (1986) observed that male speakers rated as old from sustained vowel productions had higher levels of intensity variability (standard deviation of the coefficient of variation [CV SD]) than speakers judged as young. It appears, therefore, that listeners respond to gross variability in both F_0 and amplitude when judging age from voice samples of both men and of women.

If listeners respond to high F_0 SD and CV SD values in judging speakers as old, what exactly is the perceptual phenomenon to which they are responding? Is this a different perceptual phenomenon than perceived roughness associated with high jitter/shimmer values? Perhaps listeners perceive fluctuations in F_0 SD and CV SD as relatively long-term, systematic variations in frequency or amplitude, as opposed to random, cycle-to-cycle variations (Linville & Fisher, 1985). That is, listeners may perceive progressive increases in frequency/amplitude followed by progressive decreases as a tremulous, or "wobbling," voice.

Spectral Noise

Spectral noise is unmodulated aperiodic energy (noise) in the spectra of vowels. The presence of such noise has been used as an indicator of hoarseness in a voice (Deal & Emanuel, 1978; Yumoto, Gould, & Baer, 1982). The fact that listeners have indicated that "old" voices seem hoarse and breathy in comparison with young voices (Hartman & Danhauer, 1976) would suggest that spectral noise levels are elevated in elderly speakers.

Despite suggestions that listeners feel that older voices are hoarse and breathy, spectral noise has not been investigated extensively as an acoustic correlate of perceived age. Ramig (1986) compared spectrograms produced by male speakers judged to be "old" with those judged to be "young" and found that vowel productions by speakers rated the "oldest" had the highest levels of spectral noise as judged from visual examination. This finding suggests that increased breathiness or some degree of hoarseness in the voice could be a perceptual cue to speaker age, at least in men. Further research is needed, however, to determine the relative importance of spectral noise as a factor in listener age judgments. Also, research is necessary to examine spectral noise as a correlate of perceived age estimates from women's voices.

Formant Frequencies

Formant frequencies of vowels reflect the resonance characteristics of the vocal tract through which sound travels after creation by the vocal folds. If vocal tracts undergo systematic changes as a consequence of aging or if elderly speakers alter their articulatory gestures in a consistent manner, such changes would be reflected in the formant frequencies produced by elderly speakers. If such systematic alterations in formant frequencies are significant enough, listeners may perceive those changes and use those resonance alterations in judging age from speakers' voices.

There is evidence that vocal resonance characteristics provide cues to listeners as to speaker age under certain circumstances, at least in women's voices. Linville and Fisher (1985) found that lower formant frequencies of women's whispered /æ/ vowels were associated with older age estimates by listeners. However, formant frequencies were not associated with age estimates from phonated vowels. It appears, therefore, that the perceptual significance of resonance cues to listeners is limited to situations in which F_0 information is unavailable to listeners, at least when sustained vowel productions are used as stimuli.

No data are currently available concerning the significance of resonance information to perceived age estimates from running speech. However, it is interesting to speculate about such an association, given reports by judges of speaker age that "imprecise articulation" is a feature of speech that marks speakers as elderly (Hartman, 1979; Ryan & Burk, 1974). Ramig (1986) found that old speakers in "good" physiological condition tend to be misidentified as young from productions of sustained phonated vowels, a task that primarily provides physiological information about speakers (information regarding the physiological competence of the laryngeal mechanism as well as supraglottic structures). However, the same speakers were correctly identified as old when listeners were presented with samples of connected speech. Since connected speech presents listeners with considerably more information about segmental and suprasegmental aspects of speech production than do sustained vowels, Ramig

(1986) hypothesized that during connected speech, old speakers in "good" condition may have revealed their chronological age through a "sociolect of age." That is, elderly speakers might have learned to use their speech mechanism in a manner consistent with social expectations for their chronological age. Modifications in articulatory placement that mark such a "sociolect" could be expected to manifest as alterations in resonance patterns for elderly speakers. Research is needed to consider acoustic correlates of such potential "sociolectal" adjustments in elderly speech patterns.

SPEECH RATE AND PERCEIVED AGE ESTIMATES

It is well documented that speech rate slows with advancing age in both men and women (Hartman & Danhauer, 1976; Mysak, 1959; Ramig, 1983; Ryan & Capadano, 1978; Smith, Wasowicz, & Preston, 1987). Such slowing may result from a number of physical or sociological factors, as outlined in previous chapters. In male speakers, slower speech rates are associated with older perceived age estimates. Shipp and his associates (1992) found that men perceived as old demonstrate slower speech rate (syllables/second) and longer total utterance durations than men perceived as young.

Breath management factors also have been associated with perceived age estimates in men. Specifically, a greater number of intrasentence breaths, as well as longer duration of breath pauses, have been reported in men perceived as old (Shipp et al., 1992). Listeners appear to be sensitive to changes in speech rate, as well as breathing patterns, when assessing speakers' age from connected speech.

Interestingly, when listeners are asked to estimate the liveliness of utterances, judgments of liveliness are highly dependent on articulation rate. Liveliness judgments also are affected by the perceived age of the speaker, which, in turn, is affected by the sex of the listener (Traunmuller & Eriksson, 1995).

SUMMARY

Listeners are reasonably accurate in age estimation of speakers from taped voice samples. The accuracy of age estimates declines as less acoustic information is available in the speech sample presented. That is, listeners are most accurate in judging age from connected speech and least accurate when listening to whispered vowels. Factors such as listener age, listener response bias, variability within elderly speakers, and even speaker race have been mentioned as factors that might affect listener accuracy.

Several acoustic measures have been identified as correlates of perceived age. Speaking fundamental frequency (SF_0) is a very powerful and resilient cue to perceived age. Correlations of SF_0 with perceived age estimates correspond to changes in SF_0 that occur with chronological age. However, correlations of SF_0 with perceived age do not agree entirely with listener reports of reactions to SF_0 when making age estimates.

Acoustic measures related to vocal stability vary in their importance as cues to perceived age. Jitter is not associated with perceived age estimates, at least from women's voices. However, higher F_0 SD values in both women's and men's voices tend to be associated with older age estimates by listeners. In addition, greater intensity variability has been reported in male speakers rated as old.

Spectral noise has not been investigated extensively as a cue to perceived age. However, visual examination of spectrograms produced by male speakers judged as"old"has suggested high levels of spectral noise.

Formant frequencies have been associated with age estimates of women's voices from whispered, but not phonated, vowel productions. It appears, therefore, that the perceptual significance of resonance cues to age estimates may be limited to situations in which F_0 information is unavailable to listeners, at least when sustained vowels are used as stimuli. The significance of resonance information to perceived age estimates from running speech has yet to be investigated, despite hints from listeners that "imprecise articulation" is a feature of speech that marks speakers as elderly.

Both speech rate and breath management factors have been associated with perceived age in male speakers. Specifically, slower speech rates, more breath pauses, and longer duration pauses have been reported in men perceived as old. Perceived age estimates also have been linked with liveliness judgments of connected speech.

REFERENCES

Amerman, J., & Parnell, M. (1990). Auditory impressions of the speech of normal elderly adults. *British Journal of Communication Disorders, 25,* 35–43.

Deal, R., & Emanuel, F. (1978). Some waveform and spectral features of vowel roughness. *Journal of Speech and Hearing Research, 21,* 250–264.

Deal, L., & Oyer, H. (1991). Ratings of vocal pleasantness and the aging process. *Folia Phoniatrica (Basel), 43,* 44–48.

Hartman, D. (1979). The perceptual identity and characteristics of aging in normal male adult speakers. *Journal of Communication Disorders, 12,* 53–61.

Hartman, D., & Danhauer, J. (1976). Perceptual features of speech for males in four perceived age decades. *Journal of the Acoustical Society of America, 59,* 713–715.

Hillenbrand, J. (1988). Perception of aperiodicities in synthetically generated voices. *Journal of the Acoustical Society of America, 83,* 2361–2371.

Hollien, H., & Tolhurst, G. (1978). The aging voice. In B. Weinberg (Ed.), *Transcripts of the Seventh Symposium Care of the Professional Voice* (pp. 67–73). New York: The Voice Foundation.

Horii, Y., & Ryan, W. (1981). Fundamental frequency characteristics and perceived age of adult male speakers. *Folia Phoniatrica (Basel), 33,* 227–233.

Huntley, R., Hollien, H., & Shipp, T. (1987). Influences of listener characteristics on perceived age estimations. *Journal of Voice, 1,* 49–52.

Jacques, R., & Rastatter, M. (1990). Recognition of speaker age from selected acoustic features as perceived by normal young and older listeners. *Folia Phoniatrica (Basel), 42,* 118–124.

Lass, N., Justice, L., George, B., Baldwin, L., Scherbick, K., & Wright, D. (1982). Effect of vocal disguise on estimations of speakers' ages. *Perceptual and Motor Skills, 54,* 1311–1315.

Lieberman, P. (1963). Some acoustic measures of the fundamental periodicity of normal and pathologic larynges. *Journal of the Acoustical Society of America, 35,* 344–353.

Linville, S. E., & Fisher, H. (1985). Acoustic characteristics of perceived versus actual vocal age in controlled phonation by adult females. *Journal of the Acoustical Society of America, 78,* 40–48.

Linville, S. E., & Korabic, E. (1986). Elderly listeners' estimates of vocal age in adult females. *Journal of the Acoustical Society of America, 80,* 692–694.

McCloskey, L., & Moran, M. (1988, November). Socioeconomic and racial effects on the aging male voice. Paper presented at the annual convention of the American Speech-Language-Hearing Association, Boston.

Mysak, E. (1959). Pitch and duration characteristics of older males. *Journal of Speech and Hearing Research, 2,* 46–54.

Mysak, E., & Hanley, T. (1959). Vocal aging. *Geriatrics, 14,* 652–656.

Neiman, G., & Applegate, J. (1990). Accuracy of listener judgments of perceived age relative to chronological age in adults. *Folia Phoniatrica (Basel), 42,* 327-330.

Ptacek, P., & Sander, E. (1966). Age recognition from voice. *Journal of Speech and Hearing Research, 9,* 273–277.

Ramig, L. (1983). Effects of physiological aging on speaking and reading rates. *Journal of Communication Disorders, 16,* 217–226.

Ramig, L. (1986). Aging speech: Physiological and sociological aspects. *Language and Communication, 6,* 25–34.

Ryan, E., & Capadano, H. (1978). Age perceptions and evaluative reactions toward adult speakers. *Journal of Gerontology, 33,* 98–102.

Ryan, W. (1972). Acoustic aspects of the aging voice. *Journal of Gerontology, 27,* 265–268.

Ryan, W., & Burk, K. (1974). Perceptual and acoustic correlates in the speech of males. *Journal of Communication Disorders, 7,* 181–192.

Shipp, T., & Hollien, H. (1969). Perception of the aging male voice. *Journal of Speech and Hearing Research, 12,* 703–710.

Shipp, T., Qi, Y., Huntley, R., & Hollien, H. (1992). Acoustic and temporal correlates of perceived age. *Journal of Voice, 6,* 211–216.

Smith, B., Wasowicz, J., & Preston, J. (1987). Temporal characteristics of the speech of normal elderly adults. *Journal of Speech and Hearing Research, 30,* 522–529.

Traunmuller, H., & Eriksson, A. (1995). The perceptual evaluation of F_0 excursions in speech as evidenced in liveliness estimations. *Journal of the Acoustical Society of America, 97,* 1905–1915.

Yumoto, E., Gould, W., & Baer, T. (1982). Harmonics-to-noise ratio as an index of the degree of hoarseness. *Journal of the Acoustical Society of America, 71,* 1544–1550.

CHAPTER

12

The Aging Voice: Normal Changes or Disease?

Diagnosing dysphonia is by its nature complex. However, that diagnostic process becomes increasingly complicated in the elderly. Anatomic, physiologic, and neurologic changes that occur normally with aging must be factored into the process (Sinard & Hall, 1998; Woo, Casper, Colton, & Brewer, 1992). In addition, potential interactions between normal aging and the effects of disorders of neuromotor control, respiratory function, and/or disease processes on vocal function must be considered. In essence, assessment of dysphonia in elderly patients requires clinicians to maintain a broad perspective with respect to requirements for normal phonation (Woo et al., 1992).

Often the distinction between normal and pathological vocal function in the elderly is blurred by issues of variability. A great deal of evidence has been presented in earlier chapters indicating that normal elderly speakers vary considerably across a wide range of measures involving breathing function, phonatory characteristics, and articulatory precision. This variability results from differences among people in the rate and extent of physiological aging as well as differences in variables such as lifestyle, genetics, and environmental factors.

In this chapter, issues involved in differentiating normal laryngeal aging from pathological states are explored. Pathological conditions producing laryngeal dysfunction in the elderly are examined relative to normal changes in laryngeal functioning with aging. Respiratory disorders that occur frequently in the elderly are contrasted with normal aging. Environmental factors influencing the aged voice also are described. At the heart of the discussion lies the issue of variability within the population of elderly speakers.

DIAGNOSING LARYNGEAL PATHOLOGY

Glottal Gaps

Although glottal gaps can be considered a normal laryngeal adjustment at any age, at least under certain phonatory conditions (Chapter 7), incomplete glottal closure also signals a number of pathological conditions. Neurological disease, cricoarytenoid joint disease/displacement, neoplasm formation on the vocal folds, or functional adjustments involving dominant cricothyroid activity all can compromise vocal fold closure (Hirano & Bless, 1993). Indeed, even congestive heart failure can present as vocal fold paralysis (Sinard & Hall, 1998). Clearly, the challenge to clinicians lies in differentiating normal glottal closure patterns in speakers at various ages from glottal gaps resulting from pathological conditions (Murry, Xu, & Woodson, 1998).

Södersten (1994) discussed the problem of distinguishing the normal posterior glottal chink (PGC) commonly observed in young women from functional voice disorders such as muscle tension dysphonia. In clinical practice, such distinctions often are made on the basis of the size of the gap. That is, if the PGC extends into the membranous portion of the vocal fold, the gap is considered pathological (Rammage, Peppard, & Bless, 1992). However, following stroboscopic examination of 10 young adult females, Södersten (1994) concluded that PGC extension into the membranous portion of the vocal fold does not always distinguish normal young adult female speakers from those with phonasthenia.

If distinguishing normal young women from those with voice disorders on the basis of PGC can be difficult, it stands to reason that factors involving aging of the physical structures complicate the process in elderly women. Further, the fact that aging proceeds at markedly different rates across individuals means that elderly women at a given chronological age differ in the extent of physical change to the mechanism. Therefore, it is conceivable that an 80-year-old woman demonstrates PGC for the same (as yet undetermined) reason causing PGC in a 20-year-old woman. How does a clinician determine if PGC in an 80-year-old woman reflects a variant of normal function or laryngeal pathology? The answer to this question may not be clear. Such a distinction follows a comprehensive medical evaluation and vocal history as well as additional information on phonatory function. In the last analysis, this determination comes down to clinical judgment.

In discussing glottal gaps it is important to recognize that gaps do not exist in a vacuum. Age-related changes in the laryngeal system occur in conjunction with aging changes in the pulmonary system. Changes in pulmonary function (such as alterations in vital capacity, expiratory volume, airflow rate) interact with alterations in laryngeal efficiency (such as glottal gaps) to affect the amount and force of aerodynamic energy (translaryngeal airflow/subglottal air pressure) available during voice production.

Measurement of laryngeal airway resistance (RLAW) is one method of assessing the integrity of the laryngeal valve in the elderly and ascertaining the combined impact of respiratory drive and laryngeal valving changes on the process of voice production (Chapter 6). Studies of RLAW in the elderly population have shown that RLAW decreases with advancing age in men, largely as a function of increased airflow rate, and does not differ significantly with aging in women (Hoit & Hixon, 1992; Melcon, Hoit, & Hixon, 1989). These findings fit with stroboscopic observations of an increased incidence of glottal gaps in men with aging, with no such increase in women as a function of aging. However, it is interesting that variability in RLAW among elderly women is reported to be greater than that observed among elderly men. This finding has led to speculation that elderly women may use a wider variety of strategies to control RLAW than do elderly men. For instance, when increasing vocal intensity, some elderly women may increase chest wall activity to increase respiratory drive, while others directly increase RLAW. Some elderly women may even use a combination of both strategies or some additional idiosyncratic adjustment to achieve the goal (Hoit & Hixon, 1992; Holmes, Leeper, & Nicholson, 1994). To resolve this issue, additional data is needed from simultaneous measurement of respiratory/laryngeal variables during RLAW tasks.

From a clinical perspective, RLAW findings may offer insight into the variability in vocal performance characteristic of elderly speakers. If elderly women engage in "strategy shifting" while attempting to increase respiratory drive, those shifts would be reflected in increased variability of objective measures of vocal function (such as airflow). Strategy shifts also may be reflected in greater variability in glottal closure configurations during phonation. Clinicians must consider multiple explanations for abnormal findings when interpreting evaluative voice analysis measures on elderly speakers.

Vocal Fold Atrophy

Vocal fold atrophy is usually diagnosed on laryngoscopic findings of vocal fold bowing (a spindle-shaped gap of varying degrees anteriorly in the glottis) or a thin vocal fold. The condition produces symptoms including vocal weakness, breathiness, high pitch, and vocal fatigue (Isshiki, Kojima, Shoji, & Hirano, 1996; Lindestad & Hertegård, 1994; Omori et al., 1997). A number of etiologic factors have been implicated in the development of vocal fold atrophy including vocal abuse, trauma, aging, previous laryngeal surgery, excessively high pitch associated with vocal mutation in males, familial occurrence, hormonal disease, upper respiratory tract disease, and nonspecific causes (Isshiki et al., 1996; Lindestad & Hertegård, 1994). According to Isshiki et al. (1996), interest in this condition has increased of late because of demographic trends toward an increase in the aged population worldwide.

Although vocal fold atrophy is frequently reported in elderly dysphonic patients (Lundy, Silva, Casiano, Lu, & Xue, 1998; Slavit, 1999), the extent to which such findings can be attributable solely to normal aging is unclear. It has been asserted that dysphonia in the elderly attributable solely to physiological aging is an uncommon disorder that should be diagnosed only after careful exclusion of pathological etiologies (Lundy et al., 1998; Morrison & Gore-Hickman, 1986; Woo et al., 1992). Indeed, following a chart review of dysphonic patients over the age of 60, Woo et al. (1992) found that only 6 of 151 patients had symptoms of vocal fold atrophy (bowing and breathiness) that could be attributed solely to aging. These authors concluded that dysphonia in the elderly is more likely to result from disease processes than from age-related atrophic changes in the vocal folds (Chapter 3). Studies of vocal function in dysphonic patients grouped by chronological age provide some support for this notion. Lundy et al. (1998) concluded that objective measures of vocal function (acoustic, aerodynamic, stroboscopic) did not worsen as a function of age in a group of 393 dysphonic patients ranging in age from 65 to over 80.

What is the explanation for the apparent low incidence of dysphonia in elderly patients attributable solely to age-related vocal fold atrophic changes? It is possible that atrophic changes in the vocal folds resulting from normal aging are relatively slight in a practical sense in comparison with the clinical presentation of vocal fold atrophy in a dysphonic patient. That is, perhaps normal age-related atrophic changes in the vocal folds typically are insufficient to result in voice complaints, even if voice quality has been affected. Perhaps many elderly speakers simply accept subtle changes in voice quality that accompany normal aging or never notice those changes and therefore never present for evaluation of a voice problem.

Mucosal Wave

Mucosal wave is the presence of an observable traveling wave during the vibratory cycle that emanates from the free edge of the vocal fold and moves laterally. Mucosal wave varies in extent with different phonatory conditions, but normally travels at least half the entire width of the visible portion of the vocal fold when phonation takes place at normal pitch and loudness (Hirano & Bless, 1993). Mucosal wave varies, as well, with changes in the stiffness of the mucosa and the extent of glottal closure. In the aged larynx, mucosal wave information is useful in differentiating those speakers with edematous, stiffer structures from those with atrophy of structures (Biever & Bless, 1989).

On examination of the vocal fold vibratory characteristics of normal young adult and elderly women using videostroboscopy, Biever and Bless (1989) noted mucosal wave alterations during the vibratory cycle in elderly women. However, the nature of the alterations in mucosal wave was not entirely consistent from one woman to the next. Some elderly women showed increases in mucosal wave relative to young adult women; others showed decreases. The implication of this variance is that some elderly women show signs of vocal fold edema and others display vocal fold atrophy. Of course, as noted by Biever and Bless (1989), it also is possible that edema co-occurs with increases and/or decreases in density of tissue in the lamina propria in elderly women, producing countless possibilities in terms of physical property changes in tissue that would affect mucosal wave. In addition, drying and thinning of mucosa in elderly women in conjunction with hormonal changes following menopause also could contribute to restrictions in mucosal wave. When all these interactions are considered, it probably is not surprising that elderly women display more variability in mucosal wave than do young women. Therefore, interpretation of findings of abnormal mucosal wave in an elderly woman involves sifting through any number of possible explanations. Furthermore, interpretation involves consideration of additional factors related to medical and vocal use history, additional stroboscopic findings, additional tests of vocal function, and physical findings on medical examination.

DIAGNOSING PULMONARY DISEASE

Several investigators have commented on the role of poor breath support in the occurrence of voice disorders in the elderly (Hagen, Lyons, & Nuss, 1996; Woo et al., 1992). In many cases, poor breath support accompanies age related respiratory changes and/or poor physiological conditioning in elderly speakers. However, poor breath support also is a consequence of pulmonary disease.

A number of pulmonary diseases have a higher incidence in elderly persons than in young adults including tuberculosis (Dutt & Stead, 1993; Gubser, 1998), pneumonia (LaCroix, Lipson, Miles, & White, 1989), lung cancer (Fontana et al., 1984), and chronic obstructive pulmonary disease (Mahler, 1993). Of these pulmonary diseases, perhaps chronic obstructive pulmonary disease (COPD) is the most relevant to the current discussion.

COPD is the leading respiratory cause of mortality and morbidity in the United States. Further, COPD ranks fifth among all causes of death since the late 1970s (National Center for Health Statistics, 1987). The American Thoracic Society Board of Directors (1987) defined COPD as a disorder in which tests of expiratory flow are abnormal and do not change markedly for several months. This disorder predominantly affects cigarette smokers (Petty, 1998), although only about 15% of smokers develop the problem.

The two types of COPD are chronic bronchitis and emphysema (Mahler, 1993). Chronic bronchitis involves excessive secretion of mucous into the bronchial tree on most days for a period of at least 3 months of the year over a minimum of 2 successive years (Ciba Guest Symposium Report, 1959). In chronic bronchitis, subsequent narrowing of the bronchial tree from the mucous and resultant thickening of the airway walls leads to obstruction of airflow (Mahler, 1993). In emphysema, air-spaces permanently enlarge distal to the terminal bronchiole. Such enlargement is accompanied by destruction of walls of the terminal bronchiole without fibrosis (National Heart, Lung, and Blood Institute, Division of Lung Diseases Workshop Report, 1985). The principle mechanism of airflow limitation in emphysema involves loss of elastic recoil. Of the three recognized subtypes of emphysema (centriacinar, panacinar, and distal acinar), centriacinar is associated with cigarette smoking (Mahler, 1993).

In most instances COPD is diagnosed between the ages of 55 and 65 years. The prevalence of COPD increases markedly with advancing age. As time progresses, dysfunction increases and complications frequently develop. Throughout the world, COPD is a major health problem within the elderly population. Although the incidence of COPD in women is slightly higher than in men between the ages of 55 and 64, rates for men exceed those for women by 67% between the ages of 75 and 84. At 70 years of age, men have a death rate from COPD that is more than twice that seen in women and that disparity widens further with aging. Between 1979 and 1985, men showed a slight downward trend in COPD incidence while women showed an appreciable increase in prevalence rates during this time period (Mahler, 1983, 1993). Perhaps not surprisingly, gender trends for COPD incidence are similar to trends in smoking habits. That is, men have tended to stop smoking in recent years while women have tended to take up the habit in increased numbers.

Spirometry is generally employed clinically in the diagnosis of COPD. The major spirometric value that is examined is the ratio of forced expiratory volume in 1 second (FEV_1)/ forced vital capacity (FVC) (Mahler, 1993). The diagnosis of airflow obstruction (COPD) in elderly patients requires spirometric values less than 2 standard deviations from the mean for FEV_1 and FEV_1/FVC ratio, along with supporting information from the case history, physical examination, and possibly other laboratory data (American Thoracic Society, 1991).

Norms for spirometric values are based on age. In normal elderly persons, pulmonary function tests show declines in FEV_1 and FVC in comparison to young adults, with accelerated rates of decline as aging progresses (Chapter 6). One study places the average ratio of FEV_1/FVC in normal men aged 60 to 69 at 70% with a standard deviation of 11.4%. Normal elderly women aged 70 to 79 demonstrated a similar average ratio (70%) with a standard deviation of 9.5% (Morris, Temple, & Koski, 1973).

A problem with spirometry as a diagnostic tool for COPD is excessive variability in measures of ventilatory function among asymptomatic individuals, even young adults (Morris, Koski, & Johnson, 1971). Such variability increases proportionately with advanced age. In addition, pulmonary function data for normal elderly generally have been derived from relatively small numbers of subjects (Mahler, 1983). Because of these issues, it can be difficult to determine if results of pulmonary function testing on elderly persons reflect advanced age or disease.

Current spirometric diagnostic guidelines may prove relatively clearcut with more severely involved elderly patients. However, elderly patients showing early signs of COPD having spirometric values somewhat below average but not clearly in the pathological range would be more difficult to diagnose. It is important for clinicians to recognize the limitations of spirometry as a diagnostic tool for COPD, particularly in elderly patients. The dividing line between COPD and normal aging can be fuzzy.

ENVIRONMENTAL IMPACT ON AGING VOICE

As demonstrated throughout this text, numerous physical changes interact in countless ways to produce variable performance among the aged population. However, individual difference in physical aging is not the only factor increasing variability among elderly speakers. Environmental factors can either accelerate or postpone aging effects. Although a virtually limitless combination of environmental factors may influence aging, two of the most obvious (and potentially significant) are physical fitness and cigarette smoking.

Physical Fitness

Variability in physical fitness levels among elderly individuals is extreme and the rate and extent of decline in motor/sensory performance is considerable. Variability both within and across individuals increases as a function of age (Finch & Schneider, 1985; Spirduso, 1982). Age-related declines in motor performance appear to be exacerbated by muscle disuse and, conversely, such declines can be minimized by a lifestyle that includes exercise (De Vito, Hernandez, Gonzalez, Felici, & Figura, 1997; Ringel & Chodzko-Zajko, 1987). Daily exercise appears to facilitate muscle contraction, stimulate blood flow, and enhance nerve conduction velocity (Spirduso, 1982).

Ringel and Chodzko-Zajko (1987) suggest that a healthy lifestyle including regular exercise may positively influence laryngeal performance, although they acknowledge that such a link has yet to be definitively established. They point out that laryngeal control is dependent on adequate functioning of a number of different systems (laryngeal, pulmonary, articulatory) that rely on the structural and functional integrity of a number of systems (neural, endocrine, skeletal, muscular). Disruption in any of these systems has the potential to diminish vocal quality.

Although a positive effect of healthy lifestyle has yet to be directly linked to improved laryngeal performance, it has been shown that variability on measures of phonatory function in elderly speakers is reduced greatly by controlling the physiological condition of elderly speakers. Ramig and Ringel (1983) found that elderly speakers in better physical condition (slower resting heart rates, lower resting blood pressure values, lower percentage of body fat, higher forced vital capacity adjusted for physical size) had vocal characteristics similar to young adult speakers. Elderly speakers in poor physiological condition, on the other hand, performed poorer than young adult speakers when mean fundamental frequency, jitter, and phonation range were measured during maximum performance speech tasks (phonation sustained for maximum duration at the limits of phonation range). These findings point to the importance of evaluating speakers at the limit of their ability. Breakdowns in performance may not be observed if speakers are evaluated while performing at their habitual or comfortable level. Clinicians, therefore, must be cognizant of the effort level involved in performing a given vocal task when assessing an elderly patient's vocal functioning.

Cigarette Smoking

It has been well-established that cigarette smoking is a health risk at any age. In the elderly, a history of heavy smoking is associated with an unusually high incidence of chronic respiratory disease (bronchitis, emphysema, chronic airflow obstruction) as well as excess mortality by age 70, primarily due to nonmalignant pulmonary diseases, malignant neoplasms, and cardiovascular disease. In smokers surviving beyond age 70, research predicts continued declines in pulmonary function and shortened life expectancies in comparison with nonsmoking elderly persons (Hill & Fisher, 1993).

For elderly smokers, the effects of smoking coexist with normal aging changes (Lee et al., 1999), amplifying the impact of the normal changes on function, even in the absence of identifiable pulmonary disease. In other words, cigarette smoking accelerates the decline in pulmonary function observed normally with aging. For a thorough review of the impact of smoking on the elderly, readers are referred to Hill and Fisher (1993). Older smokers suffer from reductions in peak expiratory airflow and forced expiratory volume that are significantly larger than those observed in age-matched controls (Gregg & Nunn, 1989). Age-related declines in forced vital capacity and forced expiratory volume increase more dramatically in smokers than in those who have quit smoking (Bosse, Sparrow, Rose, & Weiss, 1981). When smoking is terminated, such measures improve immediately and continue to do so for several months (Buist, Nagy, & Sexton, 1979). Improvement in these measures is proportional to pulmonary dysfunction prior to cessation of smoking, with greater improvement occurring in persons with more severe dysfunction (Mahler, 1983).

Smoking also has a decided effect on laryngeal structure and function. Women (aged 30–54) who are smokers demonstrate vocal fold thickening at a rate of 87%, in comparison with 7% in nonsmokers (Gilbert & Weismer, 1974). Similar increases in mass of the vocal folds have been reported in male smokers (Auerbach, Hammond, & Garfinkel, 1970). Tissue changes in the larynx involving thickening of tissue (and increased mass) affect the acoustic properties of the voice. Indeed, speaking fundamental frequency (SF_0) of young adult female smokers (163.75 Hz) lowers relative to nonsmokers (182.8 Hz). Since the process of aging in women (without the effects of smoking) also lowers SF_0 after menopause (Chapter 10), young adult women who smoke, and artificially lower their SF_0, risk being perceived as belonging to an older age group on the basis of the way their voice sounds (Chapter 11).

Clearly, differences among elderly speakers with regard to smoking habits increase variability across a wide range of respiratory and phonatory measures. In assessing the "normalcy" of performance in elderly patients, it is important to consider the impact of smoking history. Heavy smoking during adulthood magnifies the effects of aging, producing more marked physiologic changes during old age even in the absence of diagnosed pathology.

SUMMARY

Diagnosing dysphonia is a complex process that becomes more complicated when vocal aging is factored into the equation. Clinicians must be able to differentiate normal vocal changes with aging from pathologic vocal conditions affecting elderly patients.

Glottal gap is a frequent finding in the elderly larynx, although males and females differ in aging patterns with regard to gaps. Glottal gaps result from a number of pathological conditions as well, and on occasion differentiating gaps resulting from normal aging from those associated with pathology poses problems. It is important, as well, that the voice clinician recognize that glottal gaps do not exist in a vacuum. Changes in pulmonary function with aging interact with alterations in laryngeal efficiency to affect aerodynamic measurements (translaryngeal airflow, subglottal air pressure). Variability in aerodynamic measurements in elderly women has been observed to be particularly great, leading to speculation that elderly women use a wider variety of strategies to regulate RLAW than do even elderly men. For instance, to increase vocal intensity some elderly women may increase chest wall activity, others may directly increase RLAW, and still others may use a combination of the two strategies.

Vocal fold atrophy frequently is diagnosed in elderly dysphonic patients, although the extent to which such atrophy can be attributed solely to physiological aging is unclear. There are indications that age-related atrophic changes in the vocal folds, alone, may be insufficient to result in vocal complaints, even if voice changes have occurred. There is some evidence that complaints of dysphonia among the elderly most frequently are associated with disease processes.

Elderly women demonstrate more variable mucosal wave patterns in comparison with younger women. The implication of this variance is that some elderly women display vocal fold edema and others demonstrate atrophy, although a countless number of possibilities in terms of physical property changes in vocal fold tissue with aging are possible.

Chronic obstructive pulmonary disease is the leading respiratory cause of mortality and morbidity in the United States. COPD typically is diagnosed between the ages of 55 and 65 years and prevalence increases markedly with advancing age. Because normal elderly persons demonstrate declines in pulmonary function in comparison with young adults, it can be difficult to determine if results of pulmonary function tests on the elderly reflect advanced age or disease. This problem is exacerbated by normative data derived from a relatively small number of subjects and high intersubject variability on measures. Spirometry still is employed clinically in the diagnosis of COPD. Diagnosis typically requires spirometric values less than two standard deviations from the mean for FEV_1 and FEV_1/FVC ratio, although the dividing line between COPD and normal aging can be fuzzy.

Variability in physical fitness levels in the elderly population is extreme both within and among individuals. Age-related declines in motor performance are exacerbated by muscle disuse. A lifestyle that includes regular exercise is postulated to positively influence laryngeal performance, although such a link has yet to be definitively established. However, it has been established that variability on measures of phonatory function in elderly speakers can be reduced greatly by controlling for physiological condition.

In elderly persons the effects of smoking coexist with normal aging changes, amplifying the effects of aging. Such effects include both pulmonary and laryngeal systems. Differences among elderly speakers with regard to smoking habits increase variability across a wide range of respiratory and phonatory measures. Smoking history must be considered by clinicians in assessing normalcy of performance in elderly speakers.

REFERENCES

American Thoracic Society. (1991). Lung function testing: Selection of reference values and interpretative strategies. *American Review of Respiratory Disease, 144,* 1202–1218.

American Thoracic Society Board of Directors. (1987). Standards for the diagnosis and care of patients with chronic obstructive pulmonary disease (COPD) and asthma. *American Review of Respiratory Disease, 136,* 225–244.

Auerbach, O., Hammond, E., & Garfinkel, L. (1970). Histologic changes in the larynx in relation to smoking habits. *Cancer, 25,* 92–104.

Biever, D., & Bless, D. (1989). Vibratory characteristics of the vocal folds in young adult and geriatric women. *Journal of Voice, 3,* 120–131.

Bosse, R., Sparrow, D., Rose, C., & Weiss, S. (1981). Longitudinal effect of age and smoking cessation on pulmonary function. *American Review of Respiratory Disease, 123,* 378–381.

Buist, A. Nagy, J., & Sexton, G. (1979). The effect of smoking cessation on pulmonary function: A 30-month follow-up of two smoking cessation clinics. *American Review of Respiratory Disease, 120,* 953–957.

Ciba Guest Symposium Report. (1959). Terminology, definitions and classification of chronic pulmonary emphysema and relation conditions. *Thorax, 14,* 286–299.

DeVito, G., Hernandez, R., Gonzalez,V., Felici, F., & Figura, F. (1997). Low intensity physical training in older subjects. *Journal of Sports Medicine and Physical Fitness, 37,* 72–77.

Dutt, A., & Stead, W. (1993). Tuberculosis in the elderly. In D. Mahler (Ed.), *Pulmonary disease in the elderly patient* (pp. 323–338). New York: Marcel Dekker, Inc.

Finch, C., & Schneider, E. (Eds.) (1985). *Handbook of the biology of aging.* New York: Van Nostrand Reinhold.

Fontana, R., Sanderson, D., Taylor, W., Woolner, L., Miller, W., Muhm, J., & Uhlenhopp, M. (1984). Early lung cancer detection: Results of the initial (prevalence) radiologic and cytologic screening in the Mayo Clinic study. *American Review of Respiratory Disease, 130,* 561–565.

Gilbert, H., & Weismer, G. (1974). The effects of smoking on the speaking fundamental frequency of adult women. *Journal of Psycholinguistic Research, 3,* 225–231.

Gregg, I., & Nunn, A. (1989). Peak expiratory flow in symptomless elderly smokers and ex-smokers. *British Medical Journal, 298,* 1071–1072.

Gubser, V. (1998). Tuberculosis and the elderly. A community health perspective. *Journal of Gerontological Nursing, 24,* 36–41.

Hagen, P., Lyons, G., & Nuss, D. (1996). Dysphonia in the elderly: Diagnosis and management of age-related voice changes. *Southern Medical Journal, 89,* 204–207.

Hill, R., & Fisher, E. (1993). Smoking cessation in the older chronic smoker: A review. In C. Lenfant (Executive Ed.), *Lung biology in health and disease, Vol. 63.* D. Mahler (Ed.), *Pulmonary disease in the elderly patient* (pp. 189–218). New York: Marcel Dekker.

Hirano, M., & Bless, D. (1993). *Videostroboscopic examination of the larynx.* San Diego: Singular Publishing Group.

Hoit, J., & Hixon, T. (1992). Age and laryngeal airway resistance during vowel production in women. *Journal of Speech and Hearing Research, 35,* 309–313.

Holmes, L., Leeper, H., & Nicholson, I. (1994). Laryngeal airway resistance of older men and women as a function of vocal sound pressure level. *Journal of Speech and Hearing Research, 37,* 789–799.

Isshiki, N., Shoji, K., Kojima, H., & Hirano, S. (1996). Vocal fold atrophy and its surgical treatment. *Annals of Otology, Rhinology, and Laryngology, 105,* 182–188.

LaCroix, A., Lipson, S., Miles, T., & White, L. (1989). Prospective study of pneumonia hospitalization and mortality of U.S. older people: The role of chronic conditions, health behaviors, and nutritional status. *Public Health Reports, 104,* 350–360.

Lee, H., Lim, M., Lu, C., Liu, V., Fahn, H., Zhang, C., Nagley, P., & Wei, Y., (1999). Concurrent increase of oxidative DNA damage and lipid peroxidation together with mitochondrial DNA mutation in human lung tissues during aging—Smoking enhances oxidative stress on the aged tissues. *Archives of Biochemistry and Biophysics, 362,* 309–316.

Lindestad, P., & Hertegård, S. (1994). Spindle-shaped glottal insufficiency with and without sulcus vocalis: A retrospective study. *Annals of Otology, Rhinology, and Laryngology, 103*, 547–553.

Lundy, D., Silva, C., Casiano, R., Lu, F., & Xue, J. (1998). Cause of hoarseness in elderly patients. *Otolaryngology—Head and Neck Surgery, 118*. 481–485.

Mahler, D. (1983). Pulmonary aspects of aging. In S. Gambert (Ed.), *Contemporary geriatric medicine, Vol.1* (pp. 45–85). New York: Plenum Publishing.

Mahler, D. (1993). Chronic obstructive pulmonary disease. In D. Mahler (Ed.), *Pulmonary disease in the elderly patient (Vol. 63*, pp. 159–188). New York: Marcel Dekker.

Melcon, M., Hoit, J., & Hixon, T. (1989). Age and laryngeal airway resistance during vowel production. *Journal of Speech and Hearing Disorders, 54*, 282–286.

Morris, J., Koski, A., & Johnson, L. (1971). Spirometric standards for healthy nonsmoking adults. *American Review of Respiratory Disease, 103*, 57–67.

Morris, J., Temple, W., & Koski, A. (1973). Normal values for the ratio of one-second forced expiratory volume to forced vital capacity. *American Review of Respiratory Disease, 108*, 1000–1003.

Morrison, M., & Gore-Hickman, P. (1986). Voice disorders in the elderly. *Journal of Otolaryngology, 15*, 231–234.

Murry, T., Xu, J., & Woodson, G. (1998). Glottal configuration associated with fundamental frequency and vocal register. *Journal of Voice, 12*, 44–49.

National Center for Health Statistics. (1987). *Monthly Vital Statistics Report, 35*, (13).

National Heart, Lung, and Blood Institute, Division of Lung Diseases Workshop Report. (1985). The definition of emphysema. *American Review of Respiratory Disease, 132*, 182–185.

Omori, K., Slavit, D., Matos, C., Kojima, H., Kacker, A., & Blaugrund, S. (1997). Vocal fold atrophy: Quantitative glottic measurement and vocal function. *Annals of Otology, Rhinology, and Laryngology, 106*, 544–551.

Petty, T. (1998). Can 'old' lungs be restored? Strategies for preserving lung health and preventing and treating COPD. *Postgraduate Medicine, 104*, 173–178.

Ramig, L., & Ringel, R (1983). Effects of physiological aging on selected acoustic characteristics of voice. *Journal of Speech and Hearing Research, 26*, 22–30.

Rammage, L., Peppard, R., & Bless, D. (1992). Aerodynamic, laryngoscopic, and perceptual-acoustic characteristics in dysphonic females with posterior glottal chinks: A retrospective study. *Journal of Voice, 6*, 64–78.

Ringel, R., & Chodzko-Zajko, W. (1987). Vocal indices of biological age. *Journal of Voice, 1*, 31–37.

Sinard, R., & Hall, D. (1998). The aging voice: How to differentiate disease from normal changes. *Geriatrics, 53*, 76–79.

Slavit, D. (1999). Phonosurgery in the elderly: A review. *Ear, Nose, and Throat Journal, 78*, 505–509.

Södersten, M. (1994). Vocal fold closure during phonation: Physiological, perceptual, and acoustic studies. *Studies in Logopedics and Phoniatrics (No. 3)*. Stockholm: Huddinge University Hospital.

Spirduso, W. (1982). Physical fitness in relation to motor aging. In J. Mortimer, F. Pirozzolo, & G. Maletta (Eds.), *The aging motor system* (pp. 120–151). New York: Praeger Publishers.

Woo, P., Casper, J., Colton, R. & Brewer, D. (1992). Dysphonia in the aging: Physiology versus disease. *Laryngoscope, 102,* 139–144.

CHAPTER

13

The Aging Professional Voice

The biology of aging is nondiscriminatory in terms of occupation. Professional voice users are subject to the same biological laws as untrained voice users and face changes in laryngeal functioning as they age. Indeed, older professional singers frequently are reported to demonstrate undesirable vocal features, including reduction of range, vibrato alterations, breathiness, diminished breath control, appearance of tremolo, pitch errors, and vocal fatigue (Sataloff, Rosen, Hawkshaw, & Spiegel, 1997; Sataloff, Spiegel, & Rosen, 1997). Of course, as has been discussed in previous chapters, aging is a complex process and not all individuals undergo the same changes in function at the same chronological age. Individuals vary considerably in the extent to which they demonstrate aging effects. By virtue of their vocal training and experience, voice professionals may differ from untrained speakers in the extent to which their voices show the effects of aging. Professional voice users also may have increased sensitivity to changes in their voices with aging. Indeed, there is some evidence that professional singers are generally more sensitive to voice and more apprehensive about vocal health, in comparison with nonsingers (Hogikyan, Appel, Guinn, & Haxer, 1999; Phyland, Oates, & Greenwood, 1999; Sapir, Mathers-Schmidt, & Larson, 1996).

In this chapter the aging professional voice is investigated. Consideration is given to the possibility that professional singers show fewer aging

effects on voice than nonsingers. Vocal aging effects with potential significance to professional voice users are presented. Finally, intervention measures that might assist the voice professional in minimizing the effects of
aging are discussed.

VOICE TRAINING AS AGING PREVENTION

It is possible to speculate about the effects of training on the process of
vocal aging. It has been suggested that professional singers are more
resistant to aging effects because they have learned techniques to preserve
optimal laryngeal functioning with aging and have practiced careful vocal
hygiene (Brown, Morris, Hollien, & Howell, 1991). Certainly, there is evidence that trained singers exhibit less muscular tension while singing than
do nonsingers (Koufman, Radomski, Joharji, Russell, & Pillsbury, 1996;
Sonninen & Hurme, 1998). If professional singers do employ voice conservation strategies, perhaps they tend to sound younger as they advance
in age than their nonprofessional counterparts. However, it also is possible
that professional singers tend to "wear out" the mechanism through extensive, although not necessarily abusive, vocal use and, therefore, may tend
to sound older than nonsingers. Finally, it is possible that aging effects
occur independently of vocal training/use and the two groups do not differ
in terms of relative vocal aging.

In considering the question of age-related voice preservation in professional singers, it is important to consider the speaking voice as well as
the singing voice. That is, can it be assumed that professional singers
employ the same (presumably voice saving) strategies with their speaking
voice as used when singing? Recent findings from a questionnaire distributed to female university professional singers and nonsingers indicate
otherwise. Indeed, singers were significantly more likely to report speech
habits considered vocally abusive than were nonsingers (Sapir et al.,
1996). This finding suggests that professional singers do not necessarily
transfer vocal hygiene practices incorporated when singing into speaking
situations. If this is the case, then voice practices during speech may counteract any potential age-related benefits derived from vocal hygiene practices during singing. Interestingly, in a second study, professional singers
were readily differentiated from nonsingers (age-matched; range = 22–65
years) from samples of singing, but not from speech samples (Brown,
Rothman, Sapienza, & Jarman, 1997). Acoustic analysis of speech samples
from the two groups confirmed perceptual results. That is, measures of
speaking fundamental frequency (SF_0) and standard deviation of fundamental frequency, as well as various timing aspects of connected speech,

failed to differentiate the two groups. While validating the significance of vocal training in altering singing voice (presumably for the better), these findings do not support a model in which years of professional training insulate a singer's speaking voice from age-related change.

Investigators have made some attempt to directly address the issue of relative preservation of voice with aging in professional singers (Brown, Morris, Hicks, & Howell, 1993; Brown et al., 1991). Specifically, young and elderly professional singers and nonsingers were compared on SF_0. Findings indicate that professional singers do not follow the pattern of aging change observed in nonsingers. Rather, singers tend to maintain stable SF_0 levels throughout their adult life, suggesting that this population is somewhat "immune" from aging affects leading to alterations in nonsingers. However, smoking histories of singers and nonsingers were not reported in these investigations. Because smoking is known to lower SF_0 (Gilbert & Weismer, 1974; Sorensen & Horii, 1982), this factor could have affected the findings. Indeed, one might assume that professional singers are less likely to smoke than are nonsingers. Therefore, findings of lower SF_0 levels for nonsingers may have resulted, at least in part, from the inclusion of some smokers among the nonsinger subject pool. A definitive conclusion that professional singers are resistant to age-related changes in SF_0 is not possible until singers and nonsingers are compared with smoking history controlled.

Phonational range measures also have been examined for evidence of relative preservation in singers. Findings indicate that professional singers demonstrate the same age-related reductions in phonational range (Brown et al., 1991) observed in nonsingers (Linville, 1987; Ptacek, Sander, Maloney, & Jackson, 1966). Apparently professional voice training does not significantly impact those age-related anatomical changes within the larynx related to restriction of pitch range (such as ossification/calcification of laryngeal cartilages and weakening of the cricothyroid muscle).

AGING EFFECTS ON THE PROFESSIONAL VOICE

Breath control strategies play an important role in voice production during singing (Thomasson & Sundberg, 1999). Therefore, any changes in pulmonary function with aging in the professional singer can have particular significance. Classically trained singers typically demonstrate large vital capacity requirements, substantial deformations of the chest wall, and rapid respiratory transitions (decreases/increases in abdominal, rib cage, and lung volumes) while singing (Watson & Hixon, 1985; Watson, Hixon, Stathopoulos, & Sullivan, 1990). Indeed, requirements for control of subglottal pressure in classical singing far exceed requirements during speech production (Sundberg, 1990). With the declines in pulmonary function brought about by aging, the older professional singer's career could be jeopardized (Mitchell, 1996).

Interestingly, respiratory kinematic patterns of professional country singers appear to resemble more closely untrained singers in that patterns during singing are similar to those used during speech production (Hoit, Jenks, Watson, & Cleveland, 1996). The implications for aging professional country singers is unclear. Perhaps pulmonary-related aging implications are lessened for professional country singers, because they have managed to sustain a successful career without requiring significant pulmonary adjustments above those required for speaking. On the other hand, the cumulative effects of years of performing without adjustments in respiratory behavior may "catch up" with country singers as they age and they may experience performance difficulties earlier than classically trained singers.

Oral cavity changes with aging have particular significance for professional voice users, as well as wind instrumentalists (Sataloff et al., 1997). Tooth loss could alter articulatory precision during an acting performance or singing recital and also could impair effectiveness of an instrumental concert. Sataloff et al. (1997) recommend that professional musicians and actors have dental impressions made before dentition is impaired to maximize satisfaction with dentures that are fashioned at a later time. Age-related changes in the oral mucosa including thinning and dehydration also could have special significance for the professional voice user. Xerostomia (dryness of the mouth) is a complaint of an estimated 25% of all elderly persons (Vissink, Spijkervet, & Van Nieuw Amerongen, 1996). Although oral dryness is often related to a disease process rather than the normal aging process (Chapter 4), the sensation of a dry mouth in a healthy older professional singer could be particularly disturbing to them (Sataloff et al., 1997).

Age-related hearing loss (presbycusis) is not a focus of this text. It is mentioned here because, although presbycusis affects the quality of life in all elderly persons with such a loss, the effects on the professional voice user can be particularly devastating. Singers rely on auditory feedback to monitor the quality of their performance and significant hearing loss or excessive tinnitus can spell the end of a musician's career (Palin, 1994; Sataloff, 1991). Interestingly, recent research suggests that the process of aging increases the sensitivity of the ear to noise-induced hearing loss (Miller, Dolan, Raphael, & Altschuler, 1998). A reasonable inference to draw from these findings is that older professional singers performing with loud back-up music are at increased risk of noise-induced hearing loss, even in comparison with younger singers performing in similar settings. Therefore, although it is important to urge hearing conservation measures even in young professional singers (Mitchell, 1996), that need may be even more urgent as singers age. Some interesting inferences might be drawn, as well, from a recent large-scale ($N = 1,097$) longitudinal study (30 years in duration) limited to individuals presenting no evidence of noise-induced hearing loss (Pearson et al., 1995). Findings indicate that, across the elderly population as a whole, hearing sensitivity declines at an earlier age in men than women. Further, the rate of decline with aging is more than twice as rapid in men than women. Thus, in might be inferred that male professional voice users are more at risk for age-related hearing loss than are their female counterparts.

Psychological and cognitive changes commonly observed in elderly persons are discussed in Chapters 1 and 17. Sataloff, Spiegel, et al. (1997) note that psychological changes with aging such as mood disorders and depression may impact older professional voice users through changes in affect and behavior. Presumably, such changes also could impact performance capability or result in loss of employment opportunities. Memory changes with aging (Hartke, 1991; Smith, 1996) also may influence performance capability or necessitate compensatory strategies during a performance.

COUNTERACTING AGING EFFECTS

Not all age-related changes are viewed as inevitable in professional voice users. Indeed, it is felt that many alterations may be avoided or postponed if appropriate measures are instituted (Sataloff, Rosen, Hawkshaw, & Spiegel, 1997; Sataloff, Spiegel, & Rosen, 1997). Such measures may include medical management or physical conditioning.

Medical Management

Vocal Fold Lubrication

Mitchell (1996) points to loss of lubrication in the larynx with aging and notes that many medications have an additional drying effect on the mucosa of the throat and larynx (Chapter 14). He notes that drying effects are exacerbated in elderly singers in whom the vocal folds may have become atrophied or edematous, resulting in suboptimal voice production. He recommends the use of certain medications (guaifenesin, pilocarpine, or potassium iodine), increased water intake, and/or elimination of mouth breathing to counteract these drying effects.

Thyroid Disorders

As discussed in Chapter 15, secretion disorders involving the thyroid gland occur quite commonly in the elderly. Furthermore, diagnosing thyroid

erly patients can be difficult because of problems with
ation, other disease processes masking symptoms, and
ritional variables affecting the results of thyroid function
er singer, a missed diagnosis of a thyroid disorder can be
particularly problematic because of implications for altered vocal quality,
loss of range, and declines in vocal efficiency. However, medical management of thyroid disease generally resolves these vocal changes (Sataloff,
Spiegel, & Rosen, 1997).

Hormone Replacement Therapy

As noted in Chapter 15, hormone replacement therapy (HRT) frequently is
suggested to women after menopause to aid in the prevention of heart
disease and to prevent osteoporosis (Abrams, 1998; Handa, Landerman,
Hanlon, Harris, & Cohen, 1996; Jolleys & Olesen, 1996; Leveille, LaCroix,
Newton, & Keenan, 1997; Phillipov, Mos, Scinto, & Phillips, 1997; Rozenberg et al., 1997; Saver, Taylor, Woods, & Stevens, 1997; Thompson, 1995).
Postmenopausal voice professionals presumably are counseled similarly to
the general population as to the benefits of HRT for prevention of disease.
However, HRT may be recommended to professional voice users for additional reasons as well (Abitbol, Abitbol, & Abitbol, 1999; Boulet & Oddens,
1996). Specifically, HRT may be prescribed to forestall changes in mucous
membrane linings of the vocal tract and age-related changes in body musculature (Irving, Epstein, & Harries, 1997; Sataloff, Spiegel, & Rosen,
1997). Hormone replacement also has been recommended to maintain
vocal range (Irving et al., 1997).

The potential side effect of masculinization of the larynx from a regi-
men of HRT is of particular concern to professional singers. Recent reports
have drawn attention to vocal changes, such as hoarseness, lowered pitch,
difficulty projecting, and loss of control over singing voice, resulting from
administration of medications containing virilizing agents. These voice
changes have adversely affected women's careers and social lives. While
withdrawal of hormonal medications reduces virilization effects to some
extent, some vocal changes are permanent (Baker, 1999; Gerritsma, Brocaar, Hakkesteegt, & Birkenhäger, 1994). It is imperative, therefore, that
any medication prescribed to voice professionals be androgen-free (Sataloff, Spiegel, & Rosen, 1997).

Gastroesophageal Reflux

Gastroesophageal reflux (GER) is discussed at some length in Chapter 17.
GER is the backward flow of gastric acid into the esophagus in the absence

of vomiting. In recent years, considerable attention has been paid to this phenomenon as a factor in many problems associated with the upper airway, including the larynx (Ahuja, Yencha, & Lassen, 1999; Deveney, Benner, & Cohen, 1993; Emami, Morrison, Rammage, & Bosch, 1999; Gaynor, 1991; Giacchi, Sullivan, & Rothstein, 2000; Jasani, Piterman, & McCall, 1999; Koufman, 1991; Powell et al., 2000; Sataloff, Spiegel, & Heuer, 1994; Toohill & Kuhn, 1997). Symptoms may include heartburn, hoarseness, sore throat, chronic cough/throat clearing, pharyngitis, esophagitis, halitosis, excessive phlegm, sensation of postnasal drip, contact ulcers, and globus pharyngeus. Laryngoscopic examination may reveal erythema of the posterior larynx as well as vocal fold edema (Ahuja et al., 1999). Because GER is considered common in the elderly (Middlemiss, 1997; Richter, 2000), older voice professionals may be at increased risk of developing symptoms arising from this condition in comparison with their younger counterparts. In mature performers, lifestyle factors such as eating late in the day or drinking alcohol after a performance may exacerbate symptoms of reflux (Boone, 1997). Treatment of GER includes use of antacids, acid-blocking medications, elevation of the head while sleeping, avoidance of highly spiced food, and refraining from eating or drinking within several hours of bedtime. Many patients' symptoms resolve when they comply with a treatment plan combining behavioral changes and prescription medications (Giacchi et al., 2000).

Physical Conditioning

Sataloff, Spiegel, and Rosen (1997) discuss the notion that each professional singer has a range of performance capability from poorest to best. An excellent young adult singer may be able to perform at only 50% of full potential and do so to the satisfaction of an audience, because of excellent physical conditioning. On the other hand, at a more advanced age, that singer may not meet the expected performance standards without functioning at 80%–90% of potential because of declining physical capabilities. These authors advocate the use of aerobic conditioning in combination with singing/acting training and voice therapy to restore vocal functioning in aging professional singers. Indeed, Sataloff, Spiegel, and Rosen (1997) urge the enforcement of high standards of physical conditioning for older singers and actors. They point out that older professional voice users are less resilient than their younger counterparts and cannot as easily compensate for weaknesses or recover quickly from injuries to the vocal mechanism. Reportedly, strategies of heightened physical conditioning are sufficient in the vast majority of patients with professional singing careers who develop vocal problems associated with aging. Only occasionally is it necessary to resort to laryngeal surgery to restore satisfactory voice.

Physical conditioning strategies recommended for aging professional singers are not that different from programs recommended for elderly nonsingers. That is, aerobic exercise (walking, swimming, jogging) is suggested to improve respiratory and abdominal conditioning and allow for maintenance of good respiratory control throughout a professional singing performance. Without such conditioning, an older singer may begin to compensate by using neck and tongue musculature excessively. With a program of regular physical conditioning, along with consistent vocal technical training, tremolo in the older singer reportedly can be eliminated. Endurance, agility, and accuracy also can be improved (Sataloff, Spiegel, & Rosen, 1997).

Training Techniques

A variety of training techniques may be employed with older professional voice users. To specifically target improved respiratory control in older singers, Westerman Gregg (1997) recommends realignment of posture and/or breathing exercises. Range-of-motion exercises also have been recommended for older professional singers to increase flexibility and strength and maintain the posture necessary for adequate breath support. Further, as noted by Mitchell (1996), actors require rapid articulatory gestures while performing. Therefore, exercises are recommended to strengthen tongue muscles and counteract possible atrophy of tongue musculature and optimize articulatory function. Mitchell (1996) advocates additional practice sessions and more rest breaks for aging performers. Finally, although it is important for all professional singers to utilize warm-up and cool-down exercises, the importance of such exercises in older singers is stressed due to possible age-related arthritic changes in the cricoarytenoid and temporomandibular joints (Mitchell, 1996).

SUMMARY

Definitive conclusions as to the effects of professional voice training and experience on aging of the vocal mechanism are not yet possible. Professional voice users may be more resistant than the general population to the effects of aging on the voice. On the other hand, professional voice users could demonstrate aging effects to a greater degree because of years of extensive, although not necessarily abusive, vocal use.

There is some evidence to support the notion that professional singers are insulated from the changes in SF_0 with aging that have been documented in nonsingers. However, until SF_0 findings are replicated on a population in whom smoking history is controlled, definitive conclusions on this issue are not possible. Findings of phonational range restrictions in older professional singers suggest that professional voice users undergo the same anatomical changes in laryngeal cartilages and muscles with aging that occur in nonsingers.

Breath control strategies are important in singing. Although age-related pulmonary changes have implications for classically trained singers, implications for professional country singers are less clear. Respiratory kinematic patterns in professional country singers more closely resemble nonsingers than classically trained singers. Oral cavity changes with aging can be significant both for wind instrumentalists and professional voice users. In particular, dentition changes and xerostomia could be disturbing. Age-related hearing loss is particularly devastating for a professional singer. Recent research suggests that, with aging, sensitivity of the ear to noise-induced hearing loss increases. It appears that older professional singers performing with loud back-up music are at increased risk of hearing loss, even in comparison with younger singers. Further, findings that hearing sensitivity declines at an earlier age in men than women, and that the decline proceeds at a faster rate, suggest that male singers are more at risk for age-related hearing loss than are females. Altered mood and depression may impact older professional voice users through changes in affect and behavior. Changes in memory with aging also may impact performance capability or necessitate compensatory strategies.

Age-related vocal changes are not necessarily inevitable in professional voice users. Medical management might include medications or increased water intake to increase vocal fold lubrication, prompt treatment of thyroid dysfunction, and/or hormone replacement therapy. Medical management of GER also may be necessary. The use of aerobic conditioning in combination with singing/acting training and voice therapy is recommended for aging professional singers. Reportedly, enforcement of high standards of physical conditioning in aging singers (walking, swimming, jogging) frequently is sufficient to overcome vocal problems associated with aging. In addition, range-of-motion, breathing, and tongue-strengthening exercises might be recommended, along with additional practice sessions and extended warm-up and cool-down exercises.

REFERENCES

Abitbol, J., Abitbol, P., & Abitbol, B. (1999). Sex hormones and the female voice. *Journal of Voice, 13*, 424–446.

Abrams, J. (1998). Hormones and the cardiologist. *Clinical Cardiology, 21*, 218–222.

Ahuja, V., Yencha, M., & Lassen, L. (1999). Head and neck manifestations of gastroesophageal reflux disease. *American Family Physician, 60,* 873–880, 885–886.

Baker, J. (1999). A report on alterations to the speaking and singing voices of four women following hormonal therapy with virilizing agents. *Journal of Voice, 13,* 496–507.

Boone, D. (1997). The three ages of voice. The singing/acting voice in the mature adult. *Journal of Voice, 11,* 161–164.

Boulet, M., & Oddens, B. (1996). Female voice changes around and after the menopause: An initial investigation. *Maturitas, 23,* 15–21.

Brown, W. S., Morris, R., Hicks, D., & Howell, E. (1993). Phonational profiles of female professional singers and nonsingers. *Journal of Voice, 7,* 219–226.

Brown, W. S., Morris, R., Hollien, H., & Howell, E. (1991). Speaking fundamental frequency characteristics as a function of age and professional singing. *Journal of Voice, 5,* 310–315.

Brown, W. S., Rothman, H., Sapienza, C., & Jarman, N. (1997, June). *Perceptual and acoustic study of professionally trained versus untrained voices.* Paper presented at the 26th annual symposium: Care of the Professional Voice, Philadelphia.

Deveney, C., Benner, K., & Cohen, J. (1993). Gastroesophageal reflux and laryngeal disease. *Archives of Surgery, 128,* 1021–1027.

Emami, A., Morrison, M., Rammage, L., & Bosch, D. (1999). Treatment of laryngeal contact ulcers and granulomas: A 12-year retrospective analysis. *Journal of Voice, 13,* 612–617.

Gaynor, E. (1991). Otolaryngologic manifestations of gastroesophageal reflux. *American Journal of Gastroenterology, 86,* 801–808.

Gerritsma, E., Brocaar, M., Hakkesteegt, M., & Birkenhäger, J. (1994). Virilization of the voice in post-menopausal women due to the anabolic steroid nandrolone decanoate (Decadurabolin). The effects of medication for one year. *Clinical Otolaryngology, 19,* 79–84.

Giacchi, R., Sullivan, D., & Rothstein, S. (2000). Compliance with anti-reflux therapy in patients with otolaryngologic manifestations of gastroesophageal reflux disease. *Laryngoscope, 110,* 19–22.

Gilbert, H., & Weismer, G. (1974). The effects of smoking on the speaking fundamental frequency of adult women. *Journal of Psycholinguistic Research, 3,* 225–231.

Handa, V., Landerman, R., Hanlon, J., Harris, T., & Cohen, H. (1996). Do older women use estrogen replacement? Data from the Duke Established Populations for Epidemiologic Studies of the Elderly (EPESE). *Journal of the American Geriatrics Society, 44,* 1–6.

Hartke, R. (1991). The aging process: Cognition, personality, and coping. In R. Hartke (Ed.) *Psychological aspects of geriatric rehabilitation* (pp. 45–71). Gaithersburg, MD: Aspen Publishers.

Hogikyan, N., Appel, S., Guinn, L., & Haxer, M. (1999). Vocal fold nodules in adult singers: Regional opinions about etiologic factors, career impact, and treatment. A survey of otolaryngologists, speech pathologists, and teachers of singing. *Journal of Voice, 13,* 128–142.

Hoit, J., Jenks, C., Watson, P., & Cleveland, T. (1996). Respiratory function during speaking and singing in professional country singers. *Journal of Voice, 10,* 39–49.

Irving, R., Epstein, R., & Harries, M. (1997). Care of the professional voice. *Clinical Otolaryngology, 22,* 202–205.

Jasani, K., Piterman, L., & McCall, L. (1999). Gastroesophageal reflux and quality of life. *Australian Family Physician, 28* (Suppl. 1), S15–S18.

Jolleys, J., & Olesen, F. (1996). A comparative study of prescribing of hormone replacement therapy in USA and Europe. *Maturitas, 23,* 47–53.

Koufman, J. (1991). The otolaryngologic manifestations of gastroesophageal reflux disease (GERD): A clinical investigation of 225 patients using ambulatory 24-hour pH monitoring and an experimental investigation of the role of acid and pepsin in the development of laryngeal injury. *Laryngoscope, 101,* 1–78.

Koufman, J., Radomski, T., Joharji, G., Russell, G., & Pillsbury, D. (1996). Laryngeal biomechanics of the singing voice. *Otolaryngology—Head and Neck Surgery, 115,* 527–537.

Leveille, S., LaCroix, A., Newton, K., & Keenan, N. (1997). Older women and hormone replacement therapy: Factors influencing late life initiation. *Journal of the American Geriatrics Society, 45,* 1496–1500.

Linville, S. E. (1987). Maximum phonational frequency range capabilities of women's voices with advancing age. *Folia Phoniatrica (Basel), 39,* 297–301.

Middlemiss, C. (1997). Gastroesophageal reflux disease: A common condition in the elderly. *Nurse Practitioner, 22,* 51–52, 55–59.

Miller, J., Dolan, D., Raphael, Y., & Altschuler, R. (1998). Interactive effects of aging with noise induced hearing loss. *Scandinavian Audiology 48* (Suppl.), 53–61.

Mitchell, S. (1996). Medical problems of professional voice users. *Comprehensive Therapy, 22,* 231–238.

Palin, S. (1994). Does classical music damage the hearing of musicians? A review of the literature. *Occupational Medicine, 44,* 130–136.

Pearson, J., Morrell, C., Gordon-Salant, S., Brant, L., Metter, E., Klein, L., & Fozard, J. (1995). Gender differences in a longitudinal study of age-associated hearing loss. *Journal of the Acoustical Society of America, 97,* 1196–1205.

Phillipov, G., Mos, E., Scinto, S., & Phillips, P. (1997). Initiation of hormone replacement therapy after diagnosis of osteoporosis by bone densitometry. *Osteoporosis International, 7,* 162–164.

Phyland, D., Oates, J., & Greenwood, K. (1999). Self-reported voice problems among three groups of professional singers. *Journal of Voice, 13,* 602–611.

Powell, D., Karanfilov, B., Beechler, K., Treole, K., Trudeau, M., & Forrest, L. (2000). Paradoxical vocal cord dysfunction in juveniles. *Archives of Otolaryngology—Head and Neck Surgery, 126,* 29–34.

Ptacek, P., Sander, E., Maloney, W., & Jackson, C. (1966). Phonatory and related changes with advanced age. *Journal of Speech and Hearing Research, 9,* 353–360.

Richter, J. (2000). Gastroesophageal reflux disease in the older patient: Presentation, treatment, and complications. *American Journal of Gastroenterology, 95,* 368–373.

Rozenberg, S., Kroll, M., Vandromme, J., Paesmans, M., Lefever, A., & Ham, H. (1997). Factors influencing the prescription of hormone replacement therapy. *Obstetrics and Gynecology, 90,* 387–391.

Sapir, S., Mathers-Schmidt, B., & Larson, G. (1996). Singers' and nonsingers' vocal health, vocal behaviours, and attitudes towards voice and singing: Indirect findings from a questionnaire. *European Journal of Communication, 31,* 193–209.

Sataloff, R. (1991). Hearing loss in musicians. *American Journal of Otolaryngology, 12,* 122–127.

Sataloff, R., Rosen, D., Hawkshaw, M., & Spiegel, J. (1997). The three ages of voice: The aging adult voice. *Journal of Voice, 11,* 156–160.

Sataloff, R., Spiegel, J., & Heuer, R. (1994). "Post-intubation granuloma:" A case of reflux and voice abuse. *Ear, Nose, and Throat Journal, 73,* 299.

Sataloff, R., Spiegel, J., & Rosen, D. (1997). The effects of age on the voice. In R. Sataloff (Ed.), *Professional voice: The science and art of clinical care* (2nd ed., pp. 259–267). San Diego: Singular Publishing Group.

Saver, B., Taylor, T., Woods, N., & Stevens, N. (1997). Physician policies on the use of preventive hormone therapy. *American Journal of Preventive Medicine, 13,* 358–365.

Smith, A. (1996). Memory. In J. Birren & K. Schaie (Eds.), *Handbook of the psychology of aging* (4th ed., pp. 236–250). San Diego: Academic Press.

Sonninen, A., & Hurme, P. (1998). Vocal fold strain and vocal pitch in singing: Radiographic observations of singers and nonsingers. *Journal of Voice, 12,* 274–286.

Sorensen, D., & Horii, Y. (1982). Cigarette smoking and voice fundamental frequency. *Journal of Communication Disorders, 15,* 135–144.

Sundberg, J. (1990). What's so special about singers? *Journal of Voice, 4,* 107–119.

Thomasson, M., & Sundberg, J. (1999). Consistency of phonatory breathing patterns in professional operatic singers. *Journal of Voice, 13,* 529–541.

Thompson, W. (1995). Estrogen replacement therapy in practice: Trends and issues. *American Journal of Obstetrics and Gynecology, 173,* 990–993.

Toohill, R., & Kuhn, J. (1997). Role of refluxed acid in pathogenesis of laryngeal disorders. *American Journal of Medicine, 103* (5A), 100S–106S.

Vissink, A., Spijkervet, F. & Van Nieuw Amerongen, A. (1996). Aging and saliva: A review of the literature. *Special Care in Dentistry, 16,* 95–103.

Watson, P., & Hixon, T. (1985). Respiratory kinematics in classical (opera) singers. *Journal of Speech and Hearing Research, 28,* 104–122.

Watson, P., Hixon, T., Stathopoulos, E., & Sullivan, D. (1990). Respiratory kinematics in female classical singers. *Journal of Voice, 4,* 120–128.

Westerman Gregg, J. (1997). The three ages of voice: The singing/acting mature adult—Singing instruction perspective. *Journal of Voice, 11,* 165–170.

14

The Aging Voice: Pharmacological Effects

Whether drugs are ingested, inhaled, injected intramuscularly, or injected intravenously they eventually enter the bloodstream at some level of concentration and circulate throughout the body. Fortunately, the impact of drugs on systems far distant from the target site frequently is clinically insignificant. However, many medications in common use do have an effect on the larynx. When treating patients with voice problems, voice professionals must be aware of laryngeal side effects both from prescription and nonprescription drug use (Lawrence, 1987). Laryngeal side effects may arise from drugs prescribed by an otolaryngologist for otologic problems, allergic disorders, or management of complications from surgery (Hoffmann, 1988). Laryngeal side effects also may arise from prescriptions provided by an internist or family medicine physician for airway conditions not necessarily requiring referral to an otolaryngologist. Finally, the larynx can be affected by prescription drug use for medical problems unrelated to otolaryngology.

Attention to drug use is important in treating patients of any age. However, drug use in the elderly requires particular vigilance, because of a number of issues unique to that population. Drugs are used disproportionately by the elderly, probably as a result of a higher incidence of chronic illness. Specifically, in 1988 elderly persons made up 12% of the population but accounted for 35% of expenditures for prescription drugs that year (Chrischilles et al., 1992). When nonprescription drugs are considered as well, it is estimated that elderly persons as a group use 50% of the drugs marketed in the United States and account for 30% of total drug costs (Lichtman, 1995). Nonetheless, the bulk of studies assessing drug efficacy are conducted on young patients (Girgis & Brooks, 1994; Yuen, 1990), despite the fact that many drugs have a differential effect on older persons and require alterations in dosage levels or dosage intervals to avoid negative side effects (Bressler & Katz, 1993; Greenblatt, Sellers, & Shader, 1982; Hurwitz, 1969; Kitts et al., 1990; Leventhal, 1999; Morris, 1994; Naranjo, Herrmann, Mittmann, & Brenner, 1995). Further, compliance difficulties increase in the elderly because of such factors as vision and hearing impairment, memory loss, and inadequate communication with health care providers. Elderly persons also are at increased risk of drug interactions because of the number of different drugs being administered (Kroner, Kelley, & Baranowski, 1994; Lichtman, 1995). Undoubtedly as a result of these factors, it has been estimated that elderly persons are 3 to 7 times as likely as young adults to have adverse drug reactions (Schmucker, 1978). Drugs cited most frequently as responsible for adverse reactions in the elderly include analgesics, antiarthritics, anticoagulants, antacids, antihypertensives, cardiac glycosides, diuretics, antimicrobials, steroids, and central nervous system drugs (Lamy, 1980).

In this chapter the special needs of elderly patients in the use of prescription and nonprescription medications are explored. In particular, drug effects on the elderly larynx are investigated. Further, potential effects of drugs on other aspects of elderly speech are considered.

DRUGS AFFECTING SPEECH AND VOICE

A number of sources are available for comprehensive reviews of medications having an effect on the larynx (Harris, 1992; Lawrence, 1987; Martin, 1988; Sataloff, Hawkshaw, & Rosen, 1997; Thompson, 1995). A listing of such medications as well as drugs affecting other aspects of speech production are found in Table 14–1. For comprehensive information on medications affecting swallowing, the reader is referred to Alvi (1999).

Drying of Laryngeal Mucosa

Lawrence (1987) notes that agents producing a drying effect on the vocal fold mucosa are the largest group of medications affecting the larynx. Such medications include antihistamines (also found in motion sickness prepa-

Table 14–1. Medications known to affect voice and speech.

Drying Effect on the Larynx			
Antihistamines	Antidepressants	Antidiarrheal agents	Amphetamines
Antitussives	Antipsychotics	Vitamin C (large doses)	Diuretics
Antihypertensives	Ulcer medications	Anticholinergic agents	Reflux medications
Propellants	Sleeping pills		

Moistening Effects on Laryngeal Mucosa/Thinning of Secretions
Mucolytic agents   Expectorants

Thickening of Laryngeal Secretions
Decongestants

Virilization of Larynx
Androgens (such as   Certain contraceptives   Certain breast cancer
   Danazol)   drugs

Hoarseness/Vocal Fold Bowing
Inhaled corticosteroids

Laryngeal Mucosal Hemorrhage
Aspirin (particularly in conjunction with vocal fold trauma)

Oral Cavity Drying (Xerostomia)				
Antihistamines	Decongestants	Antipsychotics	Antidepressants	Diuretics
Anti-Parkinson	Antispasmodics	Tranquilizers	Antihypertensive	Antiviral
drugs			agents	agents

Speech Rate (Dosage-Dependent/Inconsistent)
Antidepressants   Sedatives   Antipsychotics

Extrapyramidal Disorders
Antipsychotics   Calcium-channel blockers   Substituted benzamides

Note: Compiled from Gershanik (1994); Lawrence (1987); Sataloff, Hawkshaw, & Rosen, (1997); Segelman (1989); Thompson, (1995); and Waskow (1966).

rations), antitussives, antihypertensive agents, propellants, antidepressants, antipsychotic agents, sleeping pills, anticholinergic agents, amphetamines, and diuretics. In addition, medications used in treating gastric ulcers/gastric reflux, antidiarrheal agents, as well as large doses of vitamin C are known to have drying effects on vocal tract secretions. Although clinicians generally consider caffeine also to have a drying effect on laryngeal mucosa, scientific evidence of mucosal drying from caffeine is lacking (Akhtar, Wood, Rubin, O'Flynn, & Ratcliffe, 1999).

Drugs also can affect the viscosity of laryngeal secretions, with negative effects on voice production. Decongestants, for instance, usually thicken laryngeal secretions. Thickening and drying of secretions of the upper respiratory tract from drug effects is compounded by exposure to dry environmental conditions (Lawrence, 1987). Drying effects are not restricted to the larynx, however. Xerostomia of the oral cavity has been reported as a side-effect of more than 200 drugs, including antihistamines, anti-Parkinson drugs, antihypertensives, antispasmodics, decongestants, diuretics, antidepressants, tranquilizers, and antipsychotics (Baum, 1983; Segelman, 1989).

Moistening of Laryngeal Mucosa

Thompson (1995) points out that most agents with beneficial laryngeal effects act by moistening the mucosa. Mucolytic agents or expectorants (guaifenesin, Humibid, Entex) are used most often for this purpose. While stressing that such agents do not substitute for good hydration, Sataloff et al. (1997) point out that expectorants and mucolytics can be helpful in counteracting mucosal dehydration resulting from (1) athletic or recreational activities, (2) antihistamine use, or (3) environmental factors. These authors also report that such agents are helpful for singers who complain of frequent throat clearing, thick secretions, or postnasal drip.

Virilization

Virilization of the larynx in women can occur as a consequence of side effects from medications containing androgens. The term androgen is generic and refers to any agent (usually a hormone) that encourages the development of male sexual characteristics (McDonough, 1994). For example, danazol is a synthetic derivative of testosterone used in the treatment of endometriosis (Wood, Wu, Flickinger, & Mikhail, 1975). Since danazol exhibits weak androgenic properties (American Hospital Formulary Service, 1997), use of this drug, particularly with female professional singers, is problematic because of potential side effects involving deepening of the voice (Barbieri, Evans, & Kistner, 1982; Buttram, Belue, & Reiter, 1982; Mercaitis, Peaper, & Schwartz, 1985). Similarly, women requiring treatment for breast cancer should be counseled about potential virilizing effects on the larynx of drugs they are administered (Lawrence, 1987). Early contraceptive medications also produced some virilizing effects due to relatively high progesterone content. However, modifications in birth control preparations appear to have successfully eliminated this undesirable side effect. Nonetheless, women who are professional voice users may be advised to undergo regular voice evaluations when taking oral contraceptives (Wendler et al., 1995).

Lawrence (1987) reported that permanent, structural alterations in the laryngeal mechanism occur only rarely in women as a consequence of androgenic medication, although the permanence of such changes is open to debate (Baker, 1999; Brodnitz, 1971; Damste, 1964, 1967). Indeed, Lawrence (1987) concedes that factors such as patient age, treatment duration, and dosage are factors that influence the permanency of observed laryngeal effects. Presumably, the younger the woman, the greater the likelihood of intractable laryngeal changes.

Laryngeal Effects From Steroids

Steroidal medications are prescribed to manage a variety of otolaryngologic conditions, including infections, trauma, and immunologic disorders. Steroids are used primarily for their anti-inflammatory properties, which result in decreased edema and cellular destruction. These effects are palliative, however, and do not treat the underlying cause of the inflammation. Steroid dosage is essentially empirical, and misuse of steroids can lead to serious complications in many body systems (Hoffmann, 1988).

Among the body systems adversely affected by steroids is the larynx. Specifically, bowing of the vocal folds with accompanying dysphonia has been reported as a side effect of inhaled corticosteroids prescribed in the treatment of asthma. Fungal growth on the vocal folds (laryngeal candidiasis) also can occur as a side effect of inhaled steroids, either with or without the apparent vocal fold myopathy evidenced by vocal fold bowing (Shenoi & Williams, 1984; Williams et al., 1983).

Interestingly, even patients receiving placebo inhalers occasionally demonstrate hoarseness, suggesting that propellants, in general, are irritating to vocal fold tissues (Campbell, 1984). Indeed, even automobile exhaust fumes have been mentioned as a source of irritation to the tissues of the larynx (Lawrence, 1987). Although these nonsteroidal agents can produce dysphonia, they have not been associated with glottal gap. Further, glottal gap observed in association with inhaled corticosteroids has been found to eventually resolve if the steroidal component of the inhaled preparation is eliminated, even if use of inhalants is continued (Williams et al., 1983). This observation suggests that steroids, rather than inhalants in general, show a capacity for myopathy within the larynx.

In elderly patients, steroids might be prescribed in the treatment of chronic obstructive pulmonary disease (Morris, 1994). At present no information is available on possible increased risk for laryngeal side effects from steroid use in the elderly population. However, there is evidence that age-related factors exacerbate the effects of some drugs in the elderly. It would seem prudent, therefore, for physicians to exercise caution in prescribing steroids to elderly patients. Further, careful monitoring of older patients while receiving treatment with these agents would appear wise.

Other Drug Effects

Limited information is available on drugs producing effects on nonphonatory aspects of speech production. Waskow (1966) reviewed such effects and noted that certain antidepressant drugs (pipradrol), sedatives (sodium pentobarbital) and antipsychotics (chlorpromazine, phenothiazine) affect speech rate. However, those effects may be dosage dependent and are inconsistent from patient to patient (Ostwald, 1961; Starkweather & Hargreaves, 1964). In addition, Waskow (1966) pointed out that methodological factors, such as the type of speech sample elicited and instructions given to patients, may have confounded results in these studies rendering valid conclusions impossible. Nonetheless, before concluding that an elderly patient's slowed speaking rate reflects normal aging (Chapter 9), clinicians need to be mindful of the potential influence of medications on speech rate.

Treatment with antipsychotic drugs, calcium-channel blockers, and substituted benzamides has been linked with extrapyramidal disorders that adversely affect speech and voice. Specifically, drug-induced Parkinsonism and tardive dyskinesia have developed in some patients receiving these medications. Antipsychotic drugs are prescribed for a number of different psychiatric illnesses, including dementia, schizophrenia, delirium, delusions, and mood disorders (Pollock & Mulsant, 1995). Calcium-channel blocking agents are used in the treatment of hypertension, angina, and cardiac arrhythmias. Substituted benzamides are used in the treatment of gastrointestinal disorders, including reflux (American Hospital Formulary Service, 1997; Gershanik, 1994).

It has been estimated that drug-induced Parkinsonism accounts for roughly 4% of all cases of Parkinsonism treated in neurology clinics and is substantially more common among institutionalized psychiatric patients (Gershanik, 1994; Stacy & Jankovic, 1992). Although dependent on the potency, dose, and duration of drug treatment, drug-induced Parkinsonism resulting from antipsychotics may occur in up to 75% of patients (Ganzini, Heintz, Hoffman, Keepers, & Casey, 1991) and can persist for a significant period of time after the medication is withdrawn. Estimates in earlier investigations placed resolution of symptoms at up to 36 weeks after discontinuation of drug treatment (Peabody, Warner, Whiteford, & Hollister, 1987; Wilson & MacLennan, 1989). More recently, complete remission of symptoms was estimated at 26 to 78 weeks (Gershanik, 1994).

Elderly persons are particularly prone to drug-induced extrapyramidal disorders (Gershanik, 1994; Pollock & Mulsant, 1995). For instance, tardive dyskinesia occurs very frequently in elderly patients with antipsychotic drug treatment, even at relatively low dosages, for relatively short periods of time (Jeste, Lacro, Gilbert, Kline, & Kline, 1993; Saltz et al., 1991).

Because of the increased potential for adverse reactions to antipsychotics in older patients, physicians have been advised to prescribe these drugs at lower potencies and in minimal doses in the elderly, while watching carefully for extrapyramidal symptoms. Indeed, in patients receiving any medications with antidopaminergic properties, it is important for physicians to detect extrapyramidal symptoms early and to withdraw the medication whenever possible (Gershanik, 1994; Pollock & Mulsant, 1995).

DIFFERENTIAL EFFECTS OF DRUGS IN THE ELDERLY

Drug effects on elderly persons is a complex issue. Although many drugs have a differential effect on the elderly, others may not. For instance, studies of certain oral anticoagulants have yielded conflicting results. Several studies indicated that elderly patients demonstrate a greater anticoagulant response to coumarin agents than young patients (Husted & Andreasen, 1977; Levine, Hirsh, Landefeld & Raskob, 1992; van der Meer, Rosendaal, Vandenbroucke, & Briet, 1993); others showed no age-related differences (Jones, Baran, & Reidenberg, 1980). As noted previously, a number of drugs affect the larynx and, consequently, have an effect on voice. Also, medications can affect speech rate and articulatory precision. If these drugs are used by elderly patients, will speech production be differentially affected? To date, no data are available to answer that question. However, there is information on differences in drug absorption, distribution, and clearance as a function of age. Perhaps, understanding basic differences in drug processing by the elderly will shed some light on this issue.

Pharmacokinetics

Properties of a drug considered pharmacokinetic relate to the disposition of the drug in the body. Specifically, the following parameters are included in this category: (1) absorption from the administration site, (2) dispersion throughout the body, and (3) elimination from the body. In short, pharmacokinetics includes all processes that affect a drug's concentration at the target site (Goldberg & Roberts, 1983).

   Although drugs can be administered in a number of ways (for example by inhalation or injection), the most common method of administration is oral. Absorption of drugs, therefore, is most commonly accomplished through the gastrointestinal (GI) tract. With aging, changes in GI structure and function have the cumulative effect of slowing the absorption of drugs. In addition, absorption is less complete and generally less predictable and reliable in elderly persons. However, although drug absorption is slowed somewhat by age-related changes in the GI tract, those changes are felt to be less significant to changes in drug absorption in the elderly than either (1) disease processes associated with aging or (2) interaction effects resulting from simultaneous administration of multiple drugs (Goldberg & Roberts, 1983; Lichtman, 1995; Lovat, 1996).

Drug distribution throughout the body in elderly patients may be affected by age-related changes in body weight. Elderly persons, on average, have lower body weight than young adults. Therefore, an elderly person administered the same daily dose of a medication given to a young adult is likely to be receiving a higher weight-corrected dosage. An inadvertent increase in dosage level increases the likelihood of adverse reactions in the elderly patient (Greenblatt et al., 1982). This enhancement effect theoretically could be reversed, either by reducing the dosage of the drug or increasing the interval between doses for elderly patients (Schaefer & Michaelis, 1994).

Weight-related drug dosage adjustments in the elderly are complicated by age-related body composition changes. In both men and women, the proportion of total body weight composed of fat tissue increases with aging. That is, the lean body mass declines, on average, and the ratio of fat to lean body mass increases (Bruce, Andersson, Arvidsson, & Isaksson, 1980). The effect of changing body composition on drug absorption in the elderly depends on a drug's solubility. Some drugs are relatively water soluble and lipid insoluble, decreasing the distribution of these drugs in elderly patients. Other medications are lipid soluble and would tend to be more extensively distributed in the elderly and, therefore, more highly concentrated, particularly if hepatic and renal functions are impaired (Girgis & Brooks, 1994; Greenblatt et al., 1982). An additional factor complicating dosage adjustment in the elderly is the finding that men and women may differ in age-related drug distribution changes (Greenblatt et al., 1982).

It must be remembered, also, that gender differences in body composition, regardless of age, have profound influence on the variable of drug distribution. At all age levels, women have a higher percentage of body fat than do men. Therefore, women tend to more readily distribute lipid-soluble drugs in comparison with men, while demonstrating less extensive distribution of drugs that are water-soluble. These gender differences in body composition may have more profound impact on drug distribution than do trends for age-related differences (Greenblatt et al., 1982).

Elimination of a drug from the body is best indicated by a measure known as total clearance. Total clearance is the unit of time in which a hypothetical volume of blood is completely cleared of a given drug. For most drugs, total clearance is accomplished by either the kidneys or liver. In general, drug clearance in the elderly is reduced in comparison with young adults (Greenblatt et al., 1982; Rupp, Castagnoli, Fisher, & Miller, 1987). Reasons for declining drug clearance in the elderly include depression of hepatic enzyme activity (Greenblatt, Abernethy, Matlis, Harmatz, & Shader, 1984; Richardson, Blocka, Ross, & Verbeeck, 1985), reduced hepatic blood flow (Geokas & Haverback, 1969), decreased liver size (Thompson & Williams, 1965), and reduction in glomerular filtration rate (Friedman, Raizner, Rosen, Solomon, & Sy, 1972; Rowe, Andres, & Tobin, 1976). Total clearance is the primary factor determining the extent to which a drug accumulates in the body during multiple dosing. In other words, if aging reduces the efficiency of drug-clearance mechanisms, then enhancement of a drug's effects (either therapeutic or toxic) might be expected in elderly patients.

Changes in liver enzyme activity and kidney function make elderly patients more susceptible than young adults to adverse effects from a variety of drugs (Girgis & Brooks, 1994; Morris, 1994). However, just as drug distribution changes with aging may not be identical in men and women, evidence suggests that age-related changes in drug clearance differ as a function of gender. Some drugs are that are biotransformed by oxidative mechanisms, such as certain sedatives/anxiety reducing agents (diazepam, alprazolam) and pain relieving agents (antipyrine), clear much slower in men with aging. In contrast, women show much less of an aging effect (Greenblatt et al., 1982). Unfortunately, many medications commonly prescribed to elderly patients lack definitive data on age-related differences in drug clearance. For this reason physicians are urged to exercise caution in prescribing any drugs to the elderly (Greenblatt et al., 1982).

Pharmacodynamics

Pharmacodynamics pertains to the relationship between the measurable concentration of a given drug and its effect. In other words, this measure relates to the response of the intended organ system to the drug (Pollock & Mulsant, 1995; Segelman, 1989). In comparison with pharmacokinetics, relatively little attention has been given to changes in pharmacodynamic factors of drug action with aging (Goldberg & Roberts, 1983). In humans, testing of pharmacodynamics is difficult and few studies have demonstrated in a convincing manner that aging increases drug sensitivity (Greenblatt et al., 1982). It is believed, however, that advancing age is associated with increased drug intolerance because of the diminished functional capacity of many organ systems (Bender, 1964, 1969; Vestal, 1978). That is, because of an age-related decline in the general "intactness" of cells throughout the body, older tissues are less tolerant of the action of drugs at a cellular level than are the tissues in a young adult body (Exton-Smith & Windsor, 1979). In particular, transmembrane transport functions, cellular anoxia, abnormal protein synthesis, and increased DNA repair in older cells have been discussed as confounding factors affecting pharmacodynamics in the elderly (Balducci & Mowry, 1992). The practical significance of these differences to drug tolerance in elderly patients may be minimal, however, at least with respect to anticancer drugs (Lichtman, 1995).

SPECIAL CONSIDERATIONS: DRUG USE IN THE ELDERLY

Multiple Drug Use

In geriatric medicine, multiple pathology is the rule rather than the exception (Davison, 1978). Patients with multiple medical problems are more likely to see several physicians, increasing the likelihood of multiple drug use (Bowen & Larson, 1993). As the number of prescription medications increases, the risk of unwanted side effects increases. Many drugs alter the pharmacokinetics of other drugs used concomitantly, producing unexpected results. The therapeutic effect of one or both drugs may be nullified or unforeseen unwanted effects may occur. For example, when an elderly patient is treated with warfarin, the physician must deal with the fact that there are a number of medications known to interfere with the anticoagulant action of the drug (Davison, 1978).

Negative side effects from multiple medications in the elderly are recognized as a significant medical problem. A common side effect of medications is cognitive impairment. Drug-induced cognitive impairment is an underrecognized disorder that occurs more frequently in the elderly, particularly in those with multiple diseases. The risk of drug-induced cognitive impairment increases with multiple drug use, especially if four or more medications are prescribed (Larson, Kukull, Buchner, & Reifler, 1987). Drug classes frequently found to cause confusional states include sedatives, antidepressants, antipsychotic agents, anti-Parkinsonian drugs, anticonvulsants, antihypertensives, antiarrhythmics, antibiotics, pulmonary medications, corticosteroids, and antineoplastic agents. Analgesics (pain relievers) also can cause confusional states, particularly nonsteroidal anti-inflammatory agents (NSAIDS) and aspirin. In the elderly, a safer choice of analgesic is acetaminophen, which has not been associated with confusional states (Bowen & Larson, 1993). Confusion disorders resulting from multiple drug use are particularly troubling to health care providers, because a patient in a confused state is at greater risk of additional side effects from drugs because of multiple dosing, missed dosages, or medication errors.

To minimize the likelihood of unwanted effects from multiple drug use, physicians have been warned to avoid medications in the elderly unless needed and beneficial (Bowen & Larson, 1993; Davison, 1978; Owens, Fretwell, Willey, & Murphy, 1994). Physicians have been urged to adopt a philosophy in which drugs are not viewed as a panacea in treating elderly patients. There is increasing recognition that social stress plays an important role in the problems exhibited by the elderly. Physicians have been encouraged to develop strategies of treatment in which nondrug therapies are considered (Davison, 1978). It has been recommended, as well, that physicians review drug use with elderly patients at each visit and beware of unseen drug use, such as alcohol and over-the-counter medications (Bowen & Larson, 1993).

Side effects from multiple drug use specifically pertaining to speech and voice have not been investigated to date. It is possible to speculate, however, that the potential for such effects increases as multiple drugs are consumed. Given the complex nature of speech production, it seems intuitive that drug interactions could have consequences that may interfere at some level with that process. It seems that the best advice for elderly patients is to avoid unnecessary drug use altogether, whether from prescription or over-the-counter.

Compliance Factors

Problems arising from noncompliance in drug taking involve either side effects from overdosing or failure to achieve a therapeutic aim from missed dosages. Among patients over the age of 65 years, 40%–45% fail to take their prescription drugs as prescribed (Morrow, Leirer, & Sheikh, 1988). Recent data suggests that a primary reason for poor compliance in drug usage in elderly patients is inadequate communication between patients and physicians (Kessler, 1991). As noted previously, there is a need for physicians to review dosing instructions with elderly patients. In addition, providers have been encouraged to set dosage schedules in a manner consistent with an elderly patient's lifestyle and to use explicit labeling to maximize the likelihood of compliance (Kroner et al., 1994). Arranging for friends or family members to supervise medications may be a useful strategy to avoid problems with compliance because of factors such as memory impairment (Girgis & Brooks, 1994).

SUMMARY

In treating the elderly, health care professionals need to be aware of potential side effects involving speech and voice production arising from prescription and nonprescription medications. Drying of laryngeal mucosa, virilization of voice, bowing of the vocal folds, fungal growth on the vocal folds, hoarseness, slowing of speech rate, and extrapyramidal speech and voice symptoms are effects that have been observed as a consequence of drug treatment.

Elderly patients are likely to be particularly sensitive to adverse effects of drugs because of altered drug pharmacokinetics (absorption, dispersion, and elimination) and pharmacodynamics (response to drug action). In addition, because multiple pathology in the elderly is the rule rather than the exception, multiple drug use is more common in older patients. As the number of prescription medications increases, the likelihood of unwanted side effects also increases. To minimize the likelihood of unwanted side effects in elderly patients, physicians are urged to develop strategies of treatment in which nondrug therapies are considered. Further, physicians are encouraged to review drug use with patients on a regular basis. Noncompliance in drug taking also increases in the elderly. Poor compliance is frequently linked to inadequate communications between patients and physicians. Explicit labeling of prescription medications and supervision of medications by family members are potential strategies to avoid compliance problems.

REFERENCES

Akhtar, S., Wood, G., Rubin, J., O'Flynn, P., & Ratcliffe, P. (1999). Effect of caffeine on the vocal folds: A pilot study. *Journal of Laryngology and Otology, 113,* 341–345.

Alvi, A. (1999). Iatrogenic swallowing disorders: Medications. In R. Carrau & T. Murry (Eds.), *Comprehensive management of swallowing disorders* (pp. 119–129). San Diego: Singular Publishing Group.

American Hospital Formulary Service. (1997). *Drug information.* Bethesda, MD: American Society of Health-System Pharmacists, Inc.

Baker, J. (1999). A report on alterations to the speaking and singing voices of four women following hormonal therapy with virilizing agents. *Journal of Voice, 13,* 496–507.

Balducci, L., & Mowry, K. (1992). Pharmacology and organ toxicity of chemotherapy in older patients. *Oncology, 6* (Suppl) 62–68.

Barbieri, R., Evans, S., & Kistner, R. (1982). Danazol in the treatment of endometriosis: Analysis of 100 cases with a 4-year follow-up. *Fertility and Sterility, 37,* 737–746.

Baum, B. (1983). Xerostomia is drug-related. *Dentistry Today, 4,* 25.

Bender, A. (1964). Pharmacologic aspects of aging. A survey of the effect of increasing age on drug activity in adults. *Journal of the American Geriatric Society, 12,* 114–134.

Bender, A. (1969). Geriatric pharmacology. Age and its influence on drug action in adults. *Drug Information Bulletin, 3,* 153.

Bowen, J., & Larson, E. (1993). Drug-induced cognitive impairment: Defining the problem and finding solutions. *Drugs and Aging, 3,* 349–357.

Bressler, R., & Katz, M. (1993). Drug therapy for geriatric depression. *Drugs and Aging, 3,* 195–219.

Brodnitz, F. (1971). Hormones and the human voice. *Bulletin of the New York Academy of Medicine, 47,* 183–191.

Bruce, A., Andersson, M., Arvidsson, B., & Isaksson, B. (1980). Body composition. Prediction of normal body potassium, body water and body fat in adults on the basis of body height, body weight and age. *Scandinavian Journal of Clinical Laboratory Investigation, 40,* 461–473.

Buttram, V., Belue, J., & Reiter, R. (1982). Interim report of a study of danazol for the treatment of endometriosis. *Fertility and Sterility, 37,* 478–483.

Campbell, I. (1984). Inhaled steroids and dysphonia. *Lancet, 8379,* 744.

Chrischilles, E., Foley, D., Wallace, R., Lemke, J., Semla, T., Hanlon, J., Glynn, R., Ostfeld, A., & Guralnik, J. (1992). Use of medication by persons 65 and over: Data from the established populations for epidemiologic studies of the elderly. *Journal of Gerontology Medical Sciences, 47,* M137–M144.

Damste, P. (1964). Virilization of voice due to anabolic steroids. *Folia Phoniatrica, 16,* 10–18.

Damste, P. (1967). Voice change in adult women caused by virilizing agents. *Journal of Speech and Hearing Disorders, 32,* 126–132.

Davison, W. (1978). The hazards of drug treatment in old age. In J. Brocklehurst (Ed.), *Textbook of geriatric medicine and gerontology* (2nd ed., pp. 651–669). New York: Churchill Livingstone.

Exton-Smith, A., & Windsor, A. (1979). Principles of drug treatment in the aged. In I. Rossman (Ed.), *Clinical geriatrics* (2nd ed., pp. 132–138). Philadelphia: J. B. Lippincott Company.

Friedman, S., Raizner, A., Rosen, H., Solomon, N., & Sy, W. (1972). Functional defects in the aging kidney. *Annals of Internal Medicine, 76,* 41–45.

Ganzini, L., Heintz, R., Hoffman, W., Keepers, G., & Casey, D. (1991). Acute extrapyramidal syndromes in neuroleptic-treated elders: A pilot study. *Journal of Geriatric Psychiatry and Neurology, 4,* 222–225.

Geokas, M., & Haverback, B. (1969). The aging gastrointestinal tract. *American Journal of Surgery, 117,* 881–892.

Gershanik, O. (1994). Drug-induced Parkinsonism in the aged: Recognition and prevention. *Drugs and Aging, 5,* 127–132.

Girgis, L., & Brooks, P. (1994). Nonsteroidal anti-inflammatory drugs: Differential use in older patients. *Drugs and Aging, 4,* 101–112.

Goldberg, P., & Roberts, J. (1983). Pharmacologic basis for developing rational drug regimens for elderly patients. *Symposium on Clinical Geriatric Medicine, Medical Clinics of North America, 67,* 315–331.

Greenblatt, D., Abernethy, D., Matlis, R., Harmatz, J., & Shader, R. (1984). Absorption and disposition of ibuprofen in the elderly. *Arthritis and Rheumatism, 27,* 1066–1069.

Greenblatt, D., Sellers, E., & Shader, R. (1982). Drug therapy: Drug disposition in old age. *New England Journal of Medicine, 306,* 1081–1088.

Harris, T. (1992). The pharmacological treatment of voice disorders. *Folia Phoniatrica (Basel), 44,* 143–154.

Hoffmann, D. (1988). Use of steroids in otolaryngology. *Ear, Nose and Throat Journal, 67,* 71-73, 76-78, 83.

Hurwitz, N. (1969). Predisposing factors in adverse reactions to drugs. *British Medical Journal, 1,* 536–539.

Husted, S., & Andreasen, F. (1977). The influence of age on the response to anticoagulants. *British Journal of Clinical Pharmacology, 4,* 559–565.

Jeste, D., Lacro, J., Gilbert, P., Kline, J., & Kline, N. (1993). Treatment of late-life schizophrenia with neuroleptics. *Schizophrenia Bulletin, 19,* 817–830.

Jones, B., Baran, A., & Reidenberg, M. (1980). Evaluating patients' warfarin requirements. *Journal of the American Geriatric Society, 28,* 10–12.

Kessler, D. (1991). Communicating with patients about their medications. *New England Journal of Medicine, 325,* 1650–1652.

Kitts, J., Fisher, D., Canfell, P., Spellman, M., Caldwell, J., Heier, T., Fahey, M., & Miller, R. (1990). Pharmacokinetics and pharmacodynamics of atracurium in the elderly. *Anesthesiology, 72,* 272–275.

Kroner, B., Kelley, C., & Baranowski, E. (1994). Labeling deficiencies and communication problems leading to medication misuse in the elderly. *Drugs and Aging, 5,* 403–410.

Lamy, P. (1980). *Prescribing for the elderly.* Littleton, MA: PSG Publishing Company.

Larson, E., Kukull, W., Buchner, D., & Reifler, B. (1987). Adverse drug reactions associated with global cognitive impairment in elderly persons. *Annals of Internal Medicine, 107,* 169–173.

Lawrence, V. (1987). Common medications with laryngeal effects. *Ear, Nose and Throat Journal, 66,* 318–322.

Leventhal, K. (1999). Aging & medications: An overview. *ASHA, 1,* 34–38.

Levine, M., Hirsh, J., Landefeld, S., & Raskob, G. (1992). Hemorrhagic complications of anticoagulant treatment. *Chest, 102*(Suppl.), 352–363.

Lichtman, S. (1995). Physiological aspects of aging: Implications for the treatment of cancer. *Drugs and Aging, 7,* 212–225.

Lovat, L. (1996). Age related changes in gut physiology and nutritional status. *Gut, 38,* 306–309.

Martin, F. (1988). Drugs and vocal function. *Journal of Voice, 2,* 338–344.

McDonough, J. (Ed.). (1994). *Stedman's concise medical dictionary* (2nd Ed). Baltimore: Williams & Wilkins.

Mercaitis, P., Peaper, R., & Schwartz, P. (1985). Effect of Danazol on vocal pitch: A case study. *Obstetrics and Gynecology, 65,* 131–135.

Morris, J. (1994). Physiological changes due to age: Implications for respiratory drug therapy. *Drugs and Aging, 4,* 207–220.

Morrow, D., Leirer, V., & Sheikh, J. (1988). Adherence and medication instructions: Review and recommendations. *Journal of the American Geriatric Society, 36,* 1147–1160.

Naranjo, C., Herrmann, N., Mittmann, N., & Brenner, K. (1995). Recent advances in geriatric psychopharmacology. *Drugs and Aging, 7,* 184–202.

Ostwald, P. (1961). The sounds of emotional disturbance. *Archives of General Psychiatry, 5,* 587–592.

Owens, N., Fretwell, M., Willey, C., & Murphy, S. (1994). Distinguishing between the fit and frail elderly, and optimizing pharmacotherapy. *Drugs and Aging, 4,* 47–55.

Peabody, C., Warner, M., Whiteford, H., & Hollister, L. (1987). Neuroleptics and the elderly. *Journal of the American Geriatrics Society, 35,* 233–238.

Pollock, B., & Mulsant, B. (1995). Antipsychotics in older patients: A safety perspective. *Drugs and Aging, 6,* 312–323.

Richardson, C., Blocka, K., Ross, S., & Verbeec, R. (1985). Effects of age and sex on piroxicam disposition. *Clinical Pharmacology and Therapeutics, 37,* 13–18.

Rowe, J., Andres, R., & Tobin, J. (1976). Age-adjusted standards for creatinine clearance [letter]. *Annals of Internal Medicine, 84,* 567–569.

Rupp, S., Castagnoli, K., Fisher, D., & Miller, R. (1987). Pancuronium and vercuronium pharmacokinetics and pharmacodynamics in younger and elderly adults. *Anesthesiology, 67,* 45–49.

Saltz, B., Woerner, M., Kane, J., Lieberman, J., Alvir, J., Bergmann, K., Blank, K., Koblenzer, J., & Kahaner, K. (1991). Prospective study of tardive dyskinesia incidence in the elderly. *Journal of the American Medical Association, 266,* 2402–2406.

Sataloff, R., Hawkshaw, M., & Rosen, D. (1997). Medications: Effects and side effects in professional voice users. In R. Sataloff (Ed.), *Professional voice: The science and art of clinical care* (pp. 457–470). San Diego: Singular Publishing Group.

Schaefer, H., & Michaelis, J. (1994). Biopharmaceutical aspects of anti-infective therapy at the extremes of age. *Journal of Antimicrobial Chemotherapy, 34* (Suppl. A), A33–A42.

Schmucker, D. (1978). Age-related changes in drug disposition. *Pharmacological Review, 30,* 445–456.

Segelman, A. (1989). Oral manifestations of drug therapies in the geriatric patient. *Dental Clinics of North America, 33,* 67–73.

Shenoi, P., & Williams, A. (1984). Inhaled steroids and dysphonia. *Lancet, 8376,* 577.

Stacy, M., & Jankovic, J. (1992). Differential diagnosis of Parkinson's disease and the Parkinsonism plus syndromes. *Neurology Clinics, 10,* 341–359.

Starkweather, J., & Hargreaves, W. (1964). The influence of sodium pentobarbital on vocal behavior. *Journal of Abnormal and Social Psychology, 69,* 123–126.

Thompson, A. (1995). Pharmacological agents with effects on voice. *American Journal of Otolaryngology, 16,* 12-18.

Thompson, E., & Williams, R. (1965). Effect of age on liver function with particular reference to Bromsulphalein excretion. *Gut, 6,* 266–269.

van der Meer, F., Rosendaal, F., Vandenbroucke, J., & Briet, E. (1993). Bleeding complications in oral anticoagulant therapy. *Archives of Internal Medicine, 153,* 1557–1562.

Vestal, R. (1978). Drug use in the elderly: A review of problems and special considerations. *Drugs, 16,* 358-382.

Waskow, I. (1966). The effects of drugs on speech: A review. *Psychopharmacology Bulletin, 3,* 1–20.

Wendler, J., Siegert, C., Schelhorn, P., Klinger, G., Gurr, S., Kaufmann, J., Aydinlik, S., & Braunschweig, T. (1995). The influence of microgynon and Diane-35, two sub-fifty ovulation inhibitors on voice function in women. *Contraception, 52,* 343–348.

Williams, A., Baghat, M., Stableforth, D., Cayton, R., Shenoi, P., & Skinner, C. (1983). Dysphonia caused by inhaled steroids: Recognition of a characteristic laryngeal abnormality. *Thorax, 38,* 813–821.

Wilson, J., & MacLennan, W. (1989). Drug-induced Parkinsonism in elderly patients. *Age and Ageing, 18,* 208–210.

Wood, G., Wu, C., Flickinger, G., & Mikhail, G. (1975). Hormonal changes associated with Danazol therapy, *Obstetrics and Gynecology, 45,* 302–303.

Yuen, G. (1990). Altered pharmacokinetics in the elderly. *Clinical Geriatric Medicine, 6,* 257–267.

CHAPTER

15

The Aging Voice: Endocrine Effects

The physical structure and function of the larynx is affected by the endocrine system. Therefore, normal changes in endocrine function over the life span can be expected to have an effect on voice, although the extent of vocal changes depends on the nature and extent of endocrine system alterations. At puberty, males experience dramatic changes within the larynx. Rapid growth of the larynx is triggered by activity of the sex glands. The vocal folds increase in length by approximately 1 cm in males and speaking pitch is lowered by an octave. In females, pubertal voice change is less dramatic; vocal fold length increases by only 3 to 4 mm and pitch lowers only slightly (Luchsinger & Arnold, 1965). In females, distinct hormonal shifts occur monthly following puberty and continue through middle age. Those hormonal variations are a source of temporary vocal changes, including hoarseness, lowered habitual pitch level, loss of vocal power, and vocal instability (Abitbol, Abitbol, & Abitbol, 1999; Higgins & Saxman, 1989; Sataloff, Emerich, & Hoover, 1997; Silverman & Zimmer, 1978; Smith-Frable, 1962).

The elderly also experience numerous hormonal changes (Greg-erman, 1986; Mooradian, Morley, & Korenman, 1988). Indeed, hormonal imbalances, particularly in the neuroendocrine system, are theorized to play a major role in the aging process (Chapter 1). Endocrinologists cau-tion, however, that although some hormonal changes relate directly to advancing age, others occur secondarily to other factors associated with aging, such as disease, dietary change, medications, body compositional changes, and physical activity level (Davies, 1992; Mooradian, 1993).

With the plethora of anatomic and physiologic changes in the body with advanced age, it is difficult to parcel out those aspects of senescent voice attributed solely to endocrine changes. Although reporting no data, Luchsinger & Arnold (1965) assert that reductions in hormone production with aging account for significant vocal changes. These authors view hor-monal factors as a more substantial factor in age-related voice change for women than men, with those changes occurring during middle age in association with menopause. They view hormonal alterations in men as occurring later in life, in association with what is termed the "male climac-teric." However, Luchsinger and Arnold (1965) report no data pertaining to age-related changes in hormone levels in adult males. In more recent literature, hormonal factors rarely are mentioned as a substantial factor in age-related voice change in males.

Endocrine diseases in patients of any age are of concern to voice pro-fessionals because of potential laryngeal effects from such disorders. Indeed, otolaryngologists have been urged to enlist the services of an endocrinologist to assist in the diagnosis and medical management of professional voice users with potential endocrine problems (Sataloff et al., 1997). In the elderly, disease processes affecting the endocrine system are more common than in young adults. It is a clearly established principle of geriatric endocrinology that diseases and disabilities affecting the endocrine system are more likely to develop in persons beyond the age of 75 years (frequently termed the "old old"), even in comparison with per-sons 60 to 75 years of age (Morley, 1983). Because endocrine disease is more prevalent in the elderly, voice professionals dealing with older popu-lations must be alert to vocal symptoms arising from such disorders.

In this chapter the impact of age-related changes in the endocrine system on speech and voice production is discussed. Anatomic changes in endocrine glands are summarized and changes in hormone secretion and clearance reviewed. Also, disease processes of the endocrine system hav-ing potential for laryngeal effects are discussed from the point of view of the aging process. Finally, changes in hormone action in the elderly are examined, along with potential changes in speech and voice production arising from these changes.

MECHANISMS OF ENDOCRINE DYSFUNCTION IN THE ELDERLY

Recently Mooradian (1993) summarized anatomic changes in the endocrine system with aging. Structural changes in glands include increases in connective tissue content and nodularity as well as reductions in vascularity. In addition, significant changes occur in cellular composition of glands.

Anatomic changes in the endocrine glands with aging result from three mechanisms (1) programmed cell death (apoptosis), (2) cellular destruction from autoimmune processes, and (3) increasing nodularity and development of benign and malignant tumors within the gland (Mooradian, 1993). Programmed cellular death is associated with DNA fragmentation that leads to time-dependent cellular destruction. Failure of estrogen secretion in females at menopause resulting from loss of oocytes in the ovaries is an example of an apoptotic process, although oocyte loss with age in females may be mediated by additional factors as well (Block, 1952; Costoff & Mahesh, 1975; Morradian, 1993). Autoimmune disease can affect the endocrine system at any age. Fortunately for the elderly, most endocrine autoimmune diseases decline with aging, including Type I diabetes. An exception is autoimmune disease involving the thyroid gland. In contrast, nodularity and tumor development in the endocrine glands increases with aging. The cause of this phenomenon is unknown. Advanced age also is associated with an increased incidence of tumors in the pituitary, adrenal gland, and pancreas, although these tumors usually are clinically silent (Mooradian, 1993).

It is clear that the process of aging results in structural changes within the endocrine system. A description of age-related changes to specific glands follows, along with functional implications of those changes.

Pituitary

The pituitary gland (or hypophysis) has been termed the "master gland" of the body. It regulates the functions of other endocrine glands, as well as the growth and development of the body. Because of its location in the sella turcica of the sphenoid bone in humans, direct research on the pituitary in humans has been difficult. However, research on lower vertebrates, as well as awareness of the effects of pituitary dysfunction, have provided information on the role of this gland (Zemlin, 1988).

The pituitary is composed of two lobes. The anterior lobe controls many of the body's functions and secretes thyroid-stimulating hormone (TSH), adrenocorticotropic hormone (ACTH), growth hormone (GH), prolactin, follicle-stimulating hormone (FSH), and luteinizing hormone (LH). The posterior lobe functions to maintain the correct water balance in the body (Zemlin, 1988) and is not thought to have much relevance to the aging process (Whitbourne, 1985).

Normal Aging

Given the wide-ranging control of the anterior lobe over body functions, it has been tempting for researchers to believe that this portion of the pituitary gland is particularly important in the aging process. Indeed, findings of significant structural changes in this gland with aging fuel that notion. Computerized tomographic scans (CT scans) and magnetic resonance imaging (MRI) of the pituitary indicate that aging is associated with a decline in pituitary height and volume (Hayakawa et al., 1989; Lurie et al., 1990). In contrast, autopsy evidence suggests that pituitary weight remains unchanged with aging (Andres & Tobin, 1977).

Cellular composition of the anterior lobe of the pituitary gland also changes with aging. Declines in both the number and size of cells that produce growth hormone (GH) have been reported from young adulthood into middle age (Sun et al., 1984; Zegarelli-Schmidt et al., 1985). However, despite age-related changes to cells producing GH, studies of integrated GH levels (a measure of total GH secreted) in the elderly have been inconclusive, with both lower levels and unchanged levels reported (Florini, Prinz, Vitiello, & Hintz, 1985; Ho et al., 1987).

The role of GH in the aging process has intrigued investigators for many years. It has been hypothesized that the process of aging is under the control of GH, since this hormone is known to regulate growth during the maturation process. Indeed, findings of possible lowering of GH levels with advanced age prompted initiation of GH therapy with elderly patients, on an experimental basis, in an effort to counteract the aging process (Mooradian, 1993). However, the hypothesis that high GH levels slow down the aging process may be flawed. Such reasoning is inconsistent with findings that excessive GH production in adulthood results in premature death (Whitbourne, 1985).

Pathology With Aging

Certain disease processes that involve the pituitary gland have an effect on voice production and are associated with aging. For instance, acromegaly is a disease of middle age in which the anterior lobe of the pituitary hyperfunctions, resulting in excessive production of GH (*Taber's*, 1977). Elongation and enlargement of bones of the extremities and cranial bones occurs, as well as enlargement of the nose and lips. Laryngeal changes include hypertrophy of the epiglottis, arytenoids, and aryepiglottic folds. Hypertrophy of laryngeal structures result in stridor and dyspnea as a consequence of obstruction of the laryngeal vestibule (Luchsinger & Arnold, 1965; Maceri, 1986). Vocal changes with acromegaly include lowering of fundamental frequency (F_0) and hoarseness (Luchsinger & Arnold, 1965). Interestingly, recent research indicates that lowering of F_0 in acromegaly reverses within a relatively short period of time with surgical removal of the pituitary body (Williams, Richards, Mills, & Eccles, 1994). Reversal of F_0 lowering suggests that vocal changes accompanying acromegaly result from vocal fold thickening, as opposed to enlargement of the larynx as a whole.

Thyroid

The thyroid gland is closely associated anatomically with the larynx, although it is not involved directly in voice production. The gland consists of two lobes connected by a narrow isthmus. The gland is highly variable in its structure. In some cases, the isthmus is absent altogether and in others a third lobe may be present. The glandular tissue is composed of microscopic alveoli, or follicles, that are lined with epithelial cells. The epithelial cells secrete a viscous material called colloid, which contains the thyroid hormone thyroxin (Zemlin, 1988).

Normal Aging

The primary histological changes in the thyroid gland with aging are fibrosis, increased nodularity, and infiltration of lymphocytic and plasma cells (Denham & Wills, 1980; Hodkinson & Irvine, 1985; Mooradian, 1993; Morley, 1983; Robuschi, Safran, Braverman, Gnudi, & Roti, 1987). Thyroid nodules are detected in up to 90% of women after age 72 and in 60% of men after age 80 (Hodkinson & Irvine, 1985). Studies of age-related changes in thyroid gland volume and weight have produced conflicting findings, with both increases and decreases reported (Mooradian, 1993; Robuschi et al., 1987). It is possible that contradictions in findings of volume and weight changes with aging are explained, in part, by the confounding influence of age and body weight (Hegedus et al., 1983).

Aging also alters hormone secretion by the thyroid gland (Mooradian, 1993), although altered secretion proves to have little functional significance (Robuschi et al., 1987). Interestingly, although secretion of thyroxine (T4) is reduced in the elderly, thyroid function tests demonstrate that plasma T4 concentration is unaltered in the older population (Francis & Wartofsky, 1992; Mooradian, 1993). This apparent contradiction is explained by accompanying age-related reductions in disposal rate of T4.

That is, plasma T4 levels remain unaltered in the elderly because reductions in secretion rate are counteracted by simultaneous decreases of almost 50% in clearance rate (Gregerman, Gaffney, & Shock, 1962). Thus, the reduction in T4 secretion in the elderly is felt to be a compensatory mechanism associated with age-related reductions in hormone clearance. The net effect of these changes is a stable steady-state plasma level of T4 with aging (Mooradian, 1993).

Pathology With Aging

Secretion disorders involving the thyroid gland occur quite commonly in the elderly. Approximately 5% of the elderly experience thyroid dysfunction involving either hyperthyroidism or hypothyroidism. However, diagnosing thyroid disorders in an elderly patient can be difficult in that (1) the onset of the disorder can be insidious with atypical presentation, (2) disease processes may mask symptoms, and (3) medications and nutritional variables can affect the results of thyroid function tests (Francis & Wartofsky, 1992; Morley, 1983). Because thyroid disease is a fairly common problem in the elderly, opportunistic screening of the elderly on hospital admission has been widely advocated. Routine community-based screening of the well elderly is not universally embraced, however, because of concern about false-positive thyroid function tests and subsequent development of adverse effects from inappropriate administration of T4 (Finucane & Anderson, 1995).

The prevalence of hyperthyroidism in the elderly is estimated at 0.5% to 2.3%, a rate that is 7 times higher than in younger age groups (Levy, 1991; Ronnov-Jessen & Kirkegaard, 1973). The most common causes of geriatric hyperthyroidism are Grave disease and autonomous toxic nodular disease of the thyroid gland (Francis & Wartofsky, 1992). Symptoms of hyperthyroidism related to speech production are not well documented, but include increased respiratory rate, reductions in vital capacity, tremulousness, and hoarseness (Maceri, 1986).

Finucane and Anderson (1995) discuss management of hyperthyroidism in the elderly. According to these authors, the treatment of choice involves oral administration of ^{131}I, an agent that effectively incapacitates the thyroid gland. Depending on a patient's response to the dosage administered, results vary from establishment of normal thyroid function to the development of hypothyroidism. If hypothyroidism results, the patient is given thyroxine replacement. An alternative treatment for hyperthyroidism in the elderly is thyroidectomy. Although thyroidectomy is considered well-tolerated and effective by the medical community, surgical treatment is currently less popular, with the availability of an effective nonsurgical alternative (Finucane & Anderson, 1995).

Estimates of the incidence of hypothyroidism in the elderly vary widely from 0.5% to 17.5%. This variance reflects, in part, differences in ethnicity and ambient iodine intake in the populations studied. In addition, epidemiological studies vary in the age range included as "elderly" and in the number of individuals tested (Francis & Wartofsky, 1992; Robuschi et al., 1987). Normally, symptoms of hypothyroidism include muscle weakness, lethargy, temperature intolerance, weight gain, brittle hair, dry skin, neurological dysfunction, constipation, and muscle cramps (Sataloff et al., 1997). In the elderly, however, signs of hypothyroidism often are more subtle, and symptoms frequently are attributed to normal aging. Reportedly, less than one third of elderly patients demonstrate classic indications of the disorder and two thirds present solely with apathy and weakness (Francis & Wartofsky, 1992; Robuschi et al., 1987).

Autoimmune thyroiditis (Hashimoto disease) is the most common cause of hypothroidism across all age groups. In the elderly, chronic autoimmune thyroiditis is particularly prevalent, especially among elderly women. Other possible causes of hypothyroidism in the elderly are surgical removal of the gland for disease or use of iodine-containing medications. In addition, hypothyroidism can occur as a late consequence of treatment for Grave disease (Francis & Wartofsky, 1992; Robuschi et al., 1987).

Even mild hypothyroidism is associated with vocal symptoms including vocal fatigue, muffling of voice, hoarseness, loss of range, and a feeling of a lump in the throat (Sataloff et al., 1997). Vocal consequences of more severe hypothyroidism depend on whether the condition is congenital (cretinism) or acquired (adults with myxedema). With cretinism, production of thyroid hormone is inadequate from birth and the larynx is small. Vocal quality is rough and pitch is low as a result of vocal fold hypotonia, vascular congestion, and edema. With cretinism, prognosis for vocal improvement is not particularly positive, although treatment can reverse some of the observed vocal changes. Myxedema is associated with a more positive prognosis for improved vocal quality when thyroid hormone is administered (Maceri, 1986).

The prevalence of pathological enlargement of the thyroid (goiter) increases with aging in men, with women tending to demonstrate some shrinking of the thyroid after menopause (Mooradian, 1993). Enlargement of the thyroid gland can produce vocal symptoms associated with increased pressure on the recurrent laryngeal nerve (RLN). If the pressure becomes great enough, RLN function is interrupted. The degree of disturbance in RLN function (paralysis or paresis) is not always correlated with the size of goiter, however. That is, a large tumor may produce no sign of nerve disturbance, while a small goiter can exert considerable pressure if positioned in a particular way. In addition, a small percentage of goiter patients demonstrate paralysis of RLN on the contralateral side (Judd,

1921). It may be that elderly patients with goiter are less at risk for symptoms associated with RLN disturbance than younger patients, because (1) most newly identified goiters in the elderly have been in existence for a long time and grow very slowly, and (2) goiters in the elderly rarely cause obstructive symptoms (Francis & Wartofsky, 1992).

Thyroidectomy

Thyroidectomy might be performed for a number of conditions affecting the thyroid. For example, complete or partial thyroidectomy is the treatment of choice for many forms of thyroid carcinoma. Although thyroid cancer is relatively uncommon, it is the most frequently occurring cancer involving the endocrine system. The disease affects women more often than men and occurs most frequently between the ages of 26 and 65 (National Cancer Institute, 1999). Thyroidectomy also may be performed in cases of goiter due to iodine deficiency, thyroiditis, tumors, inflammation from infection, hyperfunction, or hypofunction (*Taber's*, 1977).

Both complete and partial thyroidectomy pose a potential threat to voice from either damage to the recurrent laryngeal nerve (RLN) or the external branch of the superior laryngeal nerve (EBSLN) (Holt, McMurry, & Joseph, 1977; Lekacos, Miligos, Tzardis, Majiatis, & Patoulis, 1987; Teitelbaum & Wenig, 1995). Recent reports place the risk of RLN injury from thyroidectomy between 3.0% and 3.9% (Haider & Amin, 1997; Moulton-Barrett et al., 1997), although the risk of permanent injury is lower (2.1%). The risk of damage to EBSLN from thyroidectomy surgery (total, or subtotal involving only the superior thyroid pole) varies. Factors that determine risk include the degree to which the superior thyroid pole has been elevated by enlargement of the gland and the anatomical proximity of the nerve to the gland (Cernea, Ferraz, Furlani, et al., 1992; Cernea, Ferraz, Nishio, et al., 1992; Cernea, Nishio, & Hojaij, 1995).

Interestingly, voice changes have been reported in thyroidectomy patients, even if the procedure is deemed "uncomplicated," that is, without apparent damage to RLN or SLN. Acoustic analysis of voice in thyroidectomy patients revealed short duration lowering of F_0, reductions of pitch range in speaking, elevated jitter levels, and reduction of harmonic prominence (Debruyne, Ostyn, Delaere, & Wellens, 1997; Debruyne, Ostyn, Delaere, Wellens, & Decoster, 1997). A limitation of these studies, however, is that control groups were not tested to determine the effect of endotracheal intubation alone on acoustic parameters of voice. It is possible that subtle changes to vocal fold tissues during the process of intubation contributed to the observed voice changes, despite the fact that patients with signs of traumatic intubation were excluded from the studies. This is particularly true given the subtle nature of the voice changes observed and the temporary nature of those changes.

In addition to potential trauma to the laryngeal nerve supply, thyroidectomy also can produce damage to the laryngeal framework, although the likelihood of such a complication appears remote. Sataloff, Spiegel, Carroll, and Heuer (1992) presented a case of cricothyroid fusion following thyroidectomy resulting in a dramatic rise in speaking pitch level. Normal voice was restored following surgical separation of the cartilages.

Parathyroid

Located just behind the upper and lower poles of the thyroid gland are two pairs of pea-sized structures known as the parathyroid glands. The function of the parathyroids is to maintain the correct level of phosphorus and calcium in the blood (Zemlin, 1988).

Normal Aging

According to Mooradian (1993), the most common histological change in the parathyroid glands with aging is increased nodularity. In the elderly, large nodules made up of oxyphils (cells that react to acid dyes) may be present and may be mistaken for adenomas.

Pathology With Aging

Hypoparathyroidism is insufficient secretion of the parathyroid glands. Hypoparathyroidism is most often associated with surgery to the thyroid gland, although an idiopathic variety is recognized increasingly in the elderly. The major consequence of hypoparathyroidism is hypocalcemia, which has as its major symptom tetany. Tetany is a condition in which nerve and muscle tissue becomes hyperexcitable. In cases in which tetany affects the larynx, laryngeal spasm can cause respiratory arrest and death. In less severe cases, hypocalcemia can present with phonatory symptoms, including stridor, hoarseness, or aphonia. In the elderly, hypocalcemia also can produce reversible dementia (Belchetz, 1992; Maceri, 1986; *Taber's*, 1977; Zemlin, 1988).

Increased activity of the parathyroid glands is referred to as hyperparathyroidism. Hyperparathyroidism is a relatively rare disorder that produces hypercalcemia, or excessive calcium levels in the blood. Hypercalcemia is manifest by generalized muscular weakness and hyporeflexia. Aphonia has been reported to accompany hypercalcemia, presumably as a result of blocked neural transmission at the synapse due to an increase in calcium ion concentration (Maceri, 1986). In the elderly, alterations in mental function have been reported, even with relatively modest degrees of hypercalcemia, particularly in cases of multiple pathology (Belchetz, 1992). In the general population the most frequent cause of hyperparathyroidism is hyperplasia or parathyroid adenoma. In hospital patients, hyperparathyroidism most frequently is associated with malignancy. Hyperparathyroidism frequently occurs in association with other endocrine disorders and exemplifies the interactive nature of the endocrine glands in any given disease process (Maceri, 1986).

Gonads

The testes and ovaries have important endocrine functions. The testes produce testosterone that stimulates the acquisition of secondary sex characteristics in males. In addition, the testes produce spermatozoa. The ovary produces a battery of hormones that stimulate the onset of puberty and development of female secondary sex characteristics. In addition, hormones produced by the ovaries regulate the maturation and release of the ovum during the menstrual cycle (Zemlin, 1988).

Early studies indicated that serum testosterone levels decline in men after age 50 (Pirke & Doerr, 1973; Stearns et al., 1974; Vermeulen, Rubens, & Verdonck, 1972). However, more recent findings indicate that current health status as well as health history has a significant impact on testosterone levels in elderly men. Although it is not unusual to encounter men in this age group with low serum testosterone levels, the healthiest elderly men have testosterone levels that are comparable to younger men (Seaton, Bergman, Price, Tsitouras, & Gambert, 1986). In terms of the male voice, the most profound effects of testosterone occur at puberty, as described at the beginning of this chapter. After puberty, vocal problems associated with gonadal hormones in men are a relatively uncommon problem (Sataloff et al., 1997).

While men demonstrate unpredictable and relatively unpronounced decreases in testosterone during the aging process, women undergo monthly hormonal shifts through middle age that produce temporary voice changes (Abitbol et al., 1999), as described early in this chapter. In addition, women experience universal and dramatic declines in ovarian hormone secretions at menopause. Although the term menopause refers to a woman's final menstrual event, it is interesting that the changes in hormone secretion leading to menopause can be observed in women as early as 10 years before the termination of menstrual cycles (Seaton et al., 1986).

Numerous vocal changes in older female singers have been linked with menopause. Specifically, increased breathiness, loss of the upper end of the pitch range, altered vibrato characteristics, development of tremolo, vocal fatigue, decreased breath control, and inaccurate pitch production have been reported (Sataloff et al., 1997). What is unclear from these reports, however, is the extent to which all of these vocal changes can be directly attributable to hormonal shifts at menopause versus other age-related physiological changes in the mechanism. For instance, loss of breath control might be attributed, at least in part, to age-related declines in vital capacity associated with loss of elastic recoil in the pulmonary system (Chapters 2 and 6). In addition, the timing of some of these voice changes may not coincide with menopause, but rather occur well after middle age. For example, loss of the upper end of the physiological pitch range, at least in nonsingers, is a phenomenon that occurs in old age, not in middle age, and does not appear to be related to hormonal changes at menopause (Linville, 1987). Restriction of pitch range with aging (in both men and women) might better be attributed to changes in laryngeal cartilages and muscles later in life. An age-related voice change in women that can more safely be attributed to menopause is lowering of F_0. Slight lowering of F_0 has been documented following menopause, presumably as a consequence of thickening and edema of laryngeal mucosa resulting from hormonal changes (Chapter 10).

Pancreas

The pancreas produces enzymes that aid in digestion. In addition, insulin is produced by a small group of cells called the islets of Langerhans. Insulin is responsible for the retention and storage of sugar in the body. When the islets malfunction, sugar no longer is stored in the liver and other tissues, but instead is excreted via the kidneys with urine (Zemlin, 1988).

Normal Aging

With normal aging, the islets lose the compact structure observed in young adults and undergo hyalinization. Further, pathologic extracellular deposits (amyloids) are found in the islets of approximately 60% of healthy, nondiabetic elderly persons. These deposits are interesting, as evidence suggests a positive correlation between amyloid deposits and severity of diabetes in diabetics (Mooradian, 1993).

Epidemiologic surveys consistently show worsening of glucose tolerance with aging, even in the absence of a diagnosis of diabetes (Andres, 1992; Harris, 1990; Morley, Mooradian, Rosenthal, & Kaiser, 1987). Specifically, one report from the National Commission on Diabetes placed the incidence of elevated glucose levels (160 mg/dl 1 hour after an oral glucose load) in nondiabetic adults at 3% for patients aged 18 to 24 years, 16% for patients aged 45 to 54 years, 36% for patients aged 65 to 74, and 42% for patients aged 75 to 79 years (Bennett, 1976).

Normal elderly also tend to show a decrease in the insulin-to-glucose ratio, accompanied by elevated steady state serum insulin levels. This apparent contradiction suggests that the islet cells in elderly persons are more resistant than those of younger persons to releasing insulin when glucose levels rise (Morley et al., 1987). An alternative explanation is that decreased glucose tolerance in the elderly is a secondary manifestation of aging related to an increased incidence of obesity, declining physical activity, increased incidence of chronic/acute disease, increased use of medications, and dietary changes (Andres, 1992).

Diabetes Mellitus

Diabetes mellitus is a disorder arising from abnormal function of the pancreas. Manifestations of diabetes are diverse and complex and may involve disturbances in metabolism of protein and fat as well as glucose. However, at a minimum, all persons with diabetes share a pathological intolerance to glucose (Andres, 1992). Most diabetic patients with onset in middle age or old age have Type II diabetes mellitus, or diabetes uncomplicated by elevated levels of ketone bodies (ketoacidosis) in the body (Morley et al., 1987). Ketone bodies are compounds produced during the oxidation of fatty acids (*Taber's*, 1977).

Diabetes is exceedingly common in elderly persons and represents one of the major chronic disorders affecting the elderly population (Morley et al., 1987). In the United States, diabetes is diagnosed in 6.9% of men and 8.9% of women older than 65 years of age (Matz, 1986). In persons beyond the age of 80, diabetes occurs in 16% to 20% (Bennett, 1984). Because of the tendency for increased glucose intolerance with aging, an elderly patient must display a random blood glucose level of more than 200 mg/dl, or two fasting blood glucose levels of more than 140 mg/dl, to be diagnosed with diabetes (Morley et al., 1987).

At one extreme, diabetes can manifest as a chemical deviation from the norm without clinical symptomatology and at the other extreme the disorder can produce catastrophic health consequences (Andres, 1992). Indeed, diabetes mellitus is the fifth leading health-related cause of death in the United States (Maceri, 1986). Neuropathic disturbances are not uncommon in diabetic patients. Although neuropathic disturbances of diabetes most commonly affect the extremities, cranial nerves can be affected. From the perspective of voice production, diabetes mellitus can result in lesions of the vagus nerve with vocal fold paralysis. Additional potential consequences of diabetes include idiopathic facial paralysis (Bells palsy), altered swallow function, or sensorineural hearing loss (Maceri, 1986).

HORMONE REPLACEMENT THERAPY

Hormone replacement therapy (HRT) frequently is suggested to women after menopause to aid in the prevention of heart disease and to prevent osteoporosis (Abrams, 1998; Rolnick, Kopher, Compo, Kelley, & DeFor, 1999; Rozenberg et al., 1997; Saver, Taylor, Woods, & Stevens, 1997). In the United States, HRT has gained general acceptance among the medical community, evidenced by guidelines from the American College of Physicians recommending that most postmenopausal women be offered HRT. Interestingly, however, when U.S. physicians are surveyed about their policies and attitudes towards HRT, evidence indicates gynecologists believe more strongly in the benefits of HRT than do family physicians and general internists. Indeed, gynecologists ranked HRT as more important for postmenopausal women than counseling for cessation of smoking (Saver et al., 1997). It is interesting, as well, that HRT use within the United States and Europe varies widely (<1% to 20%) from country to country. Women in the United States are most likely to take HRT, while women in continental Europe have the lowest usage. Usage patterns in the UK and Scandinavia fall in the middle (Jolleys & Olesen, 1996).

Attitudes about HRT differ among individual women, also. A substantial number of women are deterred from HRT because of potential negative side effects or aversion to the notion of continued cyclic bleeding after menopause (Ettinger, Pressman, & Silver, 1999; Phillipov, Mos, Scinto, & Philips, 1997; Thompson, 1995). In addition, socioeconomic factors have been linked with HRT use. HRT users in the United States are more likely to be affluent, white, urban-dwellers with smaller families in comparison with nonusers (Handa, Landerman, Hanlon, Harris, & Cohen, 1996). However, recent reports from Finland suggest that socioeconomic differences among HRT users in that country are becoming less pronounced (Topo, Luoto, Hemminki, & Uutela, 1999). It has been established, as well, that physician counseling is an important variable in a woman's decision to use HRT. That is, noninitiators (62%) are more likely than initiators (18%) to report receiving no information on the benefits of HRT from medical providers (Leveille, LaCroix, Newton, & Keenan, 1997).

SUMMARY

Normal changes in the endocrine system over the adult lifespan have an effect on voice. However, it can be difficult to determine which age-related vocal changes are solely due to endocrine changes. In addition, voice professionals must be alert to possible vocal symptoms arising from endocrine disease, which is more prevalent in the elderly.

The anterior lobe of the pituitary gland undergoes significant structural changes with aging and researchers have been tempted to believe that this portion of the pituitary is particularly important to the aging process. In particular, the role of growth hormone (GH) in the aging process has intrigued investigators. However, studies of integrated GH levels in the elderly have been inconclusive.

Acromegaly is a disease of the pituitary associated with middle age that has voice effects. Vocal changes include lowering of F_0 and hoarseness. Recent research indicates that lowering of F_0 with acromegaly reverses within a relatively short time with surgical removal of the pituitary body, suggesting that vocal changes with this disorder result from vocal fold thickening as opposed to enlargement of the larynx.

Normally with aging the thyroid undergoes fibrosis, increased nodularity, and cellular changes. Aging also alters hormone secretion by the thyroid, although altered secretion has little functional significance. That is, although secretion of T4 is reduced with aging, thyroid function tests demonstrate that plasma T4 concentrations remain unchanged in the elderly because of accompanying reductions in T4 disposal rate.

Disorders of secretion involving the thyroid are common in the elderly, although diagnosing those disorders can be problematic. Both hyperthyroidism and hypothyroidism frequently produce vocal symptoms because of altered hormone levels. In addition, enlargement of the thyroid can produce vocal symptoms associated with increased pressure on the recurrent laryngeal nerve. Thyroidectomy is performed for a number of pathological conditions affecting the thyroid. This procedure poses a potential threat to voice from either (1) damage to the recurrent laryngeal nerve, (2) damage to the superior laryngeal nerve, or (3) damage to the laryngeal framework. Voice changes also have been reported in cases of "uncomplicated" thyroidectomy.

The parathyroid undergoes histological change with aging. Further, pathological conditions (hypoparathyroidism and hyperparathyroidism) can occur in the elderly and produce vocal symptoms. Potential vocal symptoms of hypoparathyroidism include stridor, hoarseness, or aphonia. Aphonia has been reported to accompany hyperparathyroidism as a consequence of resulting hypercalcemia.

The testes and ovaries have important endocrine functions. In elderly men, low serum testosterone levels are not uncommon, although recent findings indicate that the healthiest elderly men have testosterone levels that are comparable to younger men. In terms of male voice, problems associated with gonadal hormones are relatively uncommon after puberty. In women, numerous vocal changes have been linked with menopause, particularly in female singers. It is unclear, however, whether all reported vocal changes in older female singers can be attributed solely to hormonal shifts at menopause, versus other age-related physiological changes.

Functioning of the pancreas also is affected by aging. Epidemiologic surveys consistently show worsening of glucose tolerance with aging, even in the absence of a diagnosis of diabetes. Normal elderly persons also show a decline in the insulin to glucose ratio, accompanied by elevated steady-state serum insulin levels. This apparent contradiction suggests that pancreatic cells in elderly persons are more resistant than those in younger persons to releasing insulin when glucose levels rise. Other factors (physical activity, obesity, disease, medications, dietary changes) also relate to declining glucose tolerance in elderly persons. Diabetes is one of the major chronic disorders affecting the elderly population. Neuropathic disturbances are not uncommon in patients with diabetes and these disturbances can affect the cranial nerves. Vocal fold paralysis can result from vagus nerve lesions. In addition, idiopathic facial paralysis, altered swallow function, or sensorineural hearing loss can occur.

Hormone replacement therapy frequently is suggested to postmenopausal women to aid in preventing heart disease and osteoporosis. Attitudes about HRT differ among women; some women are reluctant to begin HRT because of potential unwanted side effects or aversion to continued cyclic bleeding. Socioeconomic factors and physician counseling also are linked with HRT use in older women.

REFERENCES

Abitbol, J., Abitbol, P., & Abitbol, B. (1999). Sex hormones and the female voice. *Journal of Voice, 13*, 424–446.

Andres, R. (1992). Diabetes and aging. In J. Brocklehurst, R. Tallis, & H. Fillit (Eds.), *Textbook of geriatric medicine and gerontology* (4th ed., pp. 724–728). United Kingdom: Churchill Livingstone.

Andres, R., & Tobin, J. (1977). Endocrine systems. In C. Finch & L. Hayflick (Eds.), *Handbook of the biology of aging* (pp. 367–387). New York: Van Nostrand Reinhold.

Belchetz, P. (1992). Disorders of the parathyroids. In J. Brocklehurst, R. Tallis, & H. Fillit (Eds.) *Textbook of geriatric medicine and gerontology* (4th ed., pp. 717–723). United Kingdom: Churchill Livingstone.

Bennett, P. (1976). *Report of work group on epidemiology* (Vol. 3, part 1, pp. 65–133) (DHEW publication No. NIH-76-1021). Washington: National Commission on Diabetes.

Bennett, P. (1984). Diabetes in the elderly: Diagnosis and epidemiology. *Geriatrics, 39,* 37–41.

Block, E. (1952). Quantitative morphological investigations of the follicular system in women. Variations at different ages. *Acta Anatomica, 14,* 108–123.

Cernea, C., Ferraz, A., Furlani, J., Monteiro, S., Nishio, S., Hojaij, F., Dutra Junior, A., Marques, L., Pontes, P., & Bevilacqua, R. (1992). Identification of the external branch of the superior laryngeal nerve during thyroidectomy. *American Journal of Surgery, 164,* 634–639.

Cernea, C., Ferraz, A., Nishio, S., Dutra, A., Hojaij, F., & dos Santo, L. (1992). Surgical anatomy of the external branch of the superior laryngeal nerve. *Head and Neck, 14,* 380–383.

Cernea, C., Nishio, S., & Hojaij, F. (1995). Identification of the external branch of the superior laryngeal nerve (EBSLN) in large goiters. *American Journal of Otolaryngology, 16,* 307–311.

Costoff, A., & Mahesh, V. (1975). Primordial follicles with normal oocytes in the ovaries of postmenopausal women. *Journal of the American Geriatrics Society, 23,* 193–196.

Davies, I. (1992). Aging and the endocrine system. In J. Brocklehurst, R. Tallis, & H. Fillit (Eds.), *Textbook of geriatric medicine and gerontology* (4th ed., pp. 666–674). United Kingdom: Churchill Livingstone.

Debruyne, F., Ostyn, F., Delaere, P., & Wellens, W. (1997). Acoustic analysis of the speaking voice after thyroidectomy. *Journal of Voice, 11,* 479–482.

Debruyne, F., Ostyn, F., Delaere, P., Wellens, W., & Decoster, W. (1997). Temporary voice changes after uncomplicated thyroidectomy. *Acta Oto-Rhino-Laryngologica (Belgium), 51,* 137–140.

Denham, M., & Wills, E. (1980). A clinico-pathological survey of thyroid glands in old age. *Gerontology, 26,* 160–227.

Ettinger, B., Pressman, A., & Silver, P. (1999). Effect of age on reasons for initiation and discontinuation of hormone replacement therapy. *Menopause, 6,* 282–289.

Finucane, P., & Anderson, C. (1995). Thyroid disease in older patients. Diagnosis and treatment. *Drugs and Aging, 6,* 268–277.

Florini, J., Prinz, P., Vitiello, M., & Hintz, R. (1985). Somatomedin-C levels in healthy young and old men: Relationship to peak and 24 hour integrated levels of growth hormone. *Journal of Gerontology, 40,* 2–7.

Francis, T., & Wartofsky, L. (1992). Common thyroid disorders in the elderly. *Postgraduate Medicine, 92,* 225–230, 233–236.

Gregerman, R. (1986). Mechanisms of age-related alterations of hormone secretion and action. An overview of 30 years of progress. *Experimental Gerontology, 21,* 345–365.

Gregerman, R., Gaffney, G., & Shock, N. (1962). Thyroxine turnover in euthyroid man with special reference to changes with age. *Journal of Clinical Investigation, 41,* 2065–2074.

Haider, A., & Amin, M. (1997). Follow up study of thyroidectomy. *Bangladesh Medical Research Council Bulletin, 23,* 51–55.

Handa, V., Landerman, R., Hanlon, J., Harris, T., & Cohen, H. (1996). Do older women use estrogen replacement? Data from the Duke Established Populations for Epidemiologic Studies of the Elderly (EPESE). *Journal of the American Geriatrics Society, 44,* 1–6.

Harris, M. (1990). Epidemiology of diabetes mellitus among the elderly in the United States. *Clinical Geriatric Medicine, 6,* 703–719.

Hayakawa, K., Konishi, Y., Matsuda, T., Kuriyama, M., Konishi, K., Yamashita, K., Okumura, R., & Hamanaka, D. (1989). Development and aging of brain midline structures: Assessment with MR imaging. *Radiology, 172,* 171–177.

Hegedus, L., Perrild, H., Poulsen, L., Andersen, J., Holm. B., Schnohr, P., Jensen, G., & Hansen, J. (1983). The determination of thyroid volume by ultrasound and its relationship to body weight, age, and sex in normal subjects. *Journal of Clinical Endocrinology and Metabolism, 56,* 260–263.

Higgins, M., & Saxman, J. (1989). Variations in vocal frequency perturbation across the menstrual cycle. *Journal of Voice, 3,* 233–243.

Ho, K., Evans, W., Blizzard, R., Veldhuis, J., Merriam, G., Samojlik, E., Furlanetto, R., Rogol, A., Kaiser, D., & Thorner, M. (1987). Effects of sex and age on the 24-hour profile of growth hormone secretion in man: Importance of endogenous estradiol concentrations. *Journal of Clinical Endocrinology and Metabolism, 64,* 51–58.

Hodkinson, H., & Irvine, R. (1985). The endocrine system. Thyroid disease in the elderly. In J. Brocklehurst (Ed.), *Textbook of geriatric medicine and gerontology* (3rd ed., pp. 686–714). Edinburgh: Churchill Livingstone.

Holt, G., McMurry, C., & Joseph, D. (1977). Recurrent laryngeal nerve injury following thyroid operations. *Surgery, Gynecology and Obstetrics, 144,* 567–570.

Jolleys, J., & Olesen, F. (1996). A comparative study of prescribing of hormone replacement therapy in USA and Europe. *Maturitas, 23,* 47–53.

Judd, E. (1921). Laryngeal function in thyroid cases. *Annals of Surgery, 73,* 321–327.

Lekacos, N., Miligos, N., Tzardis, P., Majiatis, S., & Patoulis, J. (1987). The superior laryngeal nerve in thyroidectomy. *American Surgeon, 53,* 610–612.

Leveille, S., LaCroix, A., Newton, K., & Keenan, N. (1997). Older women and hormone replacement therapy: Factors influencing late life initiation. *Journal of the American Geriatrics Society, 45,* 1496–1500.

Levy, E. (1991). Thyroid disease in the elderly. *Medical Clinics of North America, 75,* 151–167.

Linville, S. E. (1987). Maximum phonational frequency range capabilities of women's voices with advancing age. *Folia Phoniatrica (Basel), 39,* 297–301.

Luchsinger, R., & Arnold, G. (1965). *Voice, speech, language, clinical communicology: Its physiology and pathology* (G. Arnold & E. Finkbeiner, Trans.). Belmont, CA: Wadsworth Publishing Company.

Lurie, S., Doraiswamy, P., Husain, M., Boyko, O., Ellinwood, E., Figiel, G., & Krishnan, K. (1990). In vivo assessment of pituitary gland volume with magnetic resonance imaging: The effect of age. *Journal of Clinical Endocrinology and Metabolism, 71,* 505–508.

Maceri, D. (1986). Head and neck manifestations of endocrine disease. *Otolaryngologic Clinics of North America, 19,* 171–180.

Matz, R. (1986). Diabetes mellitus in the elderly. *Hospital Practice (office ed.), 21,* 195–218.

Mooradian, A. (1993). Mechanisms of age-related endocrine alterations: Part I. *Drugs and Aging, 3,* 81–97.

Mooradian, A., Morley, J., & Korenman, S. (1988). Endocrinology in aging. *Disease-A-Month, 34,* 393–461.

Morley, J. (1983). The aging endocrine system. *Postgraduate Medicine, 73,* 107–120.

Morley, J., Mooradian, A., Rosenthal, M., & Kaiser, F. (1987). Diabetes mellitus in elderly patients. Is it different? *American Journal of Medicine, 83,* 533–544.

Moulton-Barrett, R., Crumley, S., Jalilie, S., Segina, D., Allison, G., Marshak, D., & Chan, E. (1997). Complications of thyroid surgery. *International Surgery, 82,* 63–66.

National Cancer Institute. (1999). Cancernet: PDQ Information for Health Care Professionals.

Phillipov, G., Mos, E., Scinto, S., & Phillips, P. (1997). Initiation of hormone replacement therapy after diagnosis of osteoporosis by bone densitometry. *Osteoporosis International, 7,* 162–164.

Pirke, L., & Doerr, P. (1973). Age related changes and interrelationships between plasma testosterone, estradiol, and testosterone binding globulin in normal adult males. *Acta Endocrinologica (Copenhagen), 74,* 792–800.

Robuschi, G., Safran, M., Braverman, L., Gnudi, A., & Roti, E. (1987). Hypothyroidism in the elderly. *Endocrine Reviews, 8,* 142–153.

Rolnick, S., Kopher, R., Compo, R., Kelley, M., & DeFor, T. (1999). Provider attitudes and self-reported behaviors related to hormone replacement therapy. *Menopause, 6,* 257–263.

Ronnov-Jessen, V., & Kirkegaard, C. (1973). Hyperthyroidism—A disease of old age? *British Medical Journal, 1,* 41–43.

Rozenberg, S., Kroll, M., Vandromme, J., Paesmans, M., Lefever, A., & Ham, H. (1997). Factors influencing the prescription of hormone replacement therapy. *Obstetrics and Gynecology, 90,* 387–391.

Sataloff, R., Emerich, K., & Hoover, C. (1997). Endocrine dysfunction. In R. Sataloff (Ed.), *Professional voice: The science and art of clinical care* (pp. 291–297). San Diego: Singular Publishing Group.

Sataloff, R., Spiegel, J., Carroll, L., & Heuer, R. (1992). Male soprano voice: A rare complication of thyroidectomy. *Laryngoscope, 102,* 90–93.

Saver, B., Taylor, T., Woods, N., & Stevens, N. (1997). Physician policies on the use of preventive hormone therapy. *American Journal of Preventive Medicine, 13,* 358–365.

Seaton, T., Bergman, M., Price, W., Tsitouras, P., & Gambert, S. (1986). Endocrinology and metabolism in the elderly. In S. Gambert (Ed.), *Contemporary geriatric medicine* (2nd ed, pp. 273–329). New York: Plenum Publishing Corporation.

Silverman, E., & Zimmer, C. (1978). Effect of the menstrual cycle on voice quality. *Archives of Otolaryngology, 104,* 7–10.

Smith-Frable, M. (1962). Hoarseness. A symptom of premenstrual tension. *Archives of Otolaryngology, 75,* 80–82.

Stearns, E., MacDonnell, J., Kaufman, B., Padua, R., Lucman, T., Winter, J., & Faiman, C. (1974). Declining testicular function with age: Hormonal and clinical correlates. *American Journal of Medicine, 57,* 761–766.

Sun, Y., Xi, Y., Fenoglio, C., Pushparaj, N., O'Toole, K., Kledizik, G., Nette, E., & King, D. (1984). The effect of age on the number of pituitary cells immunoreactive to growth hormone and prolactin. *Human Pathology, 15,* 169–180.

Taber's cyclopedic medical dictionary (13th ed.). (1977). Philadelphia: F. A. Davis Company.

Teitelbaum, B., & Wenig, B. (1995). Superior laryngeal nerve injury from thyroid surgery. *Head and Neck, 17,* 36–40.

Thompson, W. (1995). Estrogen replacement therapy in practice: Trends and issues. *American Journal of Obstetrics and Gynecology, 173,* 990–993.

Topo, P., Luoto, R., Hemminki, E., & Uutela, A. (1999). Declining socioeconomic differences in the use of menopausal and postmenopausal hormone therapy in Finland. *Maturitas, 32,* 141–145.

Vermeulen, A., Rubens, R., & Verdonck, L. (1972). Testosterone secretion and metabolism in male senescence. *Journal of Clinical Endocrinology and Metabolism, 34,* 730–735.

Whitbourne, S. (1985). *The aging body: Physiological changes and psychological consequences.* New York: Springer-Verlag.

Williams, R., Richards, S., Mills, R., & Eccles, R. (1994). Voice changes in acromegaly. *Laryngoscope, 104,* 484–487.

Zegarelli-Schmidt, E., Yu, X., Fenoglio-Preiser, C., O'Toole, K., Pushparaj, N., Kledzik, G., & King, D. (1985). Endocrine changes associated with the human aging process: II. Effect of age on the number and size of thyrotropin immunoreactive cells in the human pituitary. *Human Pathology, 16,* 277–286.

Zemlin, W. (1988). Speech and hearing science: Anatomy and physiology (3rd ed.). Englewood Cliffs, NJ: Prentice-Hall.

CHAPTER

16

Surgical Care for Voice Problems of the Elderly

In recent years there has been a rapid evolution of phonosurgical procedures designed to preserve or improve the voice. These procedures are used to correct dysphonias resulting from structural abnormalities of the vocal folds as well as neuromuscular disorders of the larynx. Phonosurgical procedures have been developed for: (1) removal of vocal fold lesions (phonomicrosurgery); (2) medialization, lateralization, lengthening, or shortening of the vocal folds through laryngeal framework surgery; (3) augmentation of vocal fold tissue through injection techniques; (4) treatment of laryngeal dystonias through injection techniques; and (5) reinnervation of vocal fold musculature. As a result of these recent advances, an increasing number of voice disordered individuals are undergoing surgical procedures aimed at improving voice.

In the elderly, phonosurgery might be considered to treat glottal insufficiency brought about by pathological processes (vocal fold paralysis/paresis, neurologic disease, laryngeal trauma) or atrophic changes in the vocal folds resulting from any of several possible etiologies (Chapter 12). Glottal insufficiency could involve asymmetries in vocal fold height or deficiencies in vocal fold adduction. Phonosurgical procedures also might be used to treat vocal fold segmental problems related to scar tissue from previous surgery.

Glottal insufficiency compromises the ability of the larynx to serve as a sphincter during swallowing and/or a vibrator during phonation because of incomplete closure of the glottis (Bielamowicz, Berke, & Gerratt, 1995; Tanaka, Hirano, & Chijiwa, 1994). Clinically, the voice ascribed to glottic incompetence is weak and breathy, with a tendency to fatigue easily (Hagen, Lyons, & Nuss, 1996; Tucker, 1988). Female patients complain of a low speaking pitch with male patients feeling that their speaking pitch is too high. In addition, difficulties involving restricted pitch range have been reported (Bielamowicz et al., 1995; Hagen et al., 1996; Isshiki, Kojima, Shoji, & Hirano, 1996). Visual examination of the larynx confirms glottal insufficiency. In cases of vocal fold atrophy, bowing of the vocal folds is observed, particularly during phonatory effort (Tanaka et al., 1994; Tucker, 1988). Acoustic and aerodynamic assessment indicates that glottal gap size, regardless of etiology, is the primary factor influencing vocal function (Omori, Slavit, Kacker, & Blaugrund, 1998).

Typically, phonosurgery would not be the first treatment option undertaken when an elderly patient presents with symptoms of glottic dysfunction. Rather, phonosurgery is considered in only a small percentage of patients, if vocal symptoms do not respond to voice therapy (Shindo & Hanson, 1990) or in instances of severe glottal gap (Isshiki et al., 1996). In cases of vocal fold paralysis, surgical alteration is deferred as long as spontaneous recovery is a reasonable possibility (Woodson & Miller, 1981). In cases of vocal fold atrophy, laryngeal framework surgery might be performed to (1) medialize the vocal folds and improve glottal closure and/or (2) alter the tension of the vocal folds to improve vocal quality (Isshiki et al., 1996). In addition, injection techniques may be performed to improve vocal function by facilitating fold approximation (Ford, Bless, & Loftus, 1992). In this chapter, phonosurgical procedures with potential applications to aging voice are discussed.

VOCAL FOLD INJECTION

Vocal fold injection often is used to restore glottic competence in cases of unilateral vocal fold paralysis or vocal fold atrophy. Vocal fold injection in these cases is based on the principle that improved vocal quality follows if the vocal folds are more closely approximated during vibration (Chan & Titze, 1999). In such cases, a substance is injected lateral to the vibrating portion of the affected vocal fold, resulting in "plumping out" of that fold along with repositioning the medial edge closer to the midline. The concept of vocal fold augmentation through injection was introduced in the early 1900s but was not widely used until after 1950. Historically, Teflon has been the substance most commonly injected for this purpose, although other substances have been utilized as well (Dedo, Urrea, & Lawson, 1973; Kieff & Zeitels, 1996).

Vocal fold injection also is used in the management of mucosal defects (scarring, atrophy) involving the vocal fold. In these situations, a biomaterial such as collagen or fat may be implanted directly into the vocal fold mucosa to alter the mechanics of vocal fold oscillation (Chan & Titze, 1999). In instances in which the vocal fold mucosa is involved directly in vocal fold repair, knowledge of the mechanical properties of vocal fold tissues and implant materials is crucial to obtaining optimum voice results (Chan & Titze, 1998; Chan & Titze, 1999).

Teflon

Teflon was first used by Arnold (1962) and remains the most commonly used injection material worldwide in the treatment of unilateral vocal fold paralysis (Harries, 1996). Limitations of Teflon as an injection material are (1) it should not be injected into vocal folds with partial motion, or those in which motion may return, because the Teflon will interfere with normal function should motion be restored and (2) it is ineffective if the arytenoids are widely abducted (Kieff & Zeitels, 1996).

A problem often mentioned with Teflon injection is granuloma formation. Granulomas are more likely to result if too much Teflon is injected or if the Teflon is inappropriately placed. Correct placement of Teflon is deep within the muscle, lateral to the arytenoid (Kieff & Zeitels, 1996). The likelihood of granuloma formation increases with the passage of time following injection. Similarly, a lessening of mucosal wave is observed over time as the vocal fold becomes increasingly rigid (Dejonckere, 1998; Harries, 1996; Harries & Morrison, 1998). Although estimates of the incidence of granulomas following Teflon injections vary widely (Dedo, 1992; Dejonckere, 1998; Gardner & Parnes, 1991), this condition is known to disrupt normal vibratory function of the vocal folds and result in poor vocal quality. In some cases, patients also experience airway obstruction, coughing, choking, and swallowing difficulties (Dejonckere, 1998). Removal of Teflon granuloma is difficult because of infiltration into surrounding tissue. Successful results following removal have been linked with preservation of the lamina propria and limited involvement of the vocal ligament (Netterville et al., 1998).

Despite these limitations, investigators are not suggesting abandoning the use of Teflon. Indeed, Teflon is seen as an advantageous injection material for vocal fold medialization in patients with shortened life expectancy for whom there is a high risk of complications from general anesthesia because of the frail medical condition of the patient (Harries & Morrison, 1998; Havas, Lowinger, & Priestley, 1999).

Collagen

Bovine collagen also has been injected into the vocal fold for medialization (Berke, Gerratt, Kreiman, & Jackson, 1999; Ford & Bless, 1986; Ford, Bless, & Loftus, 1992; Ford, Martin, & Warner, 1984). Collagen offers the advantage of a biological implant that is histologically similar to vocal fold tissues. The biocompatibility of the substance reduces the host immune response that can produce granuloma. Some investigators have supported more widespread use of bovine collagen, noting particular success in treating patients with minimal glottic insufficiency accompanying vocal fold atrophy (Ford et al., 1992).

Bovine collagen injection offers more than just medial displacement of the vocal fold. Collagen reduces the impact of preexisting scar tissue on vocal fold function, as collagen injection is accompanied by an invasion of host fibroblasts. Invading fibroblasts tend to soften existing scar tissue, presumably due to fibroblastic production of collagenase. Once preexisting scar tissue is softened, voice quality improves because vibratory characteristics of the vocal fold more closely approximate normal (Ford et al, 1992; Kieff & Zeitels, 1996). However, attempts to use collagen injection to treat massive vocal fold scarring such as follows vocal fold stripping have been unsuccessful (Sataloff, Spiegel, Hawkshaw, Rosen, & Heuer, 1997).

The downside of bovine collagen injection is the potential for local and systemic immunologic reactions in the host. This concern delayed approval of collagen as a bioimplant substance and limited its availability (Kieff & Zeitels, 1996), although clinical trials involving newer formulations of collagen in 119 patients indicated that the substance was safe and well-tolerated (Ford et al., 1992). The use of bovine collagen also has been questioned, given the outbreak of many cases of bovine encephalopathy in Great Britain. There is fear of transmission to humans in the form of Creutzfeldt-Jakob disease (Remacle, Lawson, Keghian, & Jamart, 1999). However, that concern recently has been rendered mute by use of autologous collagen that is extracted from the skin of the patient (Ford, Staskowski, & Bless, 1995; Remacle, Lawson, Delos, & Jamart, 1999; Remacle, Lawson, Keghian, & Jamart, 1999).

Fat

Autologous fat injection also has been used to augment the vocal folds in cases of glottic incompetence (Brandenburg, Kirkham, & Koschkee, 1992; Mikaelian, Lowry, & Sataloff, 1991; Zaretsky, Shindo, deTar, & Rice, 1995). Autologous fat is less likely than bovine collagen to produce reactions in the immune system. However, there have been reports of reabsorption of fat over time both from canine vocal folds and in humans from sites in the head and neck other than the vocal folds (Boyce, Nuss, & Kluka, 1994; Mikus, Koufman, & Kilpatrick, 1995). Therefore, some investigators report overinjecting fat into the vocal fold as a compensatory adjustment. This procedure limits fine control over vocal fold positioning and results in inconsistent voice quality (Kieff & Zeitels, 1996). Findings of reabsorption of fat after vocal fold injection are not universal, however. Some investigators have found no consistent evidence of reabsorption at follow-up intervals of up to 42 months when fat was injected in small numbers of patients with unilateral vocal fold paralysis (Brandenburg et al., 1992; Mikaelian et al., 1991). Indeed, it has been suggested that factors such as handling of the graft, harvesting technique, method of insertion, and muscle atrophy might be related to observed declines in bulk and/or high graft reabsorption rates following injection into the vocal fold (Boyce et al., 1994; Mak & Toriumi, 1994; Nguyen, Pasyk, Bouvier, & Hassett, 1990; Zaretsky et al., 1995).

Fat implantation also is being tried on a preliminary basis to treat dysphonia caused by scar tissue formation following laryngeal trauma, microsurgery, or tumor resection (Sataloff et al., 1997). Fat implantation differs from injection in that a mucosal pocket is created on the vibratory margin of the scarred vocal fold via a narrow access tunnel excavated from a small incision on the superior surface of the fold. Care is taken to keep the mucosa along the medial and inferior margins of the vocal fold intact. The pocket is filled with fat using a Bruning's syringe with a large needle passed through the tunnel. When the needle is removed, the access tunnel closes spontaneously. Sataloff et al. (1997) reported improved vocal fold vibratory motion and voice quality after use of this procedure on 4 patients with severe, extensive vocal fold scarring. They concluded that fat implantation for treatment of laryngeal scarring is sufficiently promising to warrant additional research. Using a similar procedure, Woo, Rahbar, and Wang (1999) implanted fat in the right vocal fold of 6 dogs and harvested the larynges 6 weeks later. All 6 specimens had histologic evidence of viable implanted fat and/or fibrous tissue at the implant site. Further, the implanted vocal folds continued to show good vibratory function on stroboscopic examination. The authors concluded that fat implantation may be useful in humans for rehabilitation of the vocal fold.

LARYNGEAL FRAMEWORK SURGERY

Laryngeal framework surgery is another phonosurgical treatment option for dysphonias resulting from glottic incompetence. A variant of such surgery is performed to adjust vocal fold tension in instances of diminished tone or if vocal pitch is extremely disordered. Over the years, various phonosurgical techniques have been developed and modified to improve vocal functioning in such instances. Indeed, in many voice centers laryngeal framework surgery has become the treatment of choice for glottic incompetence, although a combination of different laryngeal framework procedures may be necessary to obtain optimum voice quality results (Mahieu, Norbart, & Snel, 1996).

In cases of vocal fold atrophy associated with aging, phonosurgical techniques have been advocated, if glottal gap is severe. Under such circumstances some surgeons feel that phonosurgery is more efficient and less burdensome on the patient than is therapy. Reportedly, phonosurgery also has a motivating effect on patients that improves voice therapy results postsurgery by providing patients with some initial success with voice production (Isshiki et al., 1996).

Medialization Thyroplasty

The most common laryngeal framework surgery is medialization (Type I) thyroplasty. Medialization thyroplasty is used primarily to correct glottic insufficiency secondary to vocal fold paralysis. In recent years, medialization thyroplasty has been increasingly performed in elderly patients to correct glottic insufficiency associated with vocal fold atrophy (Slavit, 1999).

Kieff and Zeitels (1996) present a comprehensive historical perspective on the development of this surgical procedure. Versions of medialization procedures using autologous cartilage were described early in the 20th century. However, reports of procedures using silicone bioimplants by Isshiki and his associates in the 1970s resulted in more widespread acceptance of this surgical technique (Isshiki, 1989; Isshiki, Morita, Okamura, & Hiramoto, 1974). Koufman (1986) has been credited with adding refinements to the surgical procedure that helped to popularize it within the United States (Netterville, Stone, Luken, Civantos, & Ossoff, 1993). With expanded use came more refinements of surgical technique. In addition, implications for use of this surgery widened to include glottic incompetence associated with aging and tissue loss following surgery for early glottic cancer (Isshiki et al., 1996; Kief & Zeitels, 1996; Koufman, 1989; Koufman & Isaacson, 1991; Maves, McCabe, & Gray, 1989; Sasaki, Leder, Petcu, & Friedman, 1990; Sakai et al., 1996). Investigators have cited several advantages of medialization thyroplasty (in comparison with Teflon injection) including (1) good quality voice results that are highly reproducible, (2) easier training of physicians in its use, (3) adjustability, and (4) reversibility (Netterville et al., 1993).

In performing medialization thyroplasty, a small rectangular window opening is created in the lamina of the thyroid cartilage lateral to the vocal

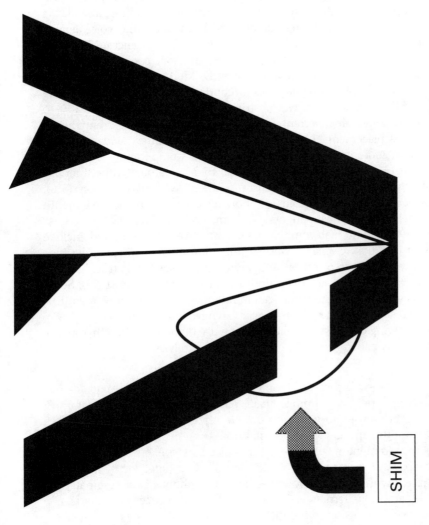

Figure 16–1. Schematic diagram of medialization thyroplasty.

fold. A synthetic shim is placed in the window that has the effect of medializing the affected vocal fold without altering its physical properties (mass, stiffness) during vibration (Figure 16–1). Avoiding contact with the medial edge of the vocal fold maintains its vibratory properties and improves voice results. Usually the procedure is carried out under local anesthesia, which reduces surgical risk. Use of local anesthesia also allows for voice monitoring during surgery which enhances the voice quality results (Mahieu et al., 1996; Tucker, Wanamaker, Trott, & Hicks, 1993).

When performed by an experienced surgeon, complications from medialization thyroplasty occur infrequently (Kieff & Zeitels, 1996). However, major complications have been reported, including extrusion of the implant (7% to 9%) and airway obstruction requiring tracheostomy (0% to 10%). In addition, inadvertent violation of the inner perichondrium during prosthesis placement (14%) has been reported (Cotter, Avidano, Crary, Cassisi, & Gorham, 1995; Tucker et al., 1993). Complications considered minor (Cotter et al., 1995) include vocal fold hematoma without airway obstruction (24%) and prosthesis movement without extrusion (5%). Reportedly, minor vocal fold irritation resolves within the first month postoperatively in most patients (Gorham, Avidano, Crary, Cotter, & Cassisi, 1998). Additional complications that have been reported include wound infection, cartilage window migration, thyroid fracture, dyspnea accompanying overcorrection, and laryngocutaneous fistula (Kieff & Zeitels, 1996; Mahieu et al., 1996; Rosen, Murry, & DeMarino, 1999). Some reports suggest that the complication rate may be higher in women than men, presumably because of smaller laryngeal size (Cotter et al., 1995). The following case histories illustrate the use of medialization thyroplasty with elderly patients experiencing vocal fold paralysis:

Mr. V (age 75) presented for a second opinion as to voice quality changes persisting from left true vocal fold paralysis suffered after surgery for an aortic aneurysm. He reported having undergone voice therapy at several hospitals following the paralysis with no improvement in voice. He felt his voice had worsened in the previous 2–3 months. Perceptually, his voice was judged to be low in pitch with decreased loudness and diplophonia. Diaphragmatic breathing patterns were observed, along with excessive musculoskeletal tension in the lower face. Videostroboscopy confirmed paralysis of the left true vocal fold in the paramedian position with bowing of the vocal fold. Incomplete closure along the length of the glottis was observed during phonation. Mobility of the right vocal fold was normal. Significant movement of the ventricular vocal folds was observed during phonation. A left medialization (Type I) thyroplasty was performed without complications. Following surgery, the patient's voice was judged to be "strong and good." Indirect laryngoscopy confirmed that medialization was excellent.

Mr. G was referred for videostroboscopy and a voice evaluation at age 78. He had experienced onset of left true vocal fold paralysis of uncertain etiology 6 months prior and had undergone voice therapy for 3 months with no improvement of voice. EMG findings indicated severe involvement of the recurrent laryngeal nerve and mild involvement of the superior laryngeal nerve. Mr. G stated that it was difficult for him to communicate in social situations and that he was frustrated by a lack of vocal intensity. He also experienced frequent coughing. Perceptually, his voice was reduced in loudness and diplophonic. Maximum phonation time was markedly short and pitch and intensity ranges were restricted. Videostroboscopy confirmed paralysis of the left vocal fold with bowing resulting in considerable mid fold gap during phonation. Mobility of the right vocal fold was normal, but approximation of the folds was absent during phonation. Mr. G underwent medialization thyroplasty (Type I) 6 weeks later. One month following surgery, Mr. G telephoned reporting difficulty breathing while eating that resulted in coughing. He reported difficulty "getting air in" for a period of 40–45 minutes. The following day, on mirror examination, good contact of the true vocal folds was observed bilaterally. Some erythema of the left vocal fold still was evident secondary to the surgery. Voice was remarkably improved in intensity. Breathing difficulties were attributed to laryngeal penetration causing cough and laryngospasm; mildly reduced superior laryngeal nerve function indicated by earlier EMG findings also may have contributed. Two months after surgery Mr. G reported satisfaction with his voice and the improvement in vocal intensity. However, he remained concerned about a persistent cough and difficulty breathing. He described breathing difficulties as occurring 1–2 times per week and involving chest constriction rather than the upper airway. During videostroboscopic examination, paralysis of the left true vocal fold again was noted. Mobility of the right vocal fold was normal. Closure was

(continued)

excellent along the entire length of the glottis during phonation. The airway was patent and adequate during quiet breathing. The left true vocal fold remained erythematous and pooling of secretions was noted in the left pyriform sinus. A bilateral mucosal wave was observed under stroboscopic light, although vibratory patterns were asymmetric. Response to vocal fold medialization was judged to be excellent. Persistent suspected laryngospasm was "difficult to sort out" because of airway findings from videostroboscopy. A chest X-ray revealed COPD and probable pulmonary hypertension, but no acute disease. A swallow study revealed abnormal esophageal motility and a small hiatal hernia with mild GERD. An echocardiogram and stress test produced abnormal findings. Pulmonary assessment concluded that breathing problems were likely related to laryngospasm. Three months after surgery Mr. G still reported experiencing some coughing, but with less frequency and intensity. He remained satisfied with vocal intensity and quality. Videostroboscopic examination again revealed good approximation of the vocal folds with a patent airway during quiet breathing. Some improvement clearing secretions from the hypopharynx also was noted. Ten months after surgery voice quality was perceived as only mildly hoarse with excellent vocal intensity. Again, vocal fold approximation was complete. Mr. G was told he did not need to return to otolaryngology unless he experienced changes in voice.

Results obtained with medialization thyroplasty depend on the cause of the glottic insufficiency requiring surgical intervention. There appears to be general agreement that the best results occur in cases of vocal fold paralysis. Results are considered generally poor in cases of vocal fold scarring accompanying glottic insufficiency or in instances of medialization surgery following previous cordial injection procedures. Similarly, vocal fold atrophy in combination with sulcus vocalis generally gives poorer results (Bielamowicz et al., 1995; Isshiki et al., 1996; Kojima, Hirano, Shoji, Omori, & Honjo, 1996; Lindestad & Hertegård, 1994; Lu, Casiano, Lundy, & Xue, 1998). Variations in tissue healing also affect voice quality results, particularly during the 3 months immediately following surgery. Although physicians generally note improvement in voice quality immediately following placement of the implant, vocal quality may deteriorate markedly in the immediate postoperative period and require varying time intervals (up to 3 months) to restabilize to the improved levels observed during surgery (Gorham et al., 1998; Tucker et al., 1993).

The success of medialization thyroplasty in the treatment of vocal fold atrophy in the elderly is open to some question. Some reports suggest that the degree of voice quality improvement is variable in elderly patients who require bilateral implants because of vocal fold bowing (Netterville et al., 1993). Similarly, Berke (1995) estimated that the incidence of voice improvement following thyroplasty in patients with vocal fold bowing is 60% with only 1 patient in 4 demonstrating dramatic improvement. Furthermore, the risk of shim migration increases when medialization surgery is performed on mobile vocal folds. Therefore, additional procedures are necessary to hold the shim in position. Also, more medialization is required in cases involving mobile vocal folds in comparison with paralytic glottic insufficiency (Isshiki et al., 1996; Mahieu et al., 1996).

Despite these issues, Isshiki et al. (1996) report that surgical medialization greatly improves the quality of life in elderly persons experiencing vocal fatigue and a weak voice due to vocal fold atrophy. Furthermore, Postma, Blalock, and Koufman (1998) report encouraging results in a recent retrospective investigation of long-term outcomes ($M = 17$ months) following bilateral medialization laryngoplasty on 16 elderly patients diagnosed with vocal fold atrophy. These investigators found significant improvement in voice/swallowing function and concluded that bilateral medialization laryngoplasty is an effective treatment for symptomatic vocal fold bowing. They also found lipoinjection useful as an adjunct to surgical medialization (vocal "fine tuning") to improve voice outcomes in some cases.

Studies examining objective voice measures (acoustic and aerodynamic) on patients receiving medialization surgery for nonparalytic vocal fold bowing also have produced conflicting results. One investigation concluded that voice results following medialization thyroplasty are equally as good in "nontraditional" (vocal fold atrophy, sulcus vocalis, glottal gap without paralysis, and previous vocal fold surgery) and "traditional" (vocal fold paralysis) applications (Bielamowicz et al., 1995). A second study indicated that medialization surgery is more successful at restoring voice in cases of vocal fold paralysis in comparison with cases of nonparalytic vocal fold bowing (Lu et al., 1998). Direct comparison between these studies is difficult, however, given methodological differences in the timing of voice quality assessment. Bielamowicz et al. (1995) examined vocal parameters an average of 6 months following surgery, with Lu and his associates (1998) evaluating voice 1 month postoperatively. As patients vary in the length of time necessary to restabilize voice following this surgery, the voice results of Lu et al. (1998) might have been poorer simply because their patients had not yet achieved fully recovered vocal quality.

Recently, clinicians have begun investigating methods other than acoustic measures, aerodynamic evaluation, and subjective assessment to determine the effects of vocal fold medialization surgery. When poor results are obtained from this surgery, magnetic resonance imaging (MRI) has been used to evaluate the anatomical and functional status of the vocal folds. The superior contrast resolution of MRI has proven useful in showing the effects of shim shape and size on vocal fold positioning (Ford, Unger, Zundel, & Bless, 1995). It is expected that increasing use of such methods in the future will lead to further refinements of surgical technique and improved outlook for successful voice outcomes in a broader spectrum of patients, including the elderly.

Nerve-Muscle Pedicle Reinnervation

In cases of unilateral vocal fold paralysis, some surgeons advocate combining medialization thyroplasty with nerve-muscle pedicle reinnervation (Tucker, 1997). The purpose of this refinement is to avoid eventual deterioration of voice improvement due to continuing loss of vocal fold mass from denervation. Reinnervation is not necessary when vocal fold medialization surgery is performed for glottic insufficiency with mobile vocal folds (such as in vocal fold atrophy), since denervation loss is not an issue (Mahieu et al., 1996). Reportedly, combined surgical medialization and nerve-muscle pedicle reinnervation has successfully avoided further vocal fold atrophy for up to 10 years after reinnervation, with complication rates comparable to those observed for medialization alone (Tucker, 1997). However, randomized studies have yet to be conducted comparing medialization procedures with and without reinnervation for treatment of unilateral vocal fold paralysis (Berke, 1995). Also, no instances of restoration of active vocal fold movement following a reinnervation procedure have been reported to date (Havas et al., 1999).

Arytenoid Adduction

Arytenoid adduction is the procedure of choice for conditions such as abductor paralysis involving deficiencies in vocal fold length and arytenoid positioning that cannot be remediated by medialization thyroplasty and vocal fold injection techniques (Blaugrund, 1991). Specifically, arytenoid adduction is indicated if the paralyzed vocal fold is shorter than the normal fold or if the affected arytenoid cartilage is rotated outward. When the vocal folds differ in length, the patient attempts to achieve glottic symmetry and decrease perceived breathiness by shortening the good vocal fold. To accomplish shortening, the glottis is compressed in the sagittal plane. This maneuver requires compensatory hyperfunction and can eventually result in bowing of the normal vocal fold. If the affected arytenoid cartilage is rotated outward, approximation of the vocal processes is precluded, even if compensation by the normal side brings the arytenoids together. Such an adjustment produces a "posterior" glottal gap on phonation (Woodson & Murry, 1994). The decision to use arytenoid adduction is not always clear-cut, however. Netterville et al. (1993) found that medialization thyroplasty alone accomplished adequate closure of the glottis for some patients in whom the use of arytenoid adduction had been anticipated.

The arytenoid adduction procedure was first described by Isshiki, Tanabe, and Sawada (1978). This procedure mimics the action of the lateral cricoarytenoid muscle by rotating the arytenoid to medialize the vocal process. Along with approximation of the vocal processes, height of the affected fold can be adjusted. This procedure is technically difficult to perform, however, and cannot be reversed (Kieff & Zeitels, 1996; Woodson & Murry, 1994). In addition, voice improvement in cases of long-standing vocal fold paralysis (20 years or more) is minimal. These poor results are thought to reflect soft tissue contracture that interferes with vocal fold lengthening (Woodson & Murry, 1994). Results also are poor if the paralyzed vocal fold is atrophic or bowed. In such instances, medialization thyroplasty or injection techniques are recommended in conjunction with arytenoid adduction to achieve optimum vocal fold approximation along the entire length of the glottis (Blaugrund, 1991; Woodson & Murry, 1994).

Recently a new adduction procedure was introduced (Zeitels, Hochman, & Hillman, 1998). This procedure (adduction arytenopexy) aims to affix the arytenoid on the medial aspect of the cricoid facet in a position that more closely simulates its normal adduction during phonation. That is, the aim is to simulate the normal agonist-antagonist function of the interarytenoid, lateral thyroarytenoid, and posterior cricoarytenoid muscles during adduction and, in that way, avoid exaggerated medial rotation of the vocal process that can accompany the classic arytenoid adduction procedure (Zeitels et al., 1998). When compared with classic arytenoid adduction on 10 fresh cadaver larynges, the adduction arytenopexy procedure reportedly resulted in greater lengthening of the vocal fold, higher vocal fold positioning, and a more normally contoured arytenoid. When adduction arytenopexy was combined with medialization thyroplasty in a clinical trial on 12 patients, complications were reported to be minimal. In addition, results were positive in terms of visual assessment of function and objective/subjective vocal assessment measures (Zeitels et al., 1998). Clearly, additional experience with this procedure both by these investigators and others will provide more insight into the usefulness of this procedure.

Vocal Fold Tension Adjustment

Various laryngeal framework surgical procedures have been developed to either lengthen or shorten the vocal folds passively, thereby altering their tension without invading the vocal fold tissues themselves. Surgically altering vocal fold tension has a direct effect on the pitch of the voice. When the vocal folds are lengthened (increased tension), pitch rises. When the vocal folds are shortened (decreased tension), pitch lowers. Therefore, tension-adjusting procedures have applications for a variety of disorders involving vocal pitch deviation, including mutational voice disorders, androphonia, and transsexual voice treatment (Isshiki, Taira & Tanabe, 1988). In addition, tension-altering procedures have been used in cases of vocal fold atrophy and vocal fold paralysis, either alone or in combination with other phonosurgical procedures.

Detailed descriptions of tension-adjusting surgical procedures have been provided in earlier reports (Blaugrund, 1991; Isshiki, Taira, & Tanabe, 1983, 1988; Zeitels, Hillman, Desloge, & Bunting, 1999). All procedures are performed under local anesthesia so that the patient can phonate on request during surgery. For vocal fold relaxation and pitch lowering (thyroplasty Type III), a vertical incision is made in the ala of the thyroid cartilage lateral to the thyroid notch. A narrow strip of cartilage is removed along the incised edge. This results in shortening of the anterior-posterior length of the vocal fold. The procedure may be performed unilaterally or bilaterally depending on the degree of vocal fold relaxation required (Isshiki et al., 1988).

In 1974 Isshiki and his associates described a method for lengthening the vocal folds referred to as cricothyroid approximation (thyroplasty Type IV). This surgery simulates approximation of the cricoid and thyroid cartilages normally achieved during pitch elevation. The two cartilages are approximated as closely as possible and held together by sutures. Silicone bolsters are placed on the side of the thyroid cartilage to disperse the force exerted on that cartilage by the suturing. Vocal fold tensing also has been accomplished by creating a midline flap in the thyroid cartilage and pulling the flap forward, advancing the anterior commissure (LeJeune, Guice, & Samuels, 1983; Tucker, 1985). Most recently, vocal fold tension has been increased by placing a suture around the inferior cornu of the thyroid lamina and passing it under the cricoid anteriorly, pulling it taut (Zeitels et al., 1999).

Laryngeal framework surgery to alter the tension level of the vocal folds has been performed on elderly speakers with vocal fold atrophy. Isshiki and his associates (1996) report using either vocal fold shortening (thyroplasty Type III) or vocal fold lengthening (thyroplasty Type IV) in combination with vocal fold medialization (thyroplasty Type I) in elderly patients on a case-by-case basis. The decision to add a tension-altering procedure and deciding which one to add is made during surgery in response to intraoperative testing. Tucker (1988) and LeJeune et al. (1983) both report performing anterior commissure advancement on elderly patients, although neither combine the procedure with medialization.

Success of tension-altering procedures with vocal fold atrophy has been limited. The greatest benefit appears to occur when tension adjustment is accompanied by medialization surgery, at least in elderly patients without sulci and widespread scarring (Isshiki et al., 1996). Surgeons who attempted to counteract the effects of aging by increasing vocal fold tension alone, without medialization, also reported early success (LeJeune et al., 1983; Tucker, 1985). However, later reports indicated that voice benefits in older patients are short-lived. Tucker (1988) observed regression of voice to presurgery quality after periods of 3 weeks to 7 months in 6 of 8 elderly patients receiving advancement surgery alone. He observed that the relatively short-lived voice improvement achieved by this surgery is not unlike results of facelifts performed on older patients. That is, an apparent fundamental loss of tissue elasticity associated with aging produces only temporary improvements in tension.

SUMMARY

In the elderly, phonosurgical procedures (vocal fold injection, laryngeal framework surgery) may be used to treat glottal insufficiency resulting from pathological processes (paralysis/paresis, neurologic disease, laryngeal trauma), atrophic changes in the vocal folds, or vocal fold segmental problems associated with scar tissue from previous surgery. Typically, phonosurgery would be considered only if vocal symptoms did not respond to voice therapy or if glottal gap is severe.

Vocal fold injection most frequently is used in cases of vocal fold paralysis to reposition the paralyzed fold closer to midline. It also is used in the treatment of mucosal defects. Teflon is the substance most frequently injected in cases of unilateral vocal fold paralysis. It should not be injected into mobile vocal folds and is ineffective if the arytenoids are widely abducted. Granuloma formation is often mentioned as a possible problem with Teflon injection, although incidence estimates vary widely. Despite these limitations, Teflon is viewed as useful in patients with shortened life expectancy in whom anesthesia use poses a high risk. Bovine collagen as an injection material offers the advantage of biocompatibility and also can lessen the impact of preexisting scar tissue on a limited basis. It can produce immunologic reactions, however, although newer formulations may minimize this risk. Recent use of autologous collagen has eliminated concern over possible disease transmission to humans from use of bovine collagen. Autologous fat is less likely than bovine collagen to produce reactions in the immune system but may tend to be reabsorbed over time. Findings of reabsorption of fat are not universal, however, and may be related to factors involved in the harvesting and handling of the graft material. Fat implantation has been tried on a limited number of patients with severe, extensive vocal fold scarring and results are promising.

Laryngeal framework surgery is performed to medialize the vocal fold or to adjust vocal fold tension. In cases of apparent vocal fold atrophy associated with aging, phonosurgery is performed if glottal gap is severe. Medialization thyroplasty involves surgical placement of a shim in a window in the lamina of the thyroid cartilage to reposition the vocal fold closer to midline. Avoiding contact with the medial edge of the fold maintains normal vibratory properties and improves voice quality results. Complications from medialization thyroplasty are infrequent. In cases of unilateral vocal fold paralysis, medialization might be combined with nerve-muscle pedicle reinnervation to avoid continuing denervation of the vocal fold. Results of medialization thyroplasty are best in cases of vocal fold paralysis. There is some evidence that surgical medialization may be less successful and more problematic in cases of vocal fold atrophy, although that finding is not universal. Lipoinjection may be useful to "fine tune" voice outcomes in some patients receiving bilateral medialization laryngoplasty.

Arytenoid adduction is performed in cases of abductor paralysis when vocal fold length and arytenoid positioning are deficient. Arytenoid adduction rotates the vocal process toward the midline and allows for adjustment of vocal fold height. The procedure is technically difficult, however, and minimally effective in cases of long-standing vocal fold paralysis. Results also are poor in instances of bowed vocal folds. Adduction arytenopexy aims to more closely simulate the normal adductory position of the arytenoid and avoid exaggerated medial rotation of the vocal process. While early results have been positive, conclusive evidence as to the usefulness of this procedure awaits additional clinical trials.

Surgical relaxation of the vocal fold (pitch lowering) is accomplished by removing a strip of cartilage from the ala of the thyroid, shortening the anterior-posterior length of the vocal fold. Increased vocal fold tension (pitch elevation) is accomplished by (1) approximating the cricoid and thyroid cartilages anteriorly, (2) advancing the anterior commissure, or (3) affixing a suture to the inferior cornu of the thyroid lamina and passing it under the anterior of the cricoid, pulling it tight. In the treatment of age-related vocal fold atrophy, both vocal fold shortening and vocal fold lengthening (cricothyroid approximation) have been combined with vocal fold medialization with limited success. Anterior commissure advancement has been performed alone on elderly patients with only short-lived voice improvement.

REFERENCES

Arnold, G. (1962). Vocal rehabilitation of paralytic dysphonia. IX. Technique of intracordal injection. *Archives of Otolaryngology, 76,* 358–368.

Berke, G. (1995). Phonosurgery—Outcomes of varied techniques. *Western Journal of Medicine, 163,* 156–157.

Berke, G., Gerratt, B., Kreiman, J., & Jackson, K. (1999). Treatment of Parkinson hypophonia with percutaneous collagen augmentation. *Laryngoscope, 109,* 1295–1299.

Bielamowicz, S., Berke, G., & Gerratt, B. (1995). A comparison of type I thyroplasty and arytenoid adduction. *Journal of Voice, 9,* 466–472.

Blaugrund, S. (1991). Laryngeal framework surgery. In C. Ford & D. Bless (Eds.), *Phonosurgery: Assessment and surgical management of voice disorders* (pp. 183–199). New York: Raven Press.

Boyce, R., Nuss, D., & Kluka, E. (1994). The use of autogenous fat, fascia, and non-vascularized muscle grafts in the head and neck. *Otolaryngologic Clinics of North America, 27,* 39–68.

Brandenburg, J., Kirkham, W., & Koschkee, D. (1992). Vocal cord augmentation with autogenous fat. *Laryngoscope, 102,* 495–500.

Chan, R., & Titze, I. (1998). Viscosities of implantable biomaterials in vocal fold augmentation surgery. *Laryngoscope, 108,* 725–731.

Chan, R., & Titze, I. (1999). Viscoelastic shear properties of human vocal fold mucosa: Measurement methodology and empirical results. *Journal of the Acoustical Society of America, 106,* 2008–2021.

Cotter, C., Avidano, M., Crary, M., Cassisi, N., & Gorham, M. (1995). Laryngeal complications after type I thyroplasty. *Otolaryngology Head & Neck Surgery, 113,* 671–673.

Dedo, H. (1992). Injection and removal of Teflon for unilateral vocal cord paralysis. *Annals of Otology, Rhinology, and Laryngology, 101,* 81–86.

Dedo, H., Urrea, R., & Lawson, L. (1973). Intracordal injection of Teflon in the treatment of 135 patients with dysphonia. *Annals of Otology, Rhinology, and Laryngology, 82,* 661–667.

Dejonckere, P. (1998). Teflon injection and thyroplasty: Objective and subjective outcomes. *Revue de Laryngologie-Otologie-Rhinologie (Bordeaux), 119,* 265–269.

Ford, C., & Bless, D. (1986). Clinical experience with injectable collagen for vocal fold augmentation. *Laryngoscope, 96,* 863–869.

Ford, C., Bless, D., & Loftus, J. (1992). Role of injectable collagen in the treatment of glottic insufficiency: A study of 119 patients. *Annals of Otology, Rhinology and Laryngology, 101,* 237–247.

Ford, C., Martin, D., & Warner, T. (1984). Injectable collagen in laryngeal rehabilitation. *Laryngoscope, 94,* 513–518.

Ford, C., Staskowski, P., & Bless, D. (1995). Autologous collagen vocal fold injection: A preliminary clinical study. *Laryngoscope, 105,* 944–948.

Ford, C., Unger, J., Zundel, R., & Bless, D. (1995). Magnetic resonance imaging (MRI) assessment of vocal fold medialization surgery. *Laryngoscope, 105,* 498–504.

Gardner, G., & Parnes, S. (1991). Status of the mucosal wave post vocal cord injection versus thyroplasty. *Journal of Voice, 5,* 64–73.

Gorham, M., Avidano, M., Crary, M., Cotter, C., & Cassisi, N. (1998). Laryngeal recovery following type I thyroplasty. *Archives of Otolaryngology—Head and Neck Surgery, 124,* 739–742.

Hagen, P., Lyons, G., & Nuss, D. (1996). Dysphonia in the elderly: Diagnosis and management of age-related voice changes. *Southern Medical Journal, 89,* 204–207.

Harries, M. (1996). Unilateral vocal fold paralysis: A review of the current methods of surgical rehabilitation. *Journal of Laryngology and Otology, 110,* 111–116.

Harries, M., & Morrison, M. (1998). Management of unilateral vocal cord paralysis by injection medialization with Teflon paste. Quantitative results. *Annals of Otology, Rhinology, and Laryngology, 107,* 332–336.

Havas, T., Lowinger, D., & Priestley, J. (1999). Unilateral vocal fold paralysis: Causes, options, and outcomes. *Australian and New Zealand Journal of Surgery, 69,* 509–513.

Isshiki, N. (1989). *Phonosurgery: Theory and practice.* Tokyo: Springer-Verlag.

Isshiki, N., Morita, H., Okamura, H., & Hiramoto, M. (1974). Thyroplasty as a new phonosurgical technique. *Acta Otolaryngologica, 78,* 451–457.

Isshiki, N., Shoji, K., Kojima, H., & Hirano, S. (1996). Vocal fold atrophy and its surgical treatment. *Annals of Otology, Rhinology and Laryngology, 105,* 182–188.

Isshiki, N., Taira, T., & Tanabe, M. (1983). Surgical alteration of the vocal pitch. *Journal of Otolaryngology, 12,* 335–340.

Isshiki, N., Taira, T., & Tanabe, M. (1988). Surgical treatment for vocal pitch disorders. In O. Fujimura (Ed.), *Vocal physiology: Voice production, mechanisms, and functions* (pp. 449–458). New York: Raven Press.

Isshiki, N., Tanabe, M., & Sawada, M. (1978). Arytenoid adduction for unilateral vocal cord paralysis. *Archives of Otolaryngology—Head and Neck Surgery, 14,* 555–558.

Kieff, D., & Zeitels, S. (1996). Phonosurgery. *Comprehensive Therapy, 22,* 222–230.

Kojima, H., Hirano, S., Shoji, K., Omori, K., & Honjo, I. (1996). Omohyoid muscle transposition for the treatment of bowed vocal fold. *Annals of Otology, Rhinology and Laryngology, 105,* 536–540.

Koufman, J. (1986). Laryngoplasty for vocal cord medialization: An alternative to Teflon. *Laryngoscope, 96,* 726–731.

Koufman, J. (1989). Surgical correction of dysphonia due to bowing of the vocal cords. *Annals of Otology, Rhinology and Laryngology, 98,* 41–45.

Koufman, J., & Isaacson, G. (1991). Laryngoplastic phonosurgery. *Otolaryngologic Clinics of North America, 24,* 1151–1177.

LeJeune, F., Guice, C., & Samuels, P. (1983). Early experiences with vocal ligament tightening. *Annals of Otology, Rhinology and Laryngology, 92,* 475–477.

Lindestad, P., & Hertegård, S. (1994). Spindle-shaped glottal insufficiency with and without sulcus vocalis: A retrospective study. *Annals of Otology, Rhinology and Laryngology, 103,* 547–553.

Lu, F., Casiano, R., Lundy, D., & Xue, J. (1998). Vocal evaluation of thyroplasty type I in the treatment of nonparalytic glottic incompetence. *Annals of Otology, Rhinology and Laryngology, 107,* 113–119.

Mahieu, H., Norbart, T., & Snel, F. (1996). Laryngeal framework surgery for voice improvement. *Revue de Laryngologie, Otologie, Rhinologie, 117,* 189–197.

Mak, K., & Toriumi, D. (1994). Injectable filler materials for soft tissue augmentation. *Otolaryngologic Clinics of North America, 27,* 211–222.

Maves, M., McCabe, B., & Gray, S. (1989). Phonosurgery: Indications and pitfalls. *Annals of Otology, Rhinology and Laryngology, 98,* 577–580.

Mikaelian, D., Lowry, L., & Sataloff, R. (1991). Lipoinjection for unilateral vocal cord paralysis. *Laryngoscope, 101,* 465–468.

Mikus, J., Koufman, J., & Kilpatrick, S. (1995). Fate of liposuctioned and purified autologous fat injections in the canine vocal fold. *Laryngoscope, 105,* 17–22.

Netterville, J., Coleman, J., Chang, S., Rainey, C., Reinisch, L., & Ossoff, R. (1998). Lateral laryngotomy for the removal of Teflon granuloma. *Annals of Otology, Rhinology and Laryngology, 107,* 735–744.

Netterville, J., Stone, R. E., Luken, E., Civantos, F., & Ossoff, R. (1993). Silastic medialization and arytenoid adduction: The Vanderbilt experience. A review of 116 phonosurgical procedures. *Annals of Otology, Rhinology and Laryngology, 102,* 413–424.

Nguyen, A., Pasyk, K., Bouvier, T., Hassett, C., & Argenta, L. (1990). Comparative study of survival of autologous adipose tissue taken and transplanted by different techniques. *Plastic and Reconstructive Surgery, 85,* 378–389.

Omori, K., Slavit, D., Kacker, A., & Blaugrund, S. (1998). Influence of size and etiology of glottal gap in glottic incompetence dysphonia. *Laryngoscope, 108,* 514–518.

Postma, G., Blalock, P., & Koufman, J. (1998). Bilateral medialization laryngoplasty. *Laryngoscope, 108,* 1429–1434.

Remacle, M., Lawson, G., Delos, M., & Jamart, J. (1999). Correcting vocal fold immobility by autologous collagen injection for voice rehabilitation: A short-term study. *Annals of Otology, Rhinology and Laryngology, 108,* 788–793.

Remacle, M., Lawson, G., Keghian, J., & Jamart, J. (1999). Use of injectable autologous collagen for correcting glottic gaps: Initial results. *Journal of Voice, 13,* 280–288.

Rosen, C., Murry, T., & DeMarino, D. (1999). Late complication of type 1 thyroplasty: A case report. *Journal of Voice, 13,* 417–423.

Sakai, N., Nishizawa, N., Matsushima, J., Kurihara, H., Kokubun, T., Koichi, K., Maguchi, S., & Inuyama, Y. (1996). Thyroplasty type I with ceramic shim. *Artificial Organs, 20,* 951–954.

Sasaki, C., Leder, S., Petcu, L., & Friedman, C. (1990). Longitudinal voice quality changes following Isshiki thyroplasty type I: The Yale experience. *Laryngoscope, 100,* 849–852.

Sataloff, R., Spiegel, J., Hawkshaw, M., Rosen, D., & Heuer, R. (1997). Autologous fat implantation for vocal fold scar: A preliminary report. *Journal of Voice, 11,* 238–246.

Shindo, M. & Hanson, D. (1990). Geriatric voice and laryngeal dysfunction. *Otolaryngologic Clinics of North America, 23,* 1035–1044.

Slavit, D. (1999). Phonosurgery in the elderly: A review. *Ear, Nose, and Throat Journal, 78,* 505–512.

Tanaka, S., Hirano, M., & Chijiwa, K. (1994). Some aspects of vocal fold bowing. *Annals of Otology, Rhinology and Laryngology, 103,* 357–362.

Tucker, H. (1985). Anterior commissure laryngoplasty for adjustment of vocal fold tension. *Annals of Otology, Rhinology and Laryngology, 94,* 547–549.

Tucker, H. (1988). Laryngeal framework surgery in the management of the aged larynx. *Annals of Otology, Rhinology and Laryngology, 97,* 534–536.

Tucker, H. (1997). Combined surgical medialization and nerve-muscle pedicle reinnervation for unilateral vocal fold paralysis: Improved functional results and prevention of long-term deterioration of voice. *Journal of Voice, 11,* 474–478.

Tucker, H., Wanamaker, J., Trott, M., & Hicks, D. (1993). Complications of laryngeal framework surgery (phonosurgery). *Laryngoscope, 103,* 525–528.

Woo, P., Rahbar, R., & Wang, Z. (1999). Fat implantation into Reineke's space: A histologic and stroboscopic study in the canine. *Annals of Otology, Rhinology and Laryngology, 108,* 738–744.

Woodson, G. & Miller, R. (1981). The timing of surgical intervention in vocal cord paralysis. *Otolaryngology—Head and Neck Surgery, 89,* 264–267.

Woodson, G., & Murry, T. (1994). Glottic configuration after arytenoid adduction. *Laryngoscope, 104,* 965–969.

Zaretsky, L., Shindo, M., deTar, M., & Rice, D. (1995). Autologous fat injection for vocal fold paralysis: Long-term histologic evaluation. *Annals of Otology, Rhinology and Laryngology, 104,* 1–4.

Zeitels, S., Hillman, R., Desloge, R., & Bunting, G. (1999). Cricothyroid subluxation: A new innovation for enhancing the voice with laryngoplastic phonosurgery. *Annals of Otology, Rhinology and Laryngology, 108,* 1126–1131.

Zeitels, S., Hochman, I., Hillman, R. (1998). Adduction arytenopexy: A new procedure for paralytic dysphonia with implications for implant medialization. *Annals of Otology, Rhinology and Laryngology 173* (Suppl.) 2–24.

CHAPTER

17

Voice Therapy for the Elderly Patient: Special Considerations

There is some evidence that the number of elderly patients receiving treatment for voice problems has increased in recent years. In 1970, Cooper observed that geriatric patients seldom were referred for vocal rehabilitation, even in cases of neurologic dysfunction or vocal fold pathology. At that time elderly persons complaining of vocal fatigue were "left to their own devices" (p. 109), which might involve such treatments as throat lozenges, gargling, and throat sprays. Recently, it has been estimated that up to 12% of elderly individuals receive treatment for voice disorders (Morrison & Gore-Hickman, 1986; Shindo & Hanson, 1990).

Voice disorders in the elderly might be attributed to changes in the laryngeal mechanism associated with normal aging or to pathological conditions unrelated to normal aging. However, distinguishing between normal aging and pathological processes can be difficult in some cases. Indeed, Woo, Casper, Colton, and Brewer (1992) found that the overwhelming majority of their elderly voice patients suffered from a disease process associated with aging as opposed to a disorder resulting from physiologic aging alone. Similarly, Morrison and Gore-Hickman (1986)

285

concluded that only 2 patients demonstrated dysphonia attributable solely to normal aging after reviewing the files of 121 elderly patients seen for voice disorders over a 5-year span. Clinicians warn that a thorough history and medical examination are necessary to rule out disease processes affecting voice in the elderly (Hagen, Lyons, & Nuss, 1996). In addition, a thorough visual inspection of the vocal folds using stroboscopy is recommended for older dysphonic patients to more accurately isolate problems such as sluggish mucosal wave and reduced amplitude of vocal fold motion that can contribute to voice disorders in this population (Woo et al., 1992).

In this chapter strategies for treating voice disorders in the elderly population are explored. Treatment of pathological conditions with a high frequency of occurrence in the elderly is discussed as well as intervention strategies for voice difficulties resulting from the normal aging process.

LIFESTYLE VARIABLES

Voice disorders have been characterized as particularly disabling for the elderly population because of associated lifestyle changes that frequently accompany aging. Any therapy plan for an elderly patient with disordered voice must take into account a number of such variables (Colton & Casper, 1996; Kahane & Beckford, 1991). Age-related loss of independence as well as an increased incidence of hearing loss are factors that exacerbate the impact of voice disorders in elderly persons (Shindo & Hanson, 1990). In addition, the patient's home living circumstances, availability of health care, communicative need, social activities, and availability of emotional support from family and friends influence voice rehabilitation (Kahane & Beckford, 1991). In the case of the aging professional voice user, lifestyle variables involving an increased focus on vocal function and motivation to maintain a youthful voice may positively impact therapy prognosis.

The degree to which an elderly patient engages in social activities also may predict the success of voice therapy. An elderly person living alone with limited social interaction has a relatively guarded prognosis for improvement of vocal function because of a low degree of intrinsic need to communicate. In contrast, elderly patients with a wide circle of friends engaged in numerous social activities have greater communicative need and also a more positive outlook for successful therapeutic intervention. Interestingly, elderly individuals with highly developed social networks appear to gain more than just an improved prognosis for successful vocal rehabilitation. The degree of social involvement of elderly persons also has been linked with mortality risk (Blazer, 1982; Seeman, Kaplan, Knudsen, Cohen, & Guralnik, 1987).

In the last analysis, decisions regarding therapy for voice disorders in the elderly must be tailored to the needs of the patient. As noted by Woo et al. (1992), it is not unusual for patients at any age to perceive a voice problem differently from the voice professional. Some elderly patients are satisfied with a severely dysphonic voice once they are assured they do not have cancer. Others are disturbed by relatively mild dysphonia. Acceptable voice quality at any age depends on a range of factors individual to each speaker.

PHYSIOLOGICAL CONDITIONING

Evidence indicates that physical conditioning, even in the absence of disease processes, plays an important role in maintaining vocal functioning into old age (Chapter 12). When physical condition of elderly speakers is taken into consideration, age-related changes in voice become quite dramatic in comparison with changes observed as a consequence of chronological aging alone (Ramig & Ringel, 1983). That is, elderly speakers whose blood pressure, heart rate, percentage of fat, and vital capacity indicate good physiological condition tend also to demonstrate acoustic characteristics of voice that are relatively youthful. Further, indices of simple activity level indicate that elderly speakers who are more physically active demonstrate better vocal performance overall than elderly individuals who are less active physically (Xue, 1995).

Attention to such factors as diet and exercise increases stamina and improves vocal functioning in older speakers. In many cases, modifying these factors alone satisfactorily ameliorates the voice disorder. For instance, a program of general body aerobic conditioning exercise is useful in improving pulmonary status and reducing fatigue associated with phonation (Hagen et al., 1996). Such a program may negate the necessity for additional direct therapeutic intervention. A proactive approach stressing prevention of voice problems in the elderly through maintaining optimum physiological conditioning has been recommended as the wisest course of action in dealing with issues of vocal aging (Boone & McFarlane, 1994; Colton & Casper, 1996; Luchsinger & Arnold, 1965; Woo et al., 1992). Further, providing the patient with general information on vocal hygiene is useful in improving vocal functioning in this population (Boone & McFarlane, 1994).

PSYCHOLOGICAL ISSUES

Psychopathological processes are known to affect voice production (Butcher, 1995; Gunther, Mayr-Graft, Miller, & Kinzl, 1996; Kiese-Himmel, Pralle, & Kruse, 1998; Roy et al., 1997; White, Deary, & Wilson, 1997). In elderly persons, factors such as tension, anxiety, and depression have been identified as contributing to functional misuse of the voice (Morrison & Gore-Hickman, 1986). The impact of psychological variables on elderly voice production might be predicted, given survey data suggesting a curvilinear relationship between age and indices of subclinical depression over the adult life span. That is, adults in early adulthood and those beyond the age of 75 have higher depression scores than adults in middle age. In addition, loneliness and separation from family during old age are psychological factors that tend to exacerbate voice symptoms (Gatz, Kasl-Godley, & Karel, 1996). It is telling, as well, that laryngeal contact granulomas (contact ulcers) occur most commonly (in men) after the age of 60. Psychological processes such as depression and emotional conflict have been associated with the development of this relatively rare voice disorder (Ferguson, 1955; Kiese-Himmel et al., 1998; Rubenstein, 1957; Wolcott, 1956).

Issues pertaining to state of mind and psychological adjustment must be addressed by the voice therapist when undertaking therapy with older patients. It is not unusual for elderly patients to feel self-conscious about seeking therapy services for a voice disorder (Cooper, 1970). Frequently elderly clients benefit from counseling either informally during the voice therapy session or through referral to appropriate psychological support services in cases of more significant need (Morrison, Rammage, & Nichol, 1989).

VOICE DISORDERS RESULTING FROM PATHOLOGICAL CONDITIONS

Disease processes may affect voice production in speakers at any age. However, elderly patients are more at risk for developing certain conditions simply because of advanced age. Neurologic disorders, carcinoma, trauma, benign lesions, inflammatory processes, and functional misuse all have been identified with considerable frequency among elderly patients (Morrison & Gore-Hickman, 1986; Woo et al., 1992). Additionally, elderly patients are more likely than younger patients to demonstrate multiple etiologic factors related to dysphonia. Woo et al. (1992) found that a second etiologic factor contributed to dysphonia in 34% of 151 patients over the age of 60.

Carcinoma of the Head and Neck

Although commonly diagnosed between the ages of 50 and 70, cancer of the head and neck occasionally occurs later in life. Indeed, recent findings suggest that squamous cell carcinoma of the head and neck, the most common type of head and neck cancer, develops spontaneously in some patients after the age of 70 even in the absence of known risk factors such as smoking or heavy alcohol consumption (Koch, Patel, Brennan, Boyle, & Sidransky, 1995; Leon et al., 1998). In addition, patients diagnosed with squamous cell head and neck cancer after the age of 75 are less likely to demonstrate a genetic mutation (p53) commonly observed in younger patients with the disease. The precise biologic mechanism responsible for the development of the disease in advanced old age is unknown (Koch et al., 1995).

After age 70, laryngeal cancer occurs more frequently in women, possibly as a consequence of greater longevity in women compared with men. In addition, elderly patients diagnosed with laryngeal cancer are less likely than younger patients to have a history of prominent tobacco and alcohol usage. Elderly patients also are more likely to have lesions located at the glottis and the incidence of previous morbidity is higher in this group. Interestingly, patients diagnosed at an advanced age also have a lower incidence of lymph node involvement, although the T category (primary tumor at diagnosis) does not differ as a function of age (Leon et al., 1998).

Treatment of head and neck cancer does not differ a great deal in elderly patients in comparison with younger adults. A number of excellent sources are available that discuss treatment of head and neck cancer in considerable detail (Blom, Singer, & Hamaker, 1998; Keith & Darley, 1994) including controversies concerning the treatment of early glottic carcinoma (Aref, Dworkin, Devi, Denton, & Fontanesi, 1997; Ballo et al., 1998; Burke et al., 1997; Chatani, Matayoshi, Masaki, Teshima, & Inoue, 1997; Dagli, Mahieu, & Festen, 1997; Koufman, 1986; Osguthorpe & Putney, 1997; Raitiola, Wigren, & Pukander, 2000; Yu, Shenouda, Beaudet, & Black, 1997). For more detailed information, readers are directed to these references. Interestingly, physicians frequently advocate aggressive standard therapies for elderly patients diagnosed with squamous cell carcinoma of the head and neck, noting that older patients in generally good health can tolerate such treatments (Koch et al., 1995; Leon et al., 1998). Differences in treatment of laryngeal cancer as a function of patient age include less frequent use of chemotherapy and partial laryngectomy surgery with the elderly. Disease control, incidence of metastasis, and 5-year survival rates for laryngeal cancer are similar regardless of age at diagnosis (Leon et al., 1998).

Neurologic Voice Disorders

Voice disorders with a neurologic etiology are common in the elderly, particularly in advanced old age (Morrison & Gore-Hickman, 1986; Shindo & Hanson, 1990). Damage to the peripheral nerve supply impairs intrinsic laryngeal muscle function and results in vocal fold paralysis or paresis. Vocal function may be impaired as a consequence of cerebral infarction that impairs voluntary motor function. Extrapyramidal lesions result in vocal harshness, reduced loudness, or altered pitch. Tremulous voice and voice arrests can signal essential tremor. Parkinson disease produces a range of vocal symptoms including reduced volume, breathiness, tremor, and monotone voice production (Brin, Fahn, Blitzer, Ramig, & Stewart, 1992; Canter, 1963; Morrison et al., 1989; Mutch, 1992; Perez, Ramig, Smith, & Dromey, 1996; Tatemichi, Freddo, Mohr, & Blitzer, 1992).

Peripheral Laryngeal Paralysis

In examining the charts of 151 dysphonic patients beyond the age of 60 Woo et al. (1992) found 32 cases of peripheral laryngeal nerve damage (incidence of 21%). Morrison & Gore-Hickman (1986) reported an incidence of 7% in 121 dysphonic patients over the age of 70. Peripheral paralysis in the elderly frequently results from disease processes characteristic of advanced age. For instance, Woo et al. (1992) noted an association between peripheral laryngeal paralysis in the elderly and lung neoplasm. In contrast, idiopathic laryngeal paralysis occurs infrequently in elderly patients.

In cases of peripheral paralysis, vocal fold adduction has been compromised. Loudness is reduced and voice quality is generally breathy. Diplophonia also may be evident. Voice therapy involves addressing specific deficits in laryngeal function as well as associated dysfunction in supporting areas of the speech production mechanism (Ramig & Scherer, 1992). Therapy generally focuses on increasing adductory force to maximize glottal closure. Techniques to accomplish this goal have been well-described in the literature and involve increasing intrinsic laryngeal muscle force by performing pushing or pulling maneuvers simultaneous with phonation (Aronson, 1985; Boone & McFarlane, 1994; Cooper, 1973; Stemple, Glaze, & Gerdeman, 1995). The respiratory system also may be targeted for treatment to facilitate consistent breath support, minimize fatigue, and achieve more appropriate breath phrases during speech production. The following case report illustrates some techniques that are used in treating peripheral laryngeal paralysis. This case also illustrates the spontaneous return of function that often occurs with idiopathic paralysis.

Ms. M, a 60-year-old female college instructor, was diagnosed with idiopathic left vocal fold paralysis 12 years prior to seeking treatment. At the time of diagnosis, it was suspected that paralysis resulted from viral infection of the vagus nerve in association with a particularly severe case of influenza immediately preceding onset of vocal symptoms. Ms. M declined therapy at the time of diagnosis after spontaneously regaining adequate vocal function. Twelve years later, Ms. M requested a second voice evaluation when voice symptoms recurred. She reported essentially "normal" vocal function during the 12-year interval since diagnosis, with the exception of a 3-week interval of hoarseness 8 months after diagnosis. Laryngological reexamination reconfirmed left vocal fold paralysis with fair to good right fold compensation. Voice evaluation revealed a predominantly breathy, hoarse voice with reduced loudness. Perceptually, speaking pitch was judged to be high despite fundamental frequency measurements indicating an appropriate adult female pitch level. Breathing patterns suggested inefficient inhalation (shoulder elevation, minimal abdominal expansion) and compromised breath control on exhalation (rapid rib cage descent). Therapy focused on: (1) breathing exercises to control exhalation, (2) half-swallow boom (Boone & McFarlane, 1994) to increase glottal closure and facilitate louder less breathy voice, and (3) head and neck exercises to decrease extrinsic laryngeal tension and facilitate lower pitch. These techniques produced dramatic improvement in vocal quality, loudness, and pitch. Unfortunately, Ms. M. attended only four therapy sessions because of job-related commitments. Therefore, successful reestablishment of improved voice production was not achieved. Ms. M was encouraged to seek therapy at a facility at which more flexible scheduling was possible.

Central Neurologic Disorders

Central disorders such as Parkinson disease, stroke, Alzheimer's disease, focal dystonia, and essential tremor also are prevalent in persons beyond the age of 60 (Morrison & Gore-Hickman, 1986; Woo et al., 1992). Interestingly, vocal changes frequently are among the earliest symptoms of neurologic dysfunction manifested by Parkinson disease patients (Stewart et al., 1995). Similarly, Woo et al. (1992) noted that 25% of 32 elderly patients with central neurologic disease demonstrated dysphonia as an initial symptom.

The reader is referred to Ramig and Scherer (1992) for an excellent and detailed review of treatment for neurological voice disorders. Briefly, once a definitive diagnosis of neurological dysfunction is made, treatment involves addressing specific deficits in laryngeal pathophysiology such as vocal fold adduction (hypoadduction, hyperadduction), stability of vocal fold vibration (phonatory instability), and coordination of vocal fold movements (phonatory incoordination). In addition, deficits in other components of the speech mechanism including the diaphragm, rib cage, abdomen, velopharynx, jaw, lips, and tongue must be remediated. Following evaluation of acoustic, perceptual, aerodynamic, and physiologic parameters, deficits in the various components are assessed. A comprehensive therapy plan ultimately is formulated in conjunction with otolaryngological and neurological findings. Therapy techniques that are utilized depend on the nature of the dysfunction. Strategies might involve increasing or decreasing vocal fold adduction, stabilizing posture, increasing respiratory support, maximizing respiratory/laryngeal coordination, improving velopharyngeal closure, altering prosody, or improving speech intelligibility. In some cases, a combination of medical management and speech therapy optimizes results. Augmentative communication may be required for certain cases (Ramig & Scherer, 1992).

Clinicians have a responsibility to provide thorough and comprehensive diagnosis and treatment services to all elderly patients with neurologic voice disorders. However, clinicians also must realize that voice disorders involving central neurologic dysfunction frequently are difficult to treat in patients of any age because of accompanying chronic deficits as well as the degenerative nature of such disorders (Woo et al., 1992). On a more optimistic note, recently there have been attempts to systematically investigate the efficacy of intensive voice therapy to improve functional communication in patients with neurological disorders (most notably Parkinson disease). Investigators suggest that intensive therapy improves voice production as well as overall communicative effectiveness in patients with certain neurological disorders (Dromey, Ramig, & Johnson, 1995; Ramig, 1997; Smith, Ramig, Dromey, Perez, & Samandari, 1995).

Benign Vocal Lesions

Certain benign lesions occur with particular frequency among elderly patients. These include unilateral and bilateral Reineke's edema, unilateral sessile polyp, polypoid degeneration, and benign epithelial lesions with variable dysplastic changes (Morrison & Gore-Hickman, 1986; Woo et al., 1992). Reineke's edema and polypoid degeneration are marked by chronic, diffused edema within the superficial layer of the lamina propria that extends along the entire length of one or both vocal folds. Both occur more commonly in women, at least in the United States and Europe, and usually are diagnosed after middle age (Kahane & Beckford, 1991). The etiology of these conditions is not fully understood. However, cigarette smoking, reflux, and vocal abuse/misuse have been implicated as possible contributing causes (Jackson & Jackson, 1937; Koufman, 1995; Meyerson, 1950; Putney & Clerf, 1940; Wallner, 1954). The notion that hyperfunctional voice production contributes to development of Reineke's edema has been further bolstered recently by documentation that persistent hyperfunctional vocal behaviors leads to recurrence of Reineke's edema following surgical treatment (Zeitels, Hillman, Bunting, & Vaughn, 1997).

It is interesting that diagnoses of Reineke's edema and polypoid degeneration are fairly common in the elderly, given that some degree of epithelial thickening with edema occurs normally in the larynx with aging (Eggston & Wolff, 1947; Hirano, Kurita, & Nakashima, 1983; Hirano, Kurita, & Sakaguchi, 1989; Hommerich, 1972). Of course, findings of epithelial changes in normal elderly have not been universal (Noell, 1962; Ryan, McDonald, & Devine, 1956). If thickening and edema do occur normally, at least in some individuals, at what point do these tissue changes become pathological? Also, why are elderly women at increased risk for developing pathological changes in the epithelium in comparison with elderly men? Perhaps the answer lies, in part, with vocal use patterns. Clinicians have noted that elderly women with early polypoidal change are more likely than elderly men to develop functional hypertensive dysphonia. Hypertensive phonatory mode among the elderly often results from a misplaced effort to compensate for pitch lowering that accompanies vocal fold thickening and edema (Morrison & Gore-Hickman, 1986). Because women are more likely to respond negatively to pitch lowering than are men, elderly women are at increased risk of developing compensatory behaviors that exacerbate epithelial changes. The risk of pathological epithelial changes is particularly high in elderly women who also smoke or have symptoms of reflux. Once again the caution of Woo and his associates (1992) comes to mind. It is important for clinicians to look for multiple causative factors in diagnosing vocal dysfunction in elderly patients.

Inflammatory Conditions

Inflammatory conditions also are common among the elderly. Laryngitis sicca, pachydermia, and nonspecific laryngitis due to smoking, medications, reflux, or poor hydration are diagnosed with some regularity.

Frequently, inflammatory conditions in the elderly coexist with vocal fold lesions that may be benign or malignant (Morrison & Gore-Hickman, 1986; Woo et al., 1992).

Laryngitis Sicca

Laryngitis sicca is a condition marked by atrophy of the laryngeal mucosa as a result of insufficient vocal fold lubrication. The vocal folds appear dry and thick secretions are present, which necessitate coughing for removal. Laryngeal crusting also can occur, which must be removed surgically (Colton & Casper, 1996). This condition results either from untreated chronic laryngitis or from age-related declines in the number and quality of mucous glands in the aged larynx (Colton & Casper, 1996; Gracco & Kahane, 1989; Woo et al., 1992). It appears that the disorder is not particularly common among the elderly, however, accounting for only 3% of diagnoses in elderly dysphonic patients (Woo et al., 1992).

Treatment of laryngitis sicca involves increasing hydration in patients for whom such treatment is not contraindicated. In addition, mucolytic drugs are used to thin thickened laryngeal secretions. Treatment also may include assessment of nasal airflow to rule out nasoseptal defects or obstruction that would interfere with adequate humidification of inhaled air. Use of room humidifiers also is recommended (Kahane & Beckford, 1991).

Gastroesophageal Reflux

Gastroesophageal reflux (GER) is defined as the backward flow of gastric acid from the stomach into the esophagus without vomiting. When exposure to refluxed gastric acid irritates the mucosal surfaces of the upper aerodigestive tract, symptoms of gastroesophageal reflux disease (GERD) are produced (Giacchi, Sullivan, & Rothstein, 2000). GERD is a relatively common disorder with an estimated lifetime prevalence in the United States population of 25% to 35% (Scott & Gelhot, 1999). Age appears to be an important factor in the incidence of GERD; several reports suggest that the disorder is more common among the elderly (Katz, 1998; Middlemiss, 1997; Richter, 2000).

The classic symptoms of GERD are heartburn and acid regurgitation. However, in an estimated 20% to 60% of patients with GERD these symptoms are absent (Ahuja, Yencha, & Lassen, 1999; Koufman, 1991; Weiner, Batch, & Radford, 1995). Indeed, symptoms of GERD vary widely and may include hoarseness, globus pharyngeus, sore throat, chest pain, shortness of breath, wheezing, chronic coughing/throat clearing, halitosis, excessive phlegm, sensation of postnasal drip, and dysphagia. Visual examination of the larynx in patients with GERD may reveal posterior findings ranging from slight interarytenoid edema and erythema to granuloma formation with ulceration over the vocal processes. Irritation of the vocal folds also might be observed. Posterior laryngeal findings resulting from GERD often are subtle, however, complicating the diagnosis in those patients without appreciable heartburn (Ahuja et al., 1999; de Carle, 1998; Fraser, 1994; Giacchi et al., 2000; Kahane & Beckford, 1991; Kamel, Hanson, & Kahrilas, 1994; Ross, Noordzji, & Woo, 1998; Sataloff, Spiegel, & Heuer, 1994; Weiner et al., 1995). Knowledge of the potential subtlety of laryngeal symptoms has led to increased awareness by health care providers of the potential for dysphonia resulting from GERD (Ross et al., 1998; Toohill & Kuhn, 1997; Weiner et al., 1995). In the elderly, GERD is a more complicated disease than in young adults because the disease has been present for a longer time. Although elderly patients often complain of less severe heartburn, they tend to demonstrate more severe erosive damage to the esophagus (Katz, 1998; Richter, 2000).

Treatment of GERD involves decreasing the amount or acidity of the gastric acid. This may be accomplished either by antacids that neutralize acid already present or by medications that reduce the amount of acid produced, such as proton-pump inhibitors. Indeed, treatment with the proton-pump inhibitor omeprazole is reported to produce significant improvement in all laryngeal symptoms of GERD except granulomas (Shaw & Searl, 1997). Additional treatment strategies for GERD involve keeping the head elevated somewhat while sleeping to allow gravity to assist in preventing the flow of gastric acid into the esophagus. Lifestyle changes also are recommended including avoidance of late meals, spicy foods, alcohol, caffeine, and tobacco. Finally, weight loss can reduce symptoms (Ahuja et al., 1999; Gaynor, 1991; Jasani, Piterman, & McCall, 1999; Kahane & Beckford, 1991).

Treatment of granuloma in the posterior larynx is difficult and controversial (Emami, Morrison, Rammage, & Bosch, 1999). In cases of vocal process granulomas, antireflux therapy often must be combined with voice therapy to eliminate vocal abuse/misuse factors that contribute to the condition. Specific therapy strategies vary, but might include elimination of abuse factors (hard glottal attack, loud voice, throat clearing), relaxation of cervical musculature, or pitch adjustment. However, even with combined medical/voice therapy, vocal process granulomas are difficult to cure and tend to recur in some cases (Sataloff, Spiegel, & Baroody, 1995).

Trauma

Trauma also causes voice problems in the elderly. Intubation granuloma and residual scar tissue from earlier vocal fold surgery, as well as other traumatic vocal fold injuries occur in this population (Morrison &

Gore-Hickman, 1986; Woo et al., 1992). Intubation granuloma is an uncommon cause of voice problems, although their occurrence is not rare. As noted by Kahane and Beckford (1991), elderly patients are at greater risk for intubation granulomas than young adults, because older persons often are subjected to a greater number of surgical procedures requiring general anesthesia. Intubation granuloma is more likely in females because of smaller laryngeal dimensions. Damage involves ulceration posteriorly in the glottis as a direct consequence of endotracheal tube placement or as a result of static pressure on the vocal process by the tube. Vocal fold scarring might occur in elderly patients as the result of blunt or penetrating neck trauma, burns, intubation, inflammatory processes such as GERD, or radiation therapy for glottic carcinoma. Scarring also can remain as a vestige of any previous vocal fold surgery. Indeed, the greatest single cause of poor voice following vocal fold surgery is scarring (Woo, Casper, Colton, & Brewer, 1994). Diagnosing vocal fold scarring requires measurement of aerodynamic and acoustic parameters of voice, in addition to a good history and careful physical examination. In addition, accurate visual assessment of the vibratory cycle using stroboscopy is indispensable to the diagnostic process (Benninger et al., 1996; Sataloff, Spiegel, & Hawkshaw, 1991).

Treatment of scarring includes voice therapy to maximize vocal quality improvement and avoid the development of hyperfunctional compensatory behaviors. Improvement in voice quality with therapy alone often is limited, however (Benninger et al., 1996). Colton and Casper (1996) report success using a trill technique. The trill is made by oscillation of the tongue tip while it contacts the alveolar ridge. Alternatively, the vibration can occur bilabially simultaneously with phonation. At first patients sustain the trill at a comfortable pitch and gradually pitch variability is introduced. As therapy progresses, trilling is extended into phonation (vowel prolongations) without trill. The sound ultimately is shaped into speech. Although the precise mechanism operating to improve voice using the trill has yet to be determined through empirical research, Colton and Casper (1996) speculate that the trill reduces the effect of vocal fold stiffness through increased force of vocal fold vibration. Treatment of scarring also can involve injection procedures or laryngoplasty (Chapter 16).

FUNCTIONAL HYPERTENSIVE DYSPHONIA

The prevalence of functional hypertensive dysphonia among the elderly is open to some question. Some writers stress the importance of considering functional hypertensive dysphonia as an etiologic factor. They note significant evidence of hypertensive phonatory patterns including hyperactivity of the ventricular vocal folds in this population (Hagen et al., 1996; Morrison & Gore-Hickman, 1986). In contrast, Woo et al. (1992) reported a low incidence of benign vocal fold lesions typically associated with hyperfunction, such as pedunculated polyps and vocal nodules, among the elderly patients they treated. In addition, these investigators found only 5 of 151 elderly patients with evidence of functional dysphonia in the absence of tissue changes.

Hyperfunctional patterns in elderly patients may result from unsuccessful attempts to compensate for age-related physiological changes in the vocal folds or respiratory system that have negatively affected voice production (Slavit, 1999). Elderly speakers of either gender may increase adductory force in an attempt to eliminate breathiness and increase loudness in response to anterior glottal gaps. Aged men may adjust vocal pitch downward to compensate for an age-related elevation of pitch following atrophy and thinning of vocal fold tissue. Elderly women may elevate speaking pitch to compensate for age-related lowering of pitch resulting from vocal fold edema. In either gender, altered respiratory patterns might be observed in response to negative changes in air supply for phonation.

Elderly patients need to be evaluated for evidence of hypertensive phonation. During phonation, the clinician may observe visible tension in cervical muscles or notice a pattern of glottal attack. The patient may report increased effort or tension during phonation. The laryngeal exam may reveal high laryngeal position, excessive medial compression, or anteroposterior compression of the larynx, although such signs may be absent (Colton & Casper, 1996).

Therapeutic strategies to promote more relaxed laryngeal adjustments during phonation have been described in detail elsewhere (Boone & McFarlane, 1994; Colton & Casper, 1996). Any of the strategies used successfully with younger patients also may be employed with the elderly. However, the clinician might need to adapt some techniques for use with elderly patients to accommodate sensory changes in hearing/visual acuity or to circumvent memory deficits. In addition, the clinician must keep in mind limitations related to breathing patterns imposed by changes in both the laryngeal and respiratory systems (Chapter 6). Elderly patients may need to modify phrasing patterns to accommodate possible age-related alterations in aerodynamic valving or loss of elasticity of lung tissues. In the following case reports, improved breath support and relaxation of musculature associated with voice production were the focus of therapeutic intervention. The multifactorial nature of voice disorders in the elderly also is evident from these reports:

Ms. P, aged 77, presented with vocal hoarseness of 8 months' duration. She reported a pattern of progressive hoarseness during the day, culminating in aphonia by day's end. Her history included smoking 1 pack of cigarettes a day for 62 years and a diagnosis of emphysema. Perceptually, Ms. P's voice was reduced in intensity and mildly to moderately hoarse. Intermittent diplophonia was noted. Breathing was shallow with evidence of shoulder elevation on inhalation. Oral mechanism examination was unremarkable. Videostroboscopy revealed mild bowing of the vocal folds with a spindle-shaped glottic configuration. Vocal fold mobility was normal bilaterally. Movement of the false vocal folds was noted on phonation suggesting hyperfunction. Arytenoid erythema and edema and thickening of interarytenoid tissue were observed suggesting GERD, which was later confirmed by an esophagram. Ms. P was treated medically for GERD and was enrolled in voice therapy to treat vocal hyperfunction. Therapy focused primarily on teaching proper respiratory support for voice. Following a review of the anatomy of the larynx, the relationship between respiration and phonation were explained. Abdominal expansion during inhalation was emphasized, along with increasing breathing frequency during speech production to avoid speaking on residual air. Reading aloud was used as a technique to reinforce good respiratory support. In addition, respiratory patterns were targeted during speaking situations most typical of those experienced during her day. Ms. P responded quickly to therapy and demonstrated improved breathing patterns after a month of home practice and two therapy sessions. It was noted, however, that normalization of breathing patterns was limited by the long-standing smoking history and diagnosis of emphysema.

Mr. R (age 82) presented complaining of hoarseness and a globus sensation. He reported intermittent episodes of hoarseness over the preceding 2–3 years. Mr. R worked part-time as a court commissioner, although he denied heavy vocal demands. He lived alone. Indirect laryngoscopy revealed normally mobile vocal folds approximating well at midline. A voice evaluation was recommended following a 1-month trial of medication for reflux. At the voice evaluation, Mr. R reported that his vocal symptoms had not improved with medical treatment of reflux. Perceptually, his voice was described as mildly hoarse and low pitched. Maximum phonation time was short and patterns of clavicular breathing were noted along with excessive cervical tension. Videostroboscopy revealed some pooling of secretions in the pyriform sinuses and tenacious mucous secretions in the glottic region. No lesions of the true vocal folds were observed, although the true vocal folds were somewhat edematous. Vocal fold adduction and abduction were normal although anterior-posterior squeezing of the mechanism was observed during phonation indicating hyperfunction. Vocal fold closure was complete. Voice therapy was recommended to improve breath support and promote more relaxed phonatory adjustments. Increased water intake also was recommended. An esophagram showed a small diverticulum in the distal third of the esophagus and a small esophageal hiatus hernia; no evidence of GERD was noted. One week after videostroboscopy, Mr. R attended his first voice therapy session. He reported having made a dramatic effort to increase his water intake since the videostroboscopy. He also reported substantial improvement in vocal quality for the preceding 2 days, along with a significant reduction in the globus sensation. In therapy, diaphragmatic breathing was demonstrated and relaxation of cervical, tongue, and jaw musculature was emphasized. Improvement in voice quality and maximum phonation time was observed following these exercises, along with elimination of observable neck and jaw tension. Carryover into conversational speech was also observed. Mr. R was provided with a vocal hygiene program; no further voice therapy sessions were scheduled.

Pitch as a contributing factor to functional hypertensive dysphonia in elderly speakers must be assessed on a case-by-case basis. If an elderly man is speaking low in his physiological pitch range and demonstrates considerable vocal fry, elevation of speaking pitch may produce more relaxed phonatory adjustments and allow for voice production with less effort. Further, vocal fold lengthening that accompanies a slight elevation of speaking pitch may improve vocal quality (decrease breathiness) by improving vocal fold adduction. In elderly women, hyperfunctional phonatory patterns often are exacerbated by attempts to maintain the higher pitch speaking voice they had when they were younger. Phonation becomes less effortful and quality improves if they are encouraged to adopt a lower speaking pitch that is consistent with age-related vocal fold changes. It may not be necessary to directly target lower speaking pitch with elderly women, however. On occasion, simply stressing more relaxed phonatory adjustments, in general, through various relaxation exercises facilitates lower speaking pitch.

In both men and women, vocal pitch must be evaluated based on each patient's physiological pitch range to determine if alteration of speaking pitch is indicated. Counseling regarding the need to adjust speaking pitch may be necessary, particularly if the elderly patient perceives the age-altered speaking pitch as uncharacteristic of their gender. Reference to public figures with higher vocal pitch (males) or lower vocal pitch (females) may be useful in encouraging the patient to adopt a pitch level that is more commensurate with his/her voice production capabilities. Therapeutic strategies for pitch alteration with the elderly are the same as strategies utilized with younger patients. Specifically, a new pitch level is memorized followed by practice in structured utterances with gradual incorporation into speech-like contexts (Boone & McFarlane, 1994).

ELDERLY VOICE PROBLEMS AND GENERAL HEALTH

Unfortunately, elderly patients with dysphonia tend to have a high incidence of systemic illness and frequently are in poor general health. In particular, pulmonary disease and hypertensive cardiac disease have been identified in elderly voice patients (Woo et al., 1992). Poor general health hinders the success of voice therapy, because an elderly voice patient with numerous physical problems is less motivated to comply with therapeutic regimens. Further, serious health problems may force postponement of treatment for a voice problem. Multiple medical conditions also complicate the diagnosis and treatment of voice problems in this population. The following case reports illustrate the complex issues that arise in treating voice problems in older patients. The impact of general health issues on diagnostic and treatment decisions concerning voice is evident:

At age 59, Ms. C presented for treatment of hoarseness. She reported a 40-year history of cigarette smoking, having quit 3 years prior. Vocal folds were within normal limits, although vocal abuse was suspected. She was referred for voice therapy, but did not keep therapy appointments and was discharged. A year later Ms. C sought treatment for continuing voice problems at a second facility and underwent surgical excision of vocal nodules. Five years later (age 65) Ms. C returned to the original facility with a consistently hoarse voice. Pitch and intensity range were restricted and loud voice production was difficult to maintain. All acoustic measures were abnormal. Videostroboscopy revealed a large anterior commissure web, adhesion of the right false vocal fold to the true vocal fold, an irregular glottal gap, minimal mucosal wave, asymmetric vocal fold motion, and erythema of arytenoids and interarytenoid area. Movement of ventricular vocal folds was evident on phonation. Laser division of the anterior commissure web was performed with insertion of a keel. Minimal esophagitis and a gastric ulcer also were diagnosed at this time. Ms. C underwent a course of voice therapy focused on improving breath support and reducing laryngeal musculature tension. Nine months after therapy ended Ms. C (age 66) again complained of hoarseness. Perceptually, her voice was very hoarse with intermittent aphonia. Videostroboscopy revealed indications of GERD in the arytenoid area. The vocal folds were edematous bilaterally and a small anterior web was observed. An anterior-posterior glottal gap also was visualized along with minimal mucosal wave and aperiodic vocal fold motion. GERD was treated medically. A second laser division of the web with keel placement was performed along with excision of scar tissue on the vocal fold. Following this surgery, voice was severely hoarse with decreased loudness. Videostroboscopy showed reduced vibratory activity and mucosal wave, anterior-posterior glottal gap, and evidence of hyperfunction. Another course of voice therapy ensued focusing on breath support, alteration of speaking pitch, and relaxation of oral musculature. Therapy was discontinued after two sessions, when Ms C was in a car accident and suffered a minor head injury and broken leg and hip. Three months later, Ms. C's voice had worsened and videostroboscopy indicated severe scarring of the vocal folds with a large glottal gap. Bilateral lipoinjection of the vocal folds was performed. Following lipoinjection, videostroboscopy indicated that the glottal gap was reduced, but vocal folds remained adynamic. Voice declined steadily following the lipoinjection. A year later (age 68) Ms C. was aphonic. Videostroboscopy showed a glottal gap posteriorly and hyperfunction evidenced by ventricular vocal fold movement and anterior-posterior squeezing. Vocal folds were stiff, short, and thickened with an irregular contour. Vocal fold movement was limited and mucosal wave was absent. Anterior commissure blunting was evident

(continued)

compatible with a web. A right vocal fold cordotomy was performed with lysis of adhesions in the lamina propria and steroid injection. Over the next 10 months, she underwent two additional courses of voice therapy. Following therapy, videostroboscopy revealed recurrence of the anterior web. Hyperfunction had lessened since the previous stroboscopy, although voice quality was unchanged. A biopsy of the right true vocal fold revealed squamous cell carcinoma. Ms. C was scheduled for a full course of radiation therapy.

Mr. G, age 72, presented with mild hoarseness and breathiness. He had been diagnosed with Type II diabetes mellitus, muscular myopathy, pancytopenia, right diaphragm paralysis, and congestive heart failure. He complained of a dry, nagging, unproductive cough. Fundamental frequency was unremarkable but pitch and intensity variability during speech were restricted. Respiratory support for speech (primarily rib cage expansion) was reduced. Videostroboscopy revealed a small, round, grayish-white, smooth polyp at the anterior commissure lying superior to the level of the vocal fold that interfered with glottic closure. Arytenoid cartilages were somewhat edematous, laryngeal secretions were thickened, and mucous stranding was observed. Vibratory motion was asymmetrical. Evidence of laryngeal hyperfunction was noted during pitch and intensity variations. It was recommended that surgical excision of the polyp be postponed pending resolution of the other medical problems. Three years later, Mr. G's voice was still mildly but consistently hoarse. Videostroboscopy revealed continued presence of the polyp that had not changed significantly in size or appearance from the earlier evaluation. Surgical removal of the polyp was scheduled.

SUMMARY

Lifestyle changes associated with aging such as loss of independence, home living circumstances, availability of health care, social activities, communicative need, and availability of emotional support influence voice rehabilitation in the elderly. Physiological conditioning, even in the absence of disease, plays an important role in maintaining vocal functioning into old age. Factors such as tension, anxiety, and depression also contribute to voice problems in this population.

A number of pathological conditions affecting voice are particularly prevalent in the elderly. Further, older patients are more likely than younger patients to have a second etiologic factor that contributes to dysphonia. Cancer of the head and neck presents somewhat differently in patients over the age of 70, although treatment does not differ a great deal as a function of age. Voice disorders with a neurologic etiology are common in the elderly. Peripheral paralysis frequently results from a disease process characteristic of advanced age, such as lung neoplasm, while idiopathic paralysis is less common. Therapy for voice disorders resulting from peripheral paralysis or central neurologic dysfunction involves addressing specific deficits in laryngeal pathophysiology as well as deficits in other components of the speech mechanism. Certain benign lesions such as Reineke's edema, sessile polyp, polypoid degeneration also occur with greater frequency in the elderly. It is possible that faulty compensatory vocal use patterns contribute to the development of pathological epithelial changes in the elderly, particularly women. Voice therapy is indicated to eliminate any compensatory hypertensive adjustments that are evident. Inflammatory conditions also are common among the elderly. Laryngitis sicca may result from untreated chronic laryngitis or declines in mucous glands in the elderly. Gastroesophageal reflux is a fairly common disorder in this population. Treatment involves decreasing the amount or acidity of gastric acid, sleeping with the head elevated, altering eating habits, and drug treatment. Voice therapy often is combined with antireflux therapy to eliminate vocal abuse/misuse factors contributing to granuloma associated with this condition. Trauma also can cause voice problems in the elderly. Intubation granuloma and residual scar tissue from earlier vocal fold surgery, as well as other traumatic vocal fold injuries occur in older persons. Treatment of scarring from trauma involves voice therapy to maximize vocal quality improvement and to avoid development of hyperfunctional compensatory behaviors. Improvement in voice quality with therapy alone often is limited, however. Treatment of scarring also can involve injection procedures or laryngoplasty.

Functional hypertensive dysphonia may be observed in elderly patients as a compensatory mechanism in response to anterior glottal gaps, pitch changes, or respiratory changes associated with aging. Therapeutic strategies to promote more relaxed laryngeal adjustments in the elderly are similar to those used with younger patients. However, some modifications may be needed to accommodate age-related sensory changes, memory deficits, or limitations imposed by age-related physical changes.

Pitch as a contributing factor to functional hypertensive dysphonia in elderly speakers must be assessed on a case-by-case basis. Elevation of speaking pitch in elderly men and the reverse in elderly women may promote less effortful voice production with improved vocal quality. Vocal pitch must be evaluated with consideration of the individual's physiological pitch range. Counseling may be necessary to facilitate acceptance of a new pitch.

Elderly patients with dysphonia tend to have a high incidence of systemic illness. Poor general health hinders the success of voice therapy. Health problems can compromise motivation and also may force the delay of treatment for a voice problem.

REFERENCES

Ahuja, V., Yencha, M., & Lassen, L. (1999). Head and neck manifestations of gastroesophageal reflux disease. *American Family Physician, 60,* 873–880.

Aref, A., Dworkin, J., Devi, S., Denton, L., & Fontanesi, J. (1997). Objective evaluation of the quality of voice following radiation therapy for T_1 glottic cancer. *Radiotherapy and Oncology, 45,* 149–153.

Aronson, A. (1985). *Clinical voice disorders* (2nd ed.). New York: Thieme.

Ballo, M., Garden, A., El-Naggar, A., Gillenwater, A., Morrison, W., Goepfert, H., & Ang, K. (1998). Radiation therapy for early stage (T1–T2) sarcomatoid carcinoma of true vocal cords: Outcomes and patterns of failure. *Laryngoscope, 108,* 760–763.

Benninger, M., Alessi, D., Archer, S., Bastian, R., Ford, C., Koufman, J., Sataloff, R., Spiegel, J., & Woo, P. (1996). Vocal fold scarring: Current concepts and management. *Otolaryngology—Head and Neck Surgery, 115,* 474–482.

Blazer, D. (1982). Social support and mortality in an elderly community population. *American Journal of Epidemiology, 115,* 684–694.

Blom, E., Singer, M., & Hamaker, R. (1998). *Tracheoesophageal voice restoration following total laryngectomy.* San Diego: Singular Publishing Group.

Boone, D., & McFarlane, S. (1994). *The voice and voice therapy* (5th ed.). Englewood Cliffs, NJ: Prentice Hall.

Brin, M., Fahn, S., Blitzer, A., Ramig, L., & Stewart, C. (1992). Movement disorders of the larynx. In A. Blitzer, M. Brin, C. Sasaki, S. Fahn, & K. Harris (Eds.), *Neurologic disorders of the larynx* (pp. 248–278). New York: Thieme Medical Publishers.

Burke, L., Greven, K., McGuirt, W., Case, D., Hoen, H., & Raben, M. (1997). Definitive radiotherapy for early glottic carcinoma: Prognostic factors and implications for treatment. *International Journal of Radiation Oncology, Biology, and Physics, 38,* 1001–1006.

Butcher, P. (1995). Psychological processes in psychogenic voice disorder. *European Journal of Disorders of Communication, 30,* 467–474.

Canter, G. (1963). Speech characteristics of patients with Parkinson's disease: I. Intensity, pitch, and duration. *Journal of Speech and Hearing Research, 28,* 221–229.

Chatani, M., Matayoshi, Y., Masaki, N., Teshima, T., & Inoue, T. (1997). Radiation therapy for early glottic carcinoma (T1N0M0). *Strahlentherapie und Onkologie, 173,* 502–506.

Colton, R., & Casper, J. (1996). *Understanding voice problems: A physiological perspective for diagnosis and treatment* (2nd ed.). Baltimore: Williams & Wilkins.

Cooper, M. (1970). Voice problems of the geriatric patient. *Geriatrics, 25,* 107–110.

Cooper, M. (1973). *Modern techniques of vocal rehabilitation.* Springfield, IL: Charles C. Thomas.

Dagli, A., Mahieu, H., & Festen, J. (1997). Quantitative analysis of voice quality in early glottic laryngeal carcinomas treated with radiotherapy. *European Archives of Oto-Rhino-Laryngology, 254,* 78–80.

de Carle, D. (1998). Gastro-oesophageal reflux disease. *Medical Journal of Australia, 169,* 549–554.

Dromey, C., Ramig, L., & Johnson, A. (1995). Phonatory and articulatory changes associated with increased vocal intensity in Parkinson Disease: A case study. *Journal of Speech and Hearing Research, 38,* 751–764.

Eggston, A., & Wolff, D. (1947). *Histopathology of the ear, nose and throat.* Baltimore: Williams & Wilkins.

Emami, A., Morrison, M., Rammage, L., & Bosch, D. (1999). Treatment of laryngeal contact ulcers and granulomas: A 12-year retrospective analysis. *Journal of Voice, 13,* 612–617.

Ferguson, G. (1955). Organic lesions of the larynx produced by misuse of the voice. *Laryngoscope, 65,* 327–337.

Fraser, A. (1994). Review article: Gastro-oesophageal reflux and laryngeal symptoms. *Alimentary Pharmacological Therapeutics, 8,* 265–272.

Gatz, M., Kasl-Godley, J., & Karel, M. (1996). Aging and mental disorders. In J. Birren & W. Schaie (Eds.), *Handbook of the psychology of aging* (4th ed., pp. 365–382). San Diego: Academic Press.

Gaynor, E. (1991). Otolaryngologic manifestations of gastroesophageal reflux. *American Journal of Gastroenterology, 86,* 801–808.

Giacchi, R., Sullivan, D., & Rothstein, S. (2000). Compliance with anti-reflux therapy in patients with otolaryngologic manifestations of gastroesophageal reflux disease. *Laryngoscope, 110,* 19–22.

Gracco, C., & Kahane, J. (1989). Age related changes in the vestibular folds of the human larynx: A histomorphometric study. *Journal of Voice, 3,* 204–212.

Gunther, V., Mayr-Graft, A., Miller, C., & Kinzl, H. (1996). A comparative study of psychological aspects of recurring and non-recurring functional aphonias. *European Archives of Otolaryngology, 253,* 240–244.

Hagen, P., Lyons, G., & Nuss, D. (1996). Dysphonia in the elderly: Diagnosis and management of age-related voice changes. *Southern Medical Journal, 89,* 204–207.

Hirano, M., Kurita, S., & Nakashima, T. (1983). Growth, development and aging of human vocal fold. In D. Bless & J. Abbs (Eds.), *Vocal fold physiology: Contemporary research and clinical issues.* San Diego: College-Hill Press.

Hirano, M., Kurita, S., & Sakaguchi, S. (1989). Ageing of the vibratory tissue of human vocal folds. *Acta Otolaryngologica, 107,* 428–433.

Hommerich, K. (1972). Der alternde Larynx: Morphologische Aspekte. *Hals Nasen Ohrenaerzte, 20,* 115–120.

Jackson, C., & Jackson, C. (1937). *The larynx and its diseases.* Philadelphia: W. B. Saunders.

Jasani, K., Piterman, L., & McCall, L. (1999). Gastroesophageal reflux and quality of life. Patients' knowledge, attitudes and perceptions. *American Family Physician, 28*(Suppl. 1), S15–S18.

Kahane, J., & Beckford, N. (1991). The aging larynx and voice. In D. Ripich (Ed.), *Handbook of geriatric communication disorders* (pp. 165–186). Austin, TX: PRO-ED.

Kamel, P., Hanson, D., & Kahrilas, P. (1994). Omeprazole for the treatment of posterior laryngitis. *American Journal of Medicine, 96*, 321–326.

Katz, P. (1998). Gastroesophageal reflux disease. *Journal of the American Geriatrics Society, 46*, 1558–1565.

Keith, R., & Darley, F. (Eds.). (1994). *Laryngectomee rehabilitation* (3rd ed.). Austin, TX: PRO-ED.

Kiese-Himmel, C., Pralle, L., & Kruse, E. (1998). Psychological profiles of patients with laryngeal contact granulomas. *European Archives of Otorhinolaryngology, 255*, 296–301.

Koch, W., Patel, H., Brennan, J., Boyle, J., & Sidransky, D. (1995). Squamous cell carcinoma of the head and neck in the elderly. *Archives of Otolaryngology—Head and Neck Surgery, 121*, 262–265.

Koufman, J. (1986). The endoscopic management of early squamous carcinoma of the vocal cord with the carbon dioxide surgical laser: Clinical experience and a proposed subclassification. *Otolaryngology—Head and Neck Surgery, 95*, 531–537.

Koufman, J. (1991). The otolaryngologic manifestations of gastroesophageal reflux disease (GERD): A clinical investigation of 225 patients using ambulatory 24-hour pH monitoring and an experimental investigation of the role of acid and pepsin in the development of laryngeal injury. *Laryngoscope, 101*(4, pt 2 Suppl. 53), 1–78.

Koufman, J. (1995). Gastroesophageal reflux and voice disorders. In: J. Rubin, R. Sataloff, G. Korovin, & W. Gould (Eds.), *Diagnosis and treatment of voice disorders* (pp. 161–175). New York: Igaku-Shoin.

Leon, X., Quer, M., Agudelo, D., Lopez-Pousa, A., De Juan, M., Diez, S., & Burgues, J. (1998). Influence of age on laryngeal carcinoma. *Annals of Otology, Rhinology and Laryngology, 107*, 164–169.

Luchsinger, R., & Arnold, G. (1965). *Voice, speech, language, clinical communicology: Its physiology and pathology* (G. Arnold & E. Finkbeiner, Trans.) Belmont, CA: Wadsworth Publishing Company.

Meyerson, M. (1950). Smoker's larynx. A clinical pathological entity. *Annals of Otology, Rhinology and Laryngology, 59*, 541–546.

Middlemiss, C. (1997). Gastroesophageal reflux disease: A common condition in the elderly. *Nurse Practitioner, 22*, 51–52, 55–59.

Morrison, M., & Gore-Hickman, P. (1986). Voice disorders in the elderly. *Journal of Otolaryngology, 15*, 231–234.

Morrison, M., Rammage, L., & Nichol, H. (1989). Evaluation and management of voice disorders in the elderly. In J. Goldstein, H. Kashima, & C. Koopermann (Eds.), *Geriatric otorhinolaryngology* (pp. 64–70). Philadelphia: B. C. Decker.

Mutch, W. (1992). Parkinsonism and other movement disorders. In J. Brocklehurst, R. Tallus, & H. Fillit (Eds.), *Textbook of Geriatric Medicine and Gerontology* (4th ed., pp. 411–429). London: Churchill Livingstone.

Noell, G. (1962). On the problem of age relate changes of the laryngeal mucosa. *Archiv fur klinische und experimentelle Ohren-Nasen-und Kehlkopfheilkunde, 179,* 361–365.

Osguthorpe, J. D., & Putney, F. J. (1997). Open surgical management of early glottic carcinoma. *Otolaryngologic Clinics of North America, 30,* 87–99.

Perez, K., Ramig, L., Smith, M., & Dromey, C. (1996). The Parkinson larynx: Tremor and videostroboscopic findings. *Journal of Voice, 10,* 354–361.

Putney, F., & Clerf, L. (1940). Treatment of chronic hypertrophic laryngitis. *Archives of Otolaryngology, 31,* 925–929.

Raitiola, H., Wigren, T., & Pukander, J. (2000). Radiotherapy outcome and prognostic factors in early glottic carcinoma. *Auris, Nasus, Larynx, 27,* 153–159.

Ramig, L. (1997). How effective is the Lee Silverman voice treatment? *ASHA, 39,* 34–35.

Ramig, L., & Ringel, R. (1983). Effects of physiological aging on selected acoustic characteristics of voice. *Journal of Speech and Hearing Research, 26,* 22–30.

Ramig, L., & Scherer, R. (1992). Speech therapy for neurologic disorders of the larynx. In A. Blitzer, M. Brin, C. Sasaki, S. Fahn, & K. Harris (Eds.), *Neurologic disorders of the larynx* (pp. 163–181). New York: Thieme Medical Publishers.

Richter, J. (2000). Gastroesophageal disease in the older patient: Presentation, treatment, and complications. *American Journal of Gastroenterology, 95,* 368–373.

Ross, J., Noordzji, J., & Woo, P. (1998). Voice disorders in patients with suspected laryngo-pharyngeal reflux disease. *Journal of Voice, 12,* 84–88.

Roy, N., McGrory, J., Tasko, S., Bless, D., Heisey, D., & Ford, C. (1997). Psychological correlates of functional dysphonia: An investigation using the Minnesota Multiphasic Personality Inventory. *Journal of Voice, 11,* 443–451.

Rubenstein, C. (1957). Contact ulcer of the larynx. *California Medicine, 86,* 275–276.

Ryan, R., McDonald, J., & Devine, K. (1956). Changes in laryngeal epithelium: Relation to age, sex and certain other factors. *Mayo Clinic Proceedings, 31,* 47–52.

Sataloff, R., Spiegel, J., & Baroody, M. (1995). Recurrent laryngeal granulomas. *Ear, Nose, and Throat Journal, 74,* 514.

Sataloff, R., Spiegel, J., & Hawkshaw, M. (1991). Strobovideolaryngoscopy. Results and clinical value. *Annals of Otology, Rhinology and Laryngology, 100,* 725–757.

Sataloff, R., Spiegel, J., & Heuer, R. (1994). "Post-intubation granuloma": A case of reflux and voice abuse. *Ear, Nose, and Throat Journal, 73,* 299.

Scott, M., & Gelhot, A. (1999). Gastroesophageal reflux disease: Diagnosis and management. *American Family Physician, 59,* 1161–1169, 1199.

Seeman, T., Kaplan, G., Knudsen, L., Cohen, R., & Guralnik, J. (1987). Social network ties and mortality among the elderly in the Alameda county study. *American Journal of Epidemiology, 126,* 714–723.

Shaw, G., & Searl, J. (1997). Laryngeal manifestations of gastroesophageal reflux before and after treatment with omeprazole. *Southern Medical Journal, 90,* 1115–1122.

Shindo, M., & Hanson, D. (1990). Geriatric voice and laryngeal dysfunction. *Otolaryngologic Clinics of North America, 23,* 1035–1044.

Slavit, D. (1999). Phonosurgery in the elderly: A review. *Ear, Nose, and Throat Journal, 78,* 505–509, 512.

Smith, M., Ramig, L., Dromey, C., Perez, K., & Samandari, R. (1995). Intensive voice treatment in Parkinson disease: Laryngostroboscopic findings. *Journal of Voice, 9,* 453–459.

Stemple, J., Glaze, L., & Gerdeman, B. (1995). *Clinical voice pathology: Theory and management* (2nd ed.). San Diego: Singular Publishing Group.

Stewart, C., Winfield, L., Hunt, A., Bressman, S., Fahn, S., Blitzer, A., & Brin, M. (1995). Speech dysfunction in early Parkinson's disease. *Movement Disorders, 10,* 562–565.

Tatemichi, T., Freddo, L., Mohr, J., & Blitzer, A. (1992). Pyramidal disease (Strokes). In A. Blitzer, M. Brin, C. Sasaki, S. Fahn, & K. Harris (Eds.), *Neurologic disorders of the larynx* (pp. 229–239). New York: Thieme Medical Publishers.

Toohill, R., & Kuhn, J. (1997). Role of refluxed acid in pathogenesis of laryngeal disorders. *American Journal of Medicine, 103,* 100S–106S.

Wallner, L. (1954). Smoker's larynx. *Laryngoscope, 64,* 259–270.

Weiner, G., Batch, A., & Radford, K. (1995). Dysphonia as an atypical presentation of gastro-oesophageal reflux. *Journal of Laryngology and Otology, 109,* 1195–1196.

White, A., Deary, I., & Wilson, J. (1997). Psychiatric disturbance and personality traits in dysphonic patients. *European Journal of Disorders of Communication, 32,* 307–314.

Wolcott, C. (1956). Contact ulcer of the larynx. *Annals of Otology, Rhinology and Laryngology, 65,* 816–819.

Woo, P., Casper, J., Colton, R., & Brewer, D. (1992). Dysphonia in the aging: Physiology versus disease. *Laryngoscope, 102,* 139–144.

Woo, P., Casper, J., Colton, R., & Brewer, D. (1994). Diagnosis and treatment of persistent dysphonia after laryngeal surgery: A retrospective analysis of 62 patients. *Laryngoscope, 104,* 1084–1091.

Xue, A. (1995). *A study of selected acoustic parameters of the voice of sedate and physically active elderly speakers.* Unpublished doctoral dissertation, Kent State University, Kent, OH.

Yu, E., Shenouda, G., Beaudet, M., & Black, M. (1997). Impact of radiation therapy fraction size on local control of early glottic carcinoma. *International Journal of Radiation Oncology, Biology, and Physics, 37,* 587–591.

Zeitels, S., Hillman, R., Bunting, G., & Vaughn, T. (1997). Reineke's edema: Phonatory mechanisms and management strategies. *Annals of Otology, Rhinology and Laryngology, 106,* 533–543.

Index